Variability in Human Drug Response

VARIABILITY IN HUMAN DRUG RESPONSE

Proceedings of the Esteve Foundation Symposium VIII,
Sitges, Spain, 7-10 October 1998

Editor:

Geoffrey T. Tucker
University of Sheffield
Section of Molecular Pharmacology and Pharmacogenetics
Division of Clinical Sciences
The Royal Hallamshire Hospital
Sheffield, U.K.

1999

EXCERPTA MEDICA

Amsterdam - Lausanne - New York - Oxford - Shannon - Singapore - Tokyo

ELSEVIER SCIENCE B.V.
Sara Burgerhartstraat 25
P.O. Box 211, 1000 AE Amsterdam, The Netherlands

First edition 1999

Library of Congress Cataloging in Publication Data
A catalog record from the Library of Congress has been applied for.

International Congress Series No. 1178
ISBN: 0 444 82958 X

♾The paper used in this publication meets the requirements of ANSI/NISO Z39.48-1992 (Permanence of Paper).
Printed in The Netherlands.

About the Esteve Foundation

The Esteve Foundation was established in 1983 to honour the late Dr. Antonio Esteve in the manner that would best fit his temperament, intellectual curiosity and dedication to science. Antonio Esteve was born in Manresa (Barcelona) in 1902, obtained a Doctorate in Pharmacy and in 1927 became manager of the pharmacy that his great-grandfather had founded in 1787. Having been actively involved in research during his student years, Dr. Antonio Esteve felt an urge for drug investigation that resulted in the establishment, in 1929, of what was to become one of the largest pharmaceutical firms in Spain. Dr. Antonio Esteve was actively involved in its research activities, actually heading this department, until his death in 1979.

The Esteve Foundation operates independently of any pharmaceutical enterprise and its main goal is to stimulate progress in pharmacotherapy through scientific communication and discussion. As a way to promote international cooperation in research, it organizes international multidisciplinary meetings - The Esteve Foundation Symposia - as well as meetings on topics of interest in its geographical area. The Esteve Foundation also sponsors lectures, seminars, courses and study groups on areas related to pharmacotherapy.

Introduction

The fact that every patient is different is one of the reasons why the art and science of medical diagnosis is so interesting. However, when it comes to treatment, this diversity can be viewed either as an obstacle or a challenge.

Traditionally, the pharmaceutical industry have generally considered individual variability in drug response to be a nuisance, and have endeavoured to ignore it by pursuing a 'one drug - one dose a day for all' ideal. Unfortunately, many prescribers also adopt this attitude and fail to tailor dosage adequately to individual patient need. On the other hand, clinical pharmacologists have long been at the forefront of the challenge of understanding the many sources of variability in drug response. The need for this understanding has now come into much sharper focus with the advent of molecular biology and its increasing impact on our appreciation of the genetic contribution to disease and to enzyme and receptor variability. Indeed, the captains of the pharmaceutical industry now see variability not as a threat but as a major opportunity, in the new development paradigm of drugs to treat selected patients based upon the genetic diagnosis of disease and pharmacogenetics. However, until the 'gene for non-compliance' has been sequenced, and all the 'genes that affect genes' have been unravelled, it remains important to take a balanced view of variability in drug response, as the outcome of environmental and behavioural as well as genetic factors.

The Esteve Foundation's eight Symposium held in Sitges, Spain (October 7-10, 1998) provided a timely forum to take stock of our understanding of the many aspects of variability in human drug response. With respect to sources of variability, considerations were split into those relating to drug metabolism enzymes, transporters and receptors, and their modulation by age, sex, race, disease and exercise; subjective factors (perception of treatment, pain, compliance, placebo response); and behavioural influences (particularly in the context of drug abuse). Methods of measuring variability were considered with regard to the role of phenotyping and genotyping and the use of population PK-PD modelling, overlayed with discussion of statistical and pharmacometric issues. Finally, the participants addressed questions related to the management of variability in drug response. Should we try to design it out of new chemical entities? When and how might it be minimised by pharmaceutical manipulation of the dosage form? What are the regulatory expectations with regard to variability and choice of drug dosage?

This volume represents a comprehensive account of the information shared by the participants in the Symposium, including a record of the lively debate that followed each individual presentation. On behalf of the contributors and the organisers, I hope that you enjoy reading the book as much as we enjoyed taking part in the Symposium.

Geoff Tucker

List of participants

Leon Aarons: School of Pharmacy and Pharmaceutical Sciences, University of Manchester, Oxford Road, MANCHESTER, M13 9PL (United Kingdom)

Julio Benítez: Department of Pharmacology and Psychiatry, Medical School, University of Extremadura, Avda. Elvas s/n., 06071 BADAJOZ (Spain)

Neal L. Benowitz: Division of Clinical Pharmacology and Experimental Therapeutics, University of California, San Francisco, Box 1220, SAN FRANCISCO, CA 94143-1220 (U.S.A.)

Fèlix Bosch: Esteve Foundation, Llobet i Vall-Llosera 2, 08032 BARCELONA (Spain)

D. Craig Brater: Division of Clinical Pharmacology, Department of Medicine, School of Medicine, Indiana University, Emerson Hall, Room 317, 545 Barnhill Drive, INDIANAPOLIS, IN 46202-5124 (U.S.A.)

Alasdair Breckenridge: Department of Pharmacology and Therapeutics, New Medical Building, Ashton Street, LIVERPOOL L69 3GE (United Kingdom)

Gershan K. Davis: Chorley and South Ribble District General Hospital, Euxton Lane, CHORLEY, Lancashire (United Kingdom)

Patrick du Souich: Department of Pharmacology, School of Medicine, University of Montreal, P.O. Box 6128, Stat. "Centre Ville", MONTREAL, Québec H3C 3J7 (Canada)

Sergio Erill: Esteve Foundation, Llobet i Vall-Llosera 2, 08032 BARCELONA (Spain)

Ian P. Hall: Department of Medicine, Division of Therapeutics, University Hospital Queen's Medical Centre, NOTTINGHAM NG7 2UH (United Kingdom)

Eija A. Kalso: Pain Relief Unit, Department of Anaesthesia, Helsinki University Central Hospital, Haartmaninkatu 4, P.O. Box 260, FIN-00029 HYKS (Finland)

Mark T. Kinirons: Clinical Age Research Unit, Guy's, King's & St. Thomas'School of Medicine, Dentistry & Biomedical Science, Bessemer Road, LONDON SE5 9RS (United Kingdom)

Ulrich Klotz: Department of Clinical Pharmacology, Dr. Margarete Fischer-Bosch-Institute of Clinical Pharmacology, Auerbachstrasse 112, 70376 STUTTGART (Germany)

Heyo K. Kroemer: Department of Pharmacology, Ernst Moritz Arndt-University, Friderich-Löfflerstrasse 23d, 17489 GREIFSWALD (Germany)

Malcolm Lader: Department of Psychiatry, Section of Clinical Psychopharmacology (MRC), The Maudsley, Institute of Psychiatry, De Crespigny Park, Denmark Hill, LONDON SE5 8AF (United Kingdom)

Carlos Martinez: Department of Global Pharmacoepidemiology, Hoechst Marion Roussel Inc., Route 202-206, P.O. Box 6800, BRIDGEWATER, NJ 08807 (U.S.A.)

Munir Pirmohamed: Department of Pharmacology & Therapeutics, The University of Liverpool, Ashton Street Medical School, Ashton Street, LIVERPOOL L69 3GE (United Kingdom)

Marcus M. Reidenberg: Division of Clinical Pharmacology, The New York Hospital-Cornell Medical Center, Box 70, 1300 York Avenue, NEW YORK, NY 10021 (U.S.A.)

Paul Rolan: Medeval Limited, Skelton House, Manchester Science Park, Lloyd Street North, MANCHESTER M15 6SH (United Kingdom)

Tomas Salmonson: Preclinical and Clinical Evaluation Unit 2, Medical Products Agency, Husargatan 8, Box 26, S-75103 UPPSALA (Sweden)

Edward M. Sellers: Department of Pharmacology, Room 4334, Medical Science Building, University of Toronto, 1 King's College Circle, TORONTO, Ontario M5S 1A8 (Canada)

Dennis A. Smith: Department of Drug Metabolism, Pfizer Central Research, Ramsgate Road, SANDWICH, Kent CT13 9NJ (United Kingdom)

Marià Sust: Clinical Research: Biostatistics Unit, Laboratorios Dr. Esteve S.A., Avda. Mare de Déu de Montserrat 221, 08041 BARCELONA (Spain)

Geoffrey T. Tucker: University of Sheffield, Section of Molecular Pharmacology and Pharmacogenetics, Division of Clinical Sciences, The Royal Hallamshire Hospital, Glossop Road, SHEFFIELD S10 2JF (United Kingdom)

John Urquhart: Pharmaco-epidemiology Group, University of Maastricht, P.O. Box 616, 6200 MD MAASTRICHT (The Netherlands)

Marleen A. van Baak: Department of Human Biology, Nutrition and Environment Research Institute, Faculty of Health Sciences, University of Maastricht, P.O. Box 616, 6200 MD MAASTRICHT (The Netherlands)

Paul B. Watkins: General Clinical Research Center, The University of Michigan Medical Center, A7119 University Hospital, Box 0108, ANN ARBOR, MI 48109-0108 (U.S.A.)

Alastair J.J. Wood: Division of Clinical Pharmacology, Vanderbilt University Medical Center, Vanderbilt University School of Medicine, 532 Medical Research Building, NASHVILLE, TN 37232-6602 (U.S.A.)

Contents

Pharmacokinetic / pharmacodynamic impact of genetic polymorphism of drug metabolizing enzymes

Heyo K. Kroemer and Werner Siegmund

Department of Pharmacology, Ernst Moritz Arndt-University, Greifswald, Germany.

ABSTRACT

Discovery of genetic polymorphisms in the expression of drug metabolizing enzymes has contributed to our understanding of the variable dose vs. effect relationship of drugs. Unexpected side effects were initially noticed by physicians and simple tests were developed to assign the extensive metabolizer (EM) or poor metabolizer (PM) phenotype (ie the visual expression of the genotype) to an individual patient. Later, molecular biology techniques were employed to characterize the individual gene locus and identify mutations responsible for aberrant enzyme function (assignment of genotype).

The present article highlights the pharmacokinetic and pharmacodynamic impact of genetic polymorphisms of drug metabolizing enzymes using the example of cytochrome P4502D6 (CYP2D6). This polymorphism is suitable to discuss the problem for various reasons: first it affects a substantial fraction of our population (about 7 to 10 percent of Caucasians), second the enzyme CYP2D6 oxidizes numerous frequently used drugs and third, the molecular biology underlying polymorphic CYP2D6 expression has been described in detail. The pharmacodynamic impact of the genetic polymorphism of CYP2D6 depends on the pharmacological features of the individual compound and cannot be generalized.

In summary, while the pharmacokinetic consequences are readily understood, the pharmacodynamic impact is complex and has to be evaluated for each compound.

Key words: genetic polymorphism, drug metabolizing enzymes, CYP2D6.

Correspondence: Prof. Heyo K. Kroemer, Department of Pharmacology, Ernst Moritz Arndt-University, Friderich-Löfflerstrasse 23d, 17489 Greifswald, Germany, Tel: +49-3834-86-5630, Fax: +49-3834-86-5631

INTRODUCTION

Aside from identifying new targets for yet untreatable diseases variability in response to a given dose of a drug has proven to be a major challenge for further improvement of pharmacotherapy. For example, the effects of a cancer chemotherapy treatment regimen are well established in large patient populations, while response in the individual person remains largely unpredictable.

Part of this variable response is due to inherited eg genetic factors and it was AE Garrod who postulated inborn errors of metabolism to contribute to this phenomenon [1]. His assumption was based on the observation that patients with alkaptonuria either excreted homogentisic acid in normal amounts or not at all: "its appearance in traces or in gradually increasing or diminishing quantities has never been observed". Multimodal distribution of activity of drug metabolizing enzymes has ever since been the hallmark of the new discipline of pharmacogenetics. The term itself has been coined by Vogel [2] and was intertwined with the assumption of Motulski that exaggerated response to drugs may be a consequence of genetically determined deficiencies in enzyme activities [3].

An early observation of unexpected drug effects followed the introduction of the depolarizing muscle relaxant succinylcholine. This compound was characterized by rapid onset and short duration of action. Administration of 1 mg/kg leads to complete paralysis within 2 minutes. The half life of 2 to 6 minutes guarantees complete recovery within a short period of time. Due to this favourable pharmacokinetics the drug gained widespread application. The use in large populations, however, revealed an unexpected feature of succinylcholine. Some patients remained completely paralyzed for several hours requiring mechanical ventilation. The pioneering work of Kalow [4] could identify the reason for the prolonged action of succinylcholine in these patients. Normally the drug is rapidly cleaved by butyrylcholine esterase. The patients with exaggerated effects showed reduced enzyme activity based on a genetic deficiency which was inherited in an autosomal recessive fashion. Later on the molecular bases of this enzyme deficiency has been unravelled [5]. The gene encoding for butyrylcholine esterase is located on chromosome 3. Nucleotides 208 to 210 have the sequence GAT and therefore encode aspartic acid at position 70 of the protein. Patients with decreased activity have a mutation in nucleotide 209 leading to GGT. The latter triplet encodes for the monocarbonic glycine instead of the dicarbonic aspartic acid in the wild type. The second carboxylic group is required for binding of the quarternary amine of succinylcholine and its loss leads to reduced affinity and therefore reduced clearance of the drug. As a consequence plasma concentrations remain elevated for a prolonged period of time. Later on several other mutant forms of succinylcholine esterase have been identified. Simple measures for phenotyping patients have been developed (dibucaine challenge). The current knowledge has been summarized by Lockridge [6].

Butyrylcholine esterase is an impressive example for a close chain of evidence from the molecular level to the clinical consequences of a genetically determined enzyme deficiency. A variety of such deficiencies has been described in the meantime (Table 1). While the above described defect in butyrylcholinesterase affects only a limited number of patients other enzymes match the definition of genetic polymorphisms. A genetic polymorphism is a monogenic trait which occurs in the population in at least two geno- or phenotypes, neither of which has a frequency of less than one percent [7].

Similar to the discovery of the genetic defect in succinylcholine esterase the initial observations of unexpected response to drugs came from physicians. Later on, the biochemistry and the molecular biology of each deficiency has been explored. Methods for assignment of phenotype and/or genotype to an individual patient were developed which allow to identify patients at risk and to adjust the dose in an individual manner. Although the tools for integrating pharmacogenetics into clinical practice are now available this discipline has not yet found its way into day to day pharmacotherapy. One reason may be that both the pharmacokinetic and the pharmacodynamic impact of such polymorphic drug metabolism is very complex thereby precluding any generalizations. In this article I will focus on the cytochrome P4502D6 polymorphism for several reasons: first the molecular bases for this genetic deficiency has been explored in great detail. Second, a substantial fraction of the population is affected by polymorphic expression of this enzyme, which in turn catalyzes the oxidation of more than 50 frequently used drugs. Third, although all prerequisites for a clinically relevant source of interindividual variability in drug disposition and action are present the individualization of dose based on pheno- or genotype has not been widely applied in clinics which may be due to the complex nature of the therapeutic consequences. Therefore, the CYP2D6 polymorphism appears to be a good example for potentials and pitfalls of pharmacogenetics.

Table 1.
Drug metabolizing enzymes, the activity of which is genetically determined

Type of enzyme	Enzyme affected	Clinical consequences of enzyme deficiency
Esterase	Butyrylcholinesterase	Prolonged action of succinylcholine
Transferase	N-Acetyltransferase	Enhanced side effects of isoniazide
	Methyltransferase	Enhanced toxicity of mercaptopurine
	UDP-Glucuronosyltransferase	Crigler-Najjar or Gilbert's Syndrome
Dehydrogenase	Aldehyde dehydrogenase	Flush after ethanol intake
Oxidoreductase	Flavin-containing monoxygenase	Fish odor syndrome
Monoxygenase	CYP2D6, CYP2C19	Depends on pharmacology of the compound

THE POLYMORPHISM OF CYP2D6

In 1972 the department of Internal Medicine at the University of Bonn performed a routine pharmacokinetic study to characterize the pharmacokinetics of the antiarrhythmic sparteine. The investigators identified one volunteer, who experienced serious side effects such as nausea, diplopia and blurred vision, which are hallmarks of intoxications with this type of antiarrhythmics. Analysis of urine samples identified a distinct metabolic pattern in this volunteer: he excreted almost the entire dose as unchanged sparteine in urine, while all other volunteers excreted the major portion of the dose as hydroxy metabolites. In accordance with these data was the observation of a dramatically decreased apparent oral clearance of sparteine in this volunteer which was reduced by 80 percent as compared to the other volunteers. Subsequent family studies revealed the deficient sparteine metabolism to be inherited as an autosomal recessive trait in about seven to ten percent of the Caucasian population [8]. A similar observation was reported at the same time for the antihypertensive debrisoquine [9].

Both sparteine and debrisoquine were used to assign phenotypes (ie the visual expression of genotypes) to individual patients. Patients affected are referred to as Poor Metabolizers (PM) while the remainder of the population is called Extensive Metabolizers (EM). Later on two further phenotypes have been denoted IM (intermediate metabolizer; patients whose metabolic capacity is between EM and PM) and finally the phenotype of ultra rapid metabolizer. The latter phenotype has been previously reported by Bertilsson and coworkers [10], again based on a patient with an unusually high dose requirements for the antidepressant nortriptyline.

The polymorphism of CYP2D6 would have been of rather limited clinical interest if the enzyme affected would catalyze only the oxidation of sparteine and debrisoquine. Further studies, however, identified numerous drugs from different therapeutic areas and a wide array of chemical structures to be substrates of CYP2D6 (a list is provided in Table 2).

Table 2.
Compounds whose metabolism cosegregates with that of sparteine

Cardiovascular drugs

Alprenolol, Flecainide, Metoprolol, N-Propylajmaline, Perhexiline, Propafenone, Propranolol, Timolol.

CNS drugs

Amitryptyline, Clomipramine, Clozapine, Desipramine, Imipramine, Nortriptyline, Thioridazine.

Others

Codeine, Dihydrocodeine, Dextromethorphan, Ethylmorphine, Hydrocodone, Norcodeine, Oxycodone, Tropisetrone.

The polymorphism of cytochrome P450 2D6 has been thoroughly characterized on the molecular level [11]. In brief, the wild type CYP2D6 gene is located on the long arm of chromosome 22 and is part of a gene cluster which besides CYP2D6 is thought to carry two pseudogenes (CYP2D7 and CYP2D8). The CYP2D6 gene locus has proven to be highly polymorphic eg both the EM and the PM phenotype are encoded by numerous allelic variants (a list of variants is shown in TABLE 3). These variants range from complete deletion of the entire CYP2D6 gene to gene amplification leading to up to 12 copies of the CYP2D6 gene in one individual. The latter phenomenon has been identified as the molecular base for the ultrarapid metabolizer phenotype [12].

The availability of probe drugs with exactly defined pharmacokinetics in combination with detailed knowledge about the molecular mechanisms underlying the CYP2D6 polymorphism should allow for an exact match of phenotype and genotype (predictions made based on the genotype of a patient should translate into enzyme expression and hence pharmacokinetics of a drug). A large scale study trying to combine genotype and phenotype of CYP2D6 has been recently reported in a detailed study by Griese and coworkers [13]. Most interestingly they found that the same genotype can be associated with a wide range of enzyme activity (Figure 1). Therefore "postgenomic factors" must contribute to the interindividual variability in

CYP2D6 activity. These data clearly point to the possibility of substantial gene regulation of CYP2D6. Interestingly, several recent reports indicate regulation of CYP2D6 activity and its analogue in rats CYP2D1 by xenobiotics such as clozapine or denaverine [14,15]. The aspect of environmental vs genetic factors in expression of CYP2D6 deserves further attention.

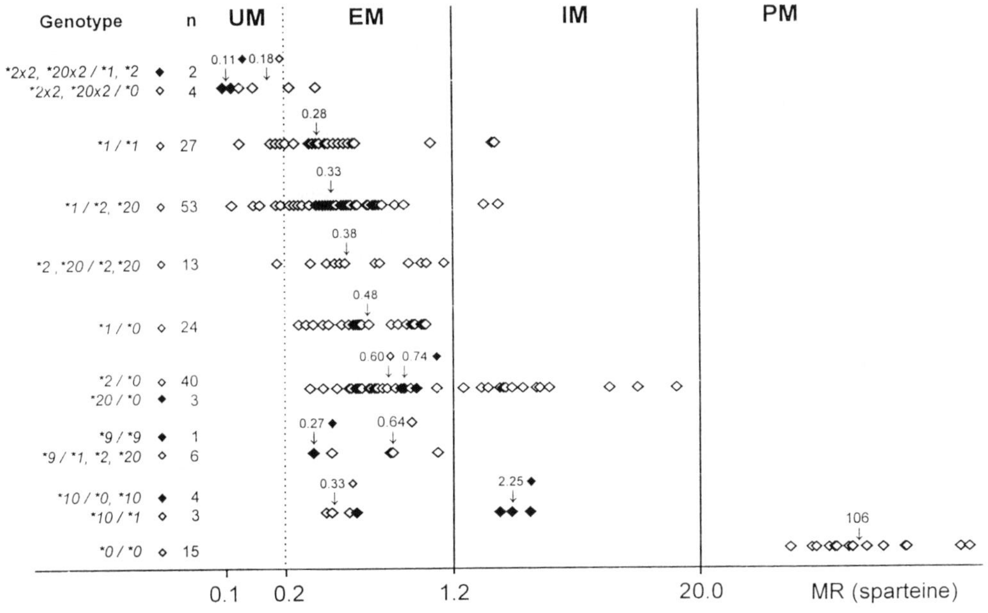

Figure 1. Distribution of sparteine metabolic ratio (MR; a measure of CYP2D6 activity) in 195 Caucasian individuals in relation to genotypes. *0 indicates the presence of any of the seven tested nonfunctional alleles. Number above the lines give the median for each group (Reproduced with permission from Griese EU *et al.* 1988 [13])

Asides from scientific interest the possibility of gene regulation supports the importance of phenotype assignment. Administration of a probe drug to an individual patient with subsequent evaluation of the excretion of parent compound and or metabolite is the only way to experimentally assess the individual enzyme function. The probe drug approach, however, carries several disadvantages. First, it is required to administer a pharmacologically active compound which always carries the potential of side effects. Second, the probe drugs used are either not widely available (eg sparteine or debrisoquine) or not specific for CYP2D6 (eg dextromethorphane or debrisoquine). Third, metabolism of the probe may be hampered by other CYP2D6 substrates concomitantly administered to the same patient thereby mimicking a reduced oxidative activity even in patients homozygous for wild type CYP2D6.

The pharmacokinetic impact of genetic polymorphism in CYP2D6 expression is readily explained. Depending on individual enzyme activity, clearance of compounds oxidized by CYP2D6 varies over a wide range. Consequently, concentrations achieved during chronic administration will show pronounced variability following administration of a fixed dose to a population of patients. In some cases, however, prediction of the pharmacokinetic consequences carried some problems, for example in the case of the antiarrhythmic flecainide.The drug has been identified as CYP2D6 substrate in panel studies (ie comparing pharmacokinetics in EM and PM volunteers) following administration of single doses [16]. Based on these data it was predicted that chronic administration of flecainide should result in accumulation of the drug in the PM phenotype. In contrast to this assumption the actual clinical experiment resulted in steady state plasma concentrations that showed no significant relationship to phenotype [17].

The pharmacodynamic impact of genetic polymorphism is even more difficult to predict. The initial observation which led to the first description of the CYP2D6 polymorphism was that of exaggerated response to regular doses. Based on this first experience it was generally assumed that patients with reduced metabolizing capacity have a high risk to experience side effects. There have been in fact numerous examples of drugs with a higher incidence of side effects in the poor metabolizer population. One example is the calcium channel antagonist perhexiline, which was associated with a high incidence of peripheral neuropathy and liver damage. Retrospective evaluation revealed about 50 percent of patients with side effects to have the PM phenotype [18]. Based on individual enzyme activity extreme dose adjustments may be necessary. One impressive example has been reported by Bertilsson *et al.* for the antidepressant nortriptyline [10]. Whereas PMs require about 10 mg per day of nortriptyline to develop therapeutic plasma concentrations ultra rapid metabolizers should be treated with 500 mg per day. The upper limit of dose recommended by the manufacturer is 150 mg and 225 mg per day for outpatients and inpatients, respectively. Thus, it is evident that this phenotype of patients has a high risk to be treated with inefficiently low doses.

A different problem occurs, when a drug which is metabolized via CYP2D6 requires metabolic activation to gain therapeutic efficacy. One example is the analgesic codeine. CYP2D6 catalyzed O-demethylation to morphine represents the analgesic mode of action [19]. Poor metabolizers were shown to form smaller amounts of morphine after administration of codeine and consequently had a reduced analgesic activity. Recent interaction studies with quinidine, a potent blocker of CYP2D6 activity, however, led to a more complex picture [20]. Although coadministration of quinidine blocked formation of morphine from codeine completely, analgesic activity of codeine was still significantly higher than in PM. It has been speculated that CYP2D6 in the CNS may locally bioactivate codeine and that this process is not blocked by quinidine.

The examples given highlight the problems of drug therapy induced by genetic polymorphism in drug oxidation. Metabolic capacity and hence concentration after administration of a given drug is an individual feature of the patient and not a characteristic disadvantage of this particular compound. Side effects due to genetically determined polymorphic oxidation (both lack of efficacy and exaggerated response) can therefore be defined as a consequence of inadequate dosing in relation to the individual metabolic capacity.

In view of the data available it has to be expected that knowledge about genetic polymorphisms in drug oxidation will be implemented into clinical practice in the near future. A recent article in the JAM states that adverse drug reactions are the fourth leading cause of death in the United States [21]. Polymorphic expression of drug metabolizing enzymes can result in adverse drug reactions and may therefore contribute to this drug-related mortality. Prospective trials are underway to proof this hypothesis.

REFERENCES

1. Garrod AE. The incidence of alcaptonuria: a study in chemical individuality. Lancet 1902;2:1616-1620.
2. Vogel F. Problem de Humangenetik. Ergebn. Inn. Med. Kinderheilk. 1959;12:52-125.
3. Motulski AG. Drug reactions, enzymes and biochemical genetics. JAMA 1957;165:835-837.
4. Kalow W. Familial incidence of low pseudocholinesterase level. Lancet 1956;2:576-577.
5. McGuire MC, Nogueira CP, Bartels CF, Lighstone H, Harja A, van de Speck AFL, Lockridge O, La Du BN. Identification of the structural mutation responsible for dibucaine resistant (atypical) form of human serum cholinesterase. PNAS 1989;86:953-957.
6. Lockridge O. Genetic variants of human serum butylcholinesterase influence the metabolism of the muscle relaxant succinylcholine. In: Kalow W (ed) Pharmacogenetics of drug metabolism. Pergamon, New York, 1992:15-50.
7. Vogel F, Motulski AG. Human Genetics. Springer. Berlin, Heidelberg, New York 1979.
8. Eichelbaum M, Spannbrucker N, Steinke B, Dengler HJ. Defective N-oxidation of sparteine in man: a new pharmacogenetic defect. Eur J Clin Pharmacol 1979;16:183-187.
9. Maghoub A, Idle JR, Dring LG, Lancaster R, Smith RL. Polymorphic hydroxylation of debrisoquine in man. Lancet 1977;2:584-586.
10. Bertilsson L, Arberd-Wistard A, Gustafsson L, Nordin C. Extremely rapid hydroxylation of debrisoquine: a case report with implication for treatment with nortriptyline and other tricyclic antidepressants. Ther Drug Monit 1985:7;478-480.
11. Kroemer HK, Eichelbaum M. "Ist the genes, stupid" Molecular bases and clinical consequences of genetic cytochrome P450 2D6 polymorphism. Life Sciences 1995;26, 2285-2298.
12. Johansson I, Lundqvist E, Bertilsson L, Dahl ML, Sjöqvist F, Ingelmann-Sundberg M. Inherited amplification of an active gene in the cytochrome P450 CYP2D locus as a cause of ultrarapid metabolism of debrisoquine. PNAS 1993;90:11825-11829.
13. Griese EU, Zanger UM, Brudermanns U, Gaedigk A, Mikus G, Morike K, Stuven T, Eichelbaum M. Assessment of the predictive power of genotypes for the in-vivo catalytic function of CYP2D6 in a German population. Pharmacogenetics 1998;8:15-26.
14. Sachse C, Frötschl R, Brockmöller J. Induction of the human CYP2D6 transcription by clozapine. Eur J Clin Pharmacol A79,1997(abstract).
15. Engel G, Walter R, Hessabi B, Scheuch H, Thümmler D, Zanger U, Siegmund W. Influence of denaverine hydrochloride on rat cytochrome P4502D enzymes. Naunyn Schmiedebergs Arch Pharmacol 1998;357:11(abstract).
16. Beckman J, Hertrampf R, Gundert-Remy U, Mikus G, Gross AS, Eichelbaum M. Is there a genetic factor in flecainide toxicity? Brit Med J 1988;297:1326.
17. Funck Brentano C, Becquemont L, Kroemer HK, Buhl K, Knebel NG,Eichelbaum M, Jaillon P. Variable disposition kinetics and electrocardiographic effects of flecainide

during repeated dosing in humans: contribution of genetic factors, dose-dependent clearance, and interaction with amiodarone. Clin Pharmacol Ther 1994;55:256-269.
18. Cooper RG, Evans DAP, Whibley EJ. Polymorphic hydroxylation of perhexiline maleate in man. J Med Genet 1984;21:27-33.
19. Sindrup SH, Brosen K, Bjerring P, Arendt-Nielssen L, Larsen U, Angelo HR, Gram LF. Codeine increases pain threshold to vapor copper laser stimuli in extensive but not in poor metabolizers of sparteine. Clin Pharmacol Ther 1990;48:686-693.
20. Eckhardt K, Li S, Ammon S, Schanzle G, Mikus G, Eichelbaum M Same incidence of adverse drug events after codeine administration irrespective of the genetically determined differences in morphine formation. Pain 1998;76:27-33.
21. Lazarou J, Pomeranz BH, Corey PN Incidence of adverse drug reactions in hospitalized patients: a meta-analysis of prospective studies. JAMA 1998 15;279:1200-1205.

Discussion: Pharmacokinetic / pharmacodynamic impact of genetic polymorphism of drug metabolizing enzymes

M.M. Reidenberg:

You pointed out how this genetic information is obtained, but not how it is utilised. What do you see as the primary barrier to the next step?

H.K. Kroemer:

I think the primary barrier to the next step is the lack of easy assays functionally measuring enzyme capacity. Easy assays for phenotyping patients should be available before administration of drugs. I think there is really a lack of good, reliable, and fast assays in terms of assessing enzyme function. If you look to the probes we are using and the ways the analytical methods are handled, there is certainly nothing a doctor in private practice can do easily.

P. Rolan:

You mentioned that, even for the same genetic expression for CYP2D6, there is quite a lot of variability in the actual phenotype, and you made a very brief comment that you think that xenobiotics may be modulating the activity there. However, I thought that CYP2D6 was relatively non-inducible and not very much affected by xenobiotics. Could you comment on this?

H.K. Kroemer:

You summarised well the current thinking on this issue. I would interpret as an induction the data of these papers where they try to induce sparteine metabolism with rifampizine. Using a statistical analysis the desired result, i.e. no induction effect, was obtained but if you look at the data there is induction. Ivar Roots group in Berlin (Sachse C *et al.*, Eur J Clin Pharmacol (Abstract), 1997) have shown that in a cell culture using clozapine, you can induce CYP2D6. Other people have used certain compounds to down-regulate CYP2D6 in cell lines. These data at least suggest, in combination with the available *in vitro* evidence, that there is some regulation of CYP2D6. Therefore we should put much more emphasis on the interaction of environment and genetics when addressing these issues.

A.J.J. Wood:

People claim that there is no effect, citing studies in which the possibility of changing poor metabolisers (PMs) into extensive metabolisers (EMs) by induction was being investigated, and this obviously was not possible. A shift to the left in EMs was achieved by induction and we have obtained similar results. I find it hard to believe that well recognised inhibitors for CYP2D6 do not also exist in the environment and that we can phenocopy an EM into a PM by giving quinidine. With respect to the effects of codeine, there is a fairly good relationship between the measurement of CYP2D6 activity and the measurement of respiratory depression, which is a much more easily measurable continuous variable. I think there is also an effect on induction in the CNS and this is particularly seen in the effect of quinidine. But certainly within the EMs, there is a fairly good relationship between CYP2D6 activity and respiratory depression produced by codeine.

H.K. Kroemer:

Aside from these global pharmacokinetic parameters like genotype or phenotype, it may be necessary to examine in greater detail the local bioactivation, for example in the CNS, or the local inactivation, for example in the lung. More studies should be done on the local area around the receptors.

M.M. Reidenberg:

I have had a patient with inflammatory bowel disease needing 600 to 900 mg of codeine a day to control the diarrhoea because other treatments did not work. This would cause CNS effects. When I added a small daily dose of quinidine to it, he was able to tolerate these doses of codeine without disabling CNS effects.

J. Benítez:

Your previous comment about statistics and sparteine induction was very interesting. Statistics can be misleading. For example, there does not necessarily exist an intermediate between an ultra-fast metaboliser and a poor metaboliser. When a patient is concerned the population data is of limited value. You have also said we lack easy essays, but I think we lack general knowledge too. For example, you have presented a graph showing a poor correlation between geno and phenotype. We have also observed this but we have not been able to interpret it. Thirdly, we have shown that maybe psychiatric patients control their treatment themselves, just by caffeine intake. Caffeine is not only a stimulating drug, but it also could block metabolism by CYP1A2, and could lead to dangerous intoxication with clozapine and with other drugs, possibly. And finally, it is not only important to take into account genetic and environmental interactions, but also interactions between different isotypes of the cytochrome P450.

G.T. Tucker:

Pregnancy is one clear example of a factor associated with up-regulation of CYP2D6. There is a very Swedish study showing that blood levels of metoprolol, a major 2D6 metabolite, are almost non-existent during pregnancy, but they return to normal levels after delivery.

J. Urquhart:

There is an incredible pricing problem that arises when you have a hundred-fold range of dose requirement. And most of the European pricing authorities still want to do milligram-based pricing, which is not possible under these circumstances.

H.K. Kroemer:

Also there can eventually be problems with the cost of treatments. But in reply to your comment, it depends on how companies should act. Tropisetron is a good example of these problems because it is under-dosed due to safety reasons.

J. Urquhart:

Treatment pricing is difficult because dosage forms are frequently cut to save money. Nevertheless, pharmaceutical companies are not alone in this. The pricing policies being set by governments also has a role.

Variability in Human Drug Response
G.T. Tucker, Editor

Clinical Aspects of Polymorphic Drug Metabolism

Geoffrey T. Tucker

University of Sheffield, Section of Molecular Pharmacology & Pharmacogenetics, Division of Clinical Sciences, The Royal Hallamshire Hospital, Sheffield, U.K.

ABSTRACT

Recent advances in our understanding of the molecular biology and genetic variability of human drug metabolizing enzymes, particularly cytochromes P450, have contributed immensely towards clarifying the pharmacokinetics and pharmacodynamics of many existing drugs, and are increasingly important in the development of new chemical entities. However, while this knowledge has implications for therapeutics, appreciation and application in clinical practice has either been limited or yet to be realised. For example, the debrisoquine polymorphism was discovered 20 years ago, but controlled prospective studies to evaluate its clinical significance are few. The clinical implications of genetic polymorphisms in drug metabolism, as they relate to drug toxicity, and therapeutic failure, are reviewed briefly with specific reference to CYP2D6.

Key words: genetic polymorphism; cytochrome P450; CYP2D6; drug interactions.

Correspondence: Prof. Geoffrey T. Tucker, Molecular Pharmacology and Pharmacogenetics, University of Sheffield, Division of Clinical Sciences, The Royal Hallamshire Hospital, Glossop Road, Sheffield S10 2JF, U.K., Tel: +44-114-271-3019, Fax: +44-114-272-0275, Email: g.t.tucker@sheffield.ac.uk

GENETIC POLYMORPHISM IN CYP2D6

It is now 20 years since the observation of distinct bimodality in the frequency distributions of log urinary drug/metabolite ratios of debrisoquine and sparteine led to the discovery of genetic polymorphism in the cytochrome P450 enzyme which was later to be designated CYP2D6 [1-4].

The term 'genetic polymorphism' refers to the inheritance of a trait controlled by a single locus with two alleles, in which the least common allele has a frequency of (arbitrarily) 1% or more. Oxidation by CYP2D6 qualifies as a genetic polymorphism since the PM (poor metaboliser) geno/phenotype occurs in about 7% of Caucasian populations, albeit to a significantly less extent in other racial groups [5,6]. Within the EM (extensive metaboliser) and PM groups further variation occurs in enzyme function as a result of allelic variants, which does not manifest as distinct modes in the frequency distribution of urinary drug/metabolite ratios [7,8]. At the extreme of the EM distribution gene amplification gives rise to so-called UM's (ultra-rapid metabolisers), these individuals being rare in most Caucasian populations but common in Ethiopians (30%) [9].

PHARMACOKINETIC AND PHARMACODYNAMIC CONSEQUENCES

The pharmacokinetic and pharmacodynamic consequences of the activity of a polymorphic enzyme depend upon whether it mediates metabolism of parent drug or primary metabolite or both, whether parent drug or metabolites or both are active, the overall contribution to clearance from the affected pathway, the potency of active species, and the patency of competing pathways of elimination [10] (Fig. 1).

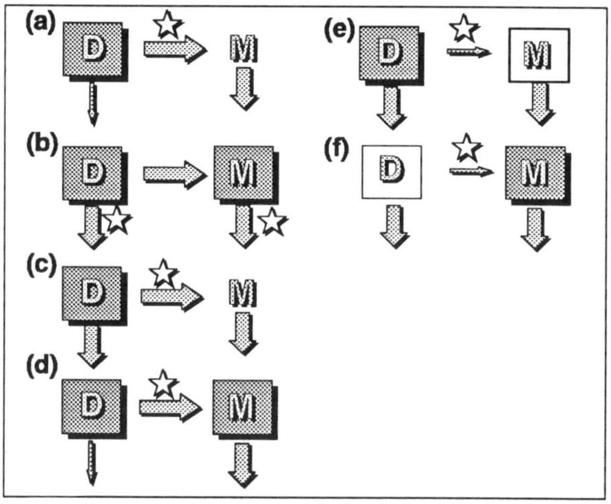

Figure 1. Precursor-product relationships illustrating different pharmacokinetic and pharmacodynamic consequences of polymorphic drug metabolism. [D = parent drug; M = metabolite; large arrow = major pathway; small arrow = minor pathway; star = polymorphic pathway; shaded box = major activity; unshaded box = minor activity; no box = no activity.]

Case (a) in Fig. 1 is where parent drug is the major active moiety and most of its clearance is effected by a polymorphic enzyme. The kinetic consequences of being a PM would be a decrease in first-pass metabolism, increased oral bioavailability and a prolonged elimination half-life. Metoprolol illustrates these features in being converted from a compound with medium to high metabolic clearance in the CYP2D6 EM to a low clearance drug in PM [11]. Accordingly, the latter individuals have more intense and more prolonged β-blockade after standard doses [12]. Case (b) (Fig. 1) is where both drug and metabolite are active and are metabolised by a polymorphic enzyme, but the conversion from drug to active metabolite is mediated largely by a non-polymorphic enzyme. Imipramine and its metabolite desipramine illustrate these features [13]. Thus, standard doses of imipramine will yield relatively high and low plasma concentrations of both active moieties in CYP2D6 PM and EM subjects, respectively, with implications for therapeutic and toxic response.

Case (c) (Fig. 1) is where the main activity resides in the parent drug and it is cleared principally by both polymorphic metabolism and renal excretion. An example of this is the antiarrhythmic flecainide, the accumulation of which will be particularly marked in PM of CYP2D6 with renal impairment [14].

Case (d) (Fig. 1) is where both drug and a major metabolite produced by a polymorphic enzyme contribute to pharmacological activity. The antiarrhythmics encainide and propafenone illustrate this possibility. Both are metabolised by CYP2D6, the former to the active O-desmethyl product [15] and the latter to the active 5-hydroxy metabolite [16]. In these cases, standard doses in both PM and EM tend to produce similar therapeutic responses because relatively high parent drug concentrations in the former are matched by relatively high active metabolite concentrations in the latter.

Case (e) (Fig. 1) is where the polymorphic enzyme catalyses metabolism through a minor pathway and most activity resides in the parent drug. Thus, although the 4-hydroxylation of propranolol is mediated partly by CYP2D6, this has little influence on the clearance of parent drug and, despite 4-hydroxypropranolol retaining some β-blocking activity, there is no significant difference in response to propranolol in PM and EM [17].

Case (f) (Fig. 1) is where drug is metabolised by a polymorphic enzyme to a quantitatively minor but much more active metabolite. Plasma concentrations of codeine are similar in EM and PM (CYP2D6), but measurable concentrations of morphine, its more analgesic O-demethylation product, are only detectable in EM [18,19].

Inhibition or induction of drug metabolising enzymes may modify the kinetic significance of a polymorphic pathway. There are many examples of drugs that inhibit CYP2D6 whereas there is little evidence, except in association with pregnancy [20], that it is significantly inducible. Clearly, EM subjects will be more susceptible to inhibition interactions than PM's and, when a potent inhibitor is administered (such as quinidine), this can lead to phenocopying (conversion into an apparent PM) [21].

DETERMINANTS OF CLINICAL RELEVANCE

The clinical relevance or otherwise of a genetic polymorphism in drug metabolism will depend upon a number of considerations:

1. For most drugs the polymorphic pathway would need to represent a major contribution to clearance for significant differences in clinical response to be apparent between phenotypes. However, as illustrated in Fig. 1, some active metabolites may be so potent or toxic that a minor polymorphic route has to be considered.

2. Variability in other pharmacokinetic processes and elimination by other routes often causes considerable overlap in unbound plasma drug concentrations between phenotypes receiving the same dose of drug [22]. A difference in genotype or a phenotypic difference in the measurement of a drug to metabolite ratio does not necessarily signify a major difference in plasma drug concentration.

3. Pharmacokinetic differences between phenotypes are most relevant for drugs with low therapeutic indices. For those where variability of plasma concentrations outside the therapeutic range is not associated with dangerous under- or overtreatment, or where usual doses produce effects at the top of the concentration-response relationship in most subjects, polymorphic metabolism will be of less or little concern. However, the perception of what is significant discomfort may differ for patient and doctor when a side-effect is not life-threatening.

4. Pharmacodynamic variability in receptor sensitivity or number or in the turnover of a natural ligand may outweigh any kinetic variability imposed by polymorphic metabolism.

5. If dosage can be titrated by direct clinical monitoring or an alternative drug is available which shows less variability in response, then polymorphic metabolism is of no practical consequence. This does, of course, assume an ideal therapeutic world where patients are not left on homeopathic or toxic doses to suffer or to become noncompliant with treatment!

6. Other risk factors such as drug interactions, the effects of disease on drug disposition and the rare combination of being a PM for more than one enzyme may elevate polymorphic metabolism in the affected individual to clinical significance.

CLINICAL RELEVANCE - IMPLICATIONS AND EVIDENCE

The potential clinical significance of the CYP2D6 polymorphism relates mainly to drugs acting on the cardiovascular and central nervous systems. Those where the implications are most well-documented are discussed below.

Perhexiline

This is a significant example of polymorphic metabolism causing the clinical demise of an otherwise useful drug. Thus, 50% of patients developing peripheral neuropathy while taking this antianginal drug were phenotyped retrospectively as PM [23].

β-Adrenoceptor Antagonists

Although there are large phenotypic differences in the pharmacokinetics and β-blocking effects of both metoprolol and timolol [24], these agents are generally considered to have high therapeutic indices and are easily titrated to response. Therefore, many dismiss the clinical relevance of polymorphic metabolism in their clinical use. However, while it is true that adverse effects are rarely life-threatening, such effects can cause discomfort leading to poor compliance, and outpatient assessment of response is not always ideal.

A retrospective analysis found no association between adverse effects from metoprolol and CYP2D6 phenotype [25], but controlled prospective studies are lacking. Lewis *et al.* [26] compared fatigue in normal subjects after single doses of metoprolol and atenolol, the biological fate of the latter being independent of polymorphic metabolism. They concluded that subjective fatigue with β-blocker treatment is unrelated to β-blockade as conventionally measured, and is determined mainly by pharmacodynamic factors with relatively little contribution from genetic variation in metabolism. Thus, in the clinical setting, genetic polymorphism may have little discernable influence on side-effects of metoprolol in cross-sectional studies. Nevertheless, the difference in exercise time and fatigue between atenolol and metoprolol, was inversely related to the ability to metabolise debrisoquine. Therefore, phenotype may have implications for the choice or dose of β-blocker in individual patients. This would also extend to the choice of dosage form. Clearly, prolonged-release preparations would not be necessary in PM subjects [27].

Inadvertent administration to asthmatics of (S)-timolol eye drops, for the treatment of open-angle glaucoma, can cause severe bronchoconstriction. However, following ocular drug administration phenotypic differences in plasma concentrations of timolol were not observed, and it was concluded that the extensive variability in systemic drug absorption from the eye outweighs any effect of oxidation phenotype as a risk factor [28]. The development of more precise ocular delivery systems might necessitate a reconsideration of this conclusion.

Antiarrhythmic Agents

These drugs have low therapeutic indices and for many of them the associated pro-arrythmic effects have rendered the cure far worse than the disease. Thus, for example, the results of the Cardiac Arrhythmia Suppression Trial (CAST) of flecainide and encainide raised substantial doubts about the clinical safety of this class of antiarrythmic [29]. Since the effects of antiarrhythmic agents are closely related to their plasma concentrations, the possibility arises that the increased mortality seen with encainide and flecainide might be related to CYP2D6 phenotype. As explained earlier, decreased renal function may increase the risk of fatal sustained ventricular tachycardia following administration of flecainide to elderly PM patients [30]. The dose of propafenone required to suppress arrhythmias is similar in EM and PM because of the activity of both drug and metabolite. However, PM have a higher incidence of adverse neurological effects. In addition, the S-isomer of propafenone has weak β-blocking activity, possibly constituting a risk in PM patients with heart failure [16].

Antidepressants and Neuroleptics

Evidence for relationships between the plasma concentrations of tricyclic antidepressants and their active metabolites and therapeutic response is contentious. To date it has not been possible to demonstrate that the higher plasma concentrations of the active species in CYP2D6 PM's are associated with greater amelioration of depression [31]. Thus, the diagnosis and severity of disease seem to be more variable than the kinetics. On the other hand, data for adverse effects associated with psychiatric drug use and CYP2D6 status are more convincing. For example, Chen *et al.* [32] found a significantly higher frequency of alleles associated with deficient CYP2D6 activity in depressed patients with adverse drug reactions than in those without such reactions and normal controls.

This issue is further compounded by polypsychopharmacy and its associated drug-drug interactions. Many antipsychotic drugs, particularly the phenothiazine neuroleptics, are potent inhibitors of CYP2D6. Thus, in a population of schizophrenic patients taking these drugs, 50% were found to have undergone phenocopying to become apparent PM's [33]. Indeed, **fixed** combination products containing both tricylic antidepressants and neuroleptics are extremely common, and there is evidence to suggest that prescribers do not lower dosage relative to single drug formulations [34,35]. Furthermore, data from therapeutic drug monitoring (TDM) of plasma nortriptyline concentrations confirm higher levels relative to dose in patients receiving certain neuroleptics compared to tricylic monotherapy. Again, and despite TDM, combination therapy was not associated with dose reduction [36]. In contrast, the effects of tricyclics on plasma concentrations of neuroleptics appear to be much less significant. Thus, for example, considerable overlap was observed in dose-corrected plasma perphenazine concentrations in EM's, co-treated EM's and PM's [37]. This probably reflects the fact that tricyclics are much weaker inhibitors of CYP2D6 and that the importance of the enzyme with respect to overall clearance of many substrates diminishes at steady-state owing to enzyme saturation.

Combined therapy with tricyclic antidepressants and the newer specific serotonin reuptake inhibitors (SSRI's) has been used in some patients who respond inadequately to tricyclics alone. However, the use of fluoxetine for this purpose has been associated with a number of case reports of massive increases in the plasma concentrations of tricyclics and severe cardiotoxicity [38]. In retrospect, such interactions are now entirely predictable based upon *in vitro* and *in vivo* studies showing that some of the SSRI's are potent CYP2D6 inhibitors [39-41]. Paroxetine has been shown to potentiate the central nervous system side effects of perphenazine
[42].

Ecstasy

The demethylenation of methylenedioxymethamphetamine (MDMA, Ecstasy) is catalysed to a large extent by CYP2D6 , and the downstream products are known to be serotoninergic and dopaminergic toxins [43]. Possible consequences of this for users of Ecstasy are that PM's may be at greater risk of acute toxicity mediated by parent drug, while EM's may be more susceptible to long-term problems because of greater formation of neurotoxic metabolites. There are also implications with regard to interactions between Ecstasy and inhibitors of CYP2D6. Thus, combination with fluoxetine allegedly increases the duration of effect [44]. Patients taking the HIV protease inhibitor ritonavir, a particularly potent inhibitor of CYP2D6 [45], are likely to be at significant risk of acute toxicity. A recent death in such a patient, who allegedly took only two Ecstasy tablets, was associated with plasma concentrations of MDMA more consistent with the ingestion of 20 tablets [46].

Analgesics and Antitussives

Codeine

Objective and subjective measurements of analgesia have shown that codeine increases experimental pain thresholds in EM's but is without effect in PM's, who do not O-demethylate it to morphine [18,19]. This implies that patients who are PM for CYP2D6 and those who are also taking potent inhibitors of the enzyme might gain no benefit from treatment with codeine. Unfortunately, studies on clinical pain to support this hypothesis are currently lacking, although there are reports indicating that the incidence of non-response to codeine is similar to the frequency of PM's [47]. Further investigations in healthy subjects suggested that PM's may be inherently less tolerant to tonic pain than EM's, possibly because of decreased endogenous synthesis of morphine by CYP2D6 in the brain [48]. However, in contrast to the findings with exogenous codeine showing pronounced phenotypic differences in morphine formation, no differences in endogenous morphine and codeine excretion were detected between EM's and PM's [49].

The diminished production of morphine from exogenous codeine in PM's is associated with significantly reduced respiratory, psychomotor and pupillary effects [50], although another study has shown no clear decrease in the frequency and intensity of adverse events in PM's [47]. A greater decrease in gastrointestinal motility following administration of codeine to EM's compared to PM's has been claimed [51], but the statistical analysis of these data is questionable.

Tyndale *et al.* [52] have shown that the PM genotype offers significant protection against the risk of developing oral opiate-dependence with codeine and its congeners oxycodone and hydrocodone. Thus, amongst 83 patients dependent on these drugs they found no PM's, compared to frequencies of 4% in 276 never-dependent controls and 6.5% in 93 multi-drug dependent patients (estimated odds ratio >7). Such 'pharmacogenetic protection' may have implications for other drugs of abuse, including many of the 'designer amphetamines' which are also substrates of CYP2D6 [43,53,54].

Dihydrocodeine

In quinidine-induced PM's a significant decrease in dihydromorphine formation was not associated with corresponding decreases in experimental pain thresholds, suggesting that this CYP2D6-mediated reaction is not of clinical importance for analgesia [55].

Tramadol

The analgesic effect of this drug in experimental pain models has been shown to be greater in EM's than in PM's, reflecting higher plasma concentrations in the former of the active (+)-O-desmethyl metabolite [56,57].

Dextromethorphan

Although much higher plasma concentrations of dextromethorphan and lower concentrations of conjugated dextrorphan have been observed in PM's compared to EM's following administration of 30mg doses of dextromethorpan, no difference in capsaicin-induced cough frequency was observed [58]. However, these studies need to be repeated using a validated cough model, shown to be responsive to change in the dose of dextromethorphan. The issue of whether the antitussive activity is mediated by parent drug or metabolite remains unresolved, and there are implications for the use of combinations of dextromethorphan (and codeine) with diphenhydramine, an inhibitor of CYP2D6 [59].

Fenfluramine and Dexfenfluramine

Evidence linking the use of these drugs to an unacceptable incidence of primary pulmonary hypertension and valvular heart disease [60] has led to their recent withdrawal. Since the clearance of dexfenfluramine in CYP2D6 PM's is half that in EM's [61], it is important to establish retrospectively whether there is an overrepresentation of PM's (real and phenocopies) in the patients who developed serious cardiovascular toxicity.

PROSPECTS

So, what are the clinical perspectives with regard to genetic polymorphism in drug metabolism, specifically with respect to CYP2D6? The issue may be separated into a consideration of old and new drugs.

Understanding the impact of genetic polymorphism in drug metabolism is clearly only part of the task of improving existing therapy. In the metabolic context, environmentally evoked variability in CYP3A4 activity is just as, if not more important than genetic control of CYP2D6 activity. Nevertheless, there is a need for prospective clinical studies to assess safety and efficacy, particularly in relation to those individuals at the extremes of the CYP2D6 spectrum of activity. The problem is that such studies are difficult to fund, and these days (at least in the UK) it is difficult to find clinical pharmacologists to do them. Perhaps a more realistic strategy is through education. Certainly, a glance through the APBI Data Sheet Compendium and the PDR will indicate significant mention of CYP2D6 polymorphism and associated drug interactions. However, whether the average physician knows what cytochrome P450 is and can relate to this information is debatable; the task of flagging it up would seem to be more appropriate for the pharmacist armed with modern information technology. Another possibility is to assess enzyme activity in the individual patient, In terms of phenotyping this would essentially be an add-on or alternative to TDM (Therapeutic Drug Monitoring). But then, of course, outside of some specialist centres, TDM has never really caught on. Alternatively, the zealots of molecular genetics would argue that everybody should be genotyped and, indeed, the technology is now available for rapid microchip typing for many of the mutations of CYPs 2D6 and 2C19. Thus, the Brave New World would involve entering genotypes on a SMART card for each person, which would then flag out recommendations for individual drug therapy to the health care system as and when needed [62]. Currently, at least with regard to CYP2D6, there are two problems with this. Firstly, the instrumentation needed to read the gene chip is affordable only by the pharmaceutical industry and, secondly, genotype does not necessarily predict phenotype and hence enzyme function and clinical outcome. Although genotyping may be prognostic with regard to the dichotomous distinction between enzyme function in EM's and PM's and with respect to gene replication [63], the ability to predict function from knowledge of allelic variants within the large EM envelope appears to be much less precise [7,8,64].

As far as new drugs are concerned, the way forward is much clearer. The *in vitro* technology is well-developed to understand the enzymology of new chemical entities at an early stage in development [65]. If, for example, CYP2D6 proves to be a major player, it might be possible to de-select the compound or to design out significant involvement of the enzyme. Where this is not feasible it is then essential that the safety and efficacy profile be evaluated with respect to geno/phenotype. Studies with tolterodine, a new antimuscarinic agent for the treatment of bladder dysfunction, illustrate this approach, showing that the clinical impact of the CYP2D6 polymorphism is likely to be minimal because of an additive action of parent drug and the active metabolite produced by the enzyme [66]. Progressing into clinical studies, an optimal way of assessing the impact of variability in drug metabolism would be to use geno/phenotypes as a covariates in sparse sampling - population kinetics methodology. Hence, it should be possible to tell the physician (and, indeed, the regulators) prospectively that genetic polymorphism and variability in drug metabolism is or is not clinically important.

REFERENCES

1. Mahgoub A, Idle JR, Dring LG, Lancaster R, Smith RL. Polymorphic hydroxylation of debrisoquine in man. Lancet 1977;1:584-586.

2. Tucker GT, Silas JH, Iyun AO, Lennard MS, Smith AJ. Polymorphic hydroxylation of debrisoquine. Lancet 1977;2:718.
3. Eichelbaum M, Spannbrucker N, Steincke B, Dengler JJ. Defective N-oxidation of sparteine in man: a new pharmacogenetic defect. Eur J Clin Pharmacol 1979;16:183-187.
4. Meyer U. The molecular basis of genetic polymorphisms of drug metabolism. J Pharm Pharmacol 1994;46(suppl.1):409-415.
5. Alvan G, Bechtel B, Iselius L, Gundert-Remy U. Hydroxylation polymorphisms of debrisoquine and mephenytoin in European populations. Eur J Clin Pharmacol 1990;39:533-537.
6. Llerena A, Cobaleda J, Martinez C, Benitez J. Inter-ethnic differences in drug metabolism: influence of genetic and environmental factors on debrisoquine hydroxylation phenotype. Eur J Drug Metab Pharmacokin 1996;21:129-138.
7. Sachse C, Brockmoller J, Bauer S, Roots I. Cytochrome P450 2D6 variants in a Caucasian population: Allele frequency and phenotypic consequences. Amer J Hum Genet 1997;60:284-295.
8. Marez D, Legrand M, Sabbagh N, Lo Guidice J-M, Spire C, Lafitte J-J, Meyer UA, Broly F. Polymorphism of the cytochrome P450 2D6 gene in a European population: characterization of 48 mutations and 53 alleles, their frequencies and evolution. Pharmacogenetics 1997;7:193-202.
9. Aklillu E, Persson I, Bertilsson L, Johansson I, Rodrigues D, Ingelman-Sundberg M. Frequent distribution of ultrarapid metabolizers of debrisoquine in an Ethiopian population carrying duplicated and multiduplicated functional CYP2D6 alleles. J Pharmacol Exp Ther 1996;278:441-446.
10. Tucker GT. Clinical implications of genetic polymorphism in drug metabolism. J Pharm Pharmacol 1994:46(suppl.1):417-424.
11. Lennard MS, Tucker GT, Silas JH, Freestone S, Ramsay LE, Woods HF. Differential stereoselective metabolism of metoprolol in extensive and poor debrisoquine metabolizers. Clin Pharmacol Ther 1983;34:732-737.
12. Lennard MS, Silas JH, Freestone S, Ramsay LE, Tucker GT, Woods HF. Oxidation phenotype - a major determinant of metoprolol metabolism and response, N Engl J Med 1982;307:1558-1560.
13. Brosen K, Otton SV, Gram LF. Imipramine demethylation and hydroxylation: impact of the sparteine oxidation phenotype. Clin Pharmacol Ther 1986;40:543-549.
14. Gross AS, Mikus G, Fischer C, Eichelbaum M. Polymorphic flecainide disposition under conditions of uncontrolled urine flow and pH. Eur J Clin Pharmacol 1991;40:155-162.
15. Woosley RL, Wood AJJ, Roden DM. Drug therapy - encainide. N Engl J Med 1988;318:1107-1115.
16. Funck-Brentano C, Kroemer HK, Lee JT, Roden DM. Drug therapy - propafenone. N Engl J Med 1990;322:518-525.
17. Lennard MS, Jackson PR, Freestone S, Tucker GT, Ramsay LE, Woods HF. The relationship between the debrisoquine oxidation phenotype and the pharmacokinetics and pharmacodynamics of propranolol. Br J Clin Pharmacol 1984;17:679-686.
18. Desmeules J, Gascon M-P, Dayer P, Magistris M. Impact of environmental and genetic factors on codeine analgesia. Eur J Clin Pharmacol 1991;41:23-26.

19. Sindrup SH, Brosen K, Bjerring P, Arendt-Nielsen L, Larsen U, Angelo HR, Gram LF. Codeine increases pain thresholds to copper vapor laser stimuli in extensive but not poor metabolizers of sparteine. Clin Pharmacol Ther 1991;49:686-693.
20. Wadelius M, Darj E, Frenne G, Rane A. Induction of CYP2D6 in pregnancy. Clin Pharmacol Ther 1997;62:400-407.
21. Speirs CJ, Murray S, Boobis AR, Seddon CE, Davies DS. Quinidine and the identification of drugs whose elimination is impaired in subjects classified as poor metabolizers of debrisoquine. Br J Clin Pharmacol 1986;22:739-743.
22. Jackson PR, Tucker GT, Lennard MS, Woods HF. Polymorphic drug oxidation: pharmacokinetic basis and comparison of experimental indices. Br J Clin Pharmacol 1986;22:541-550.
23. Shah RR, Oates N, Idle JR, Smith RL, Lockart JD. Impaired oxidation of debrisoquine in patients with perhexiline neuropathy. Br Med J 1982;284:295-299.
24. Lennard MS.,The polymorphic oxidation of beta-adrenoceptor antagonists. Pharmacol Ther 1989;41:461-477.
25. Clark DWJ, Morgan AKW, Waal-Manning H. Adverse effects from metoprolol are not generally associated with oxidation status. Br Clin Pharmacol 1984;18:965-966.
26. Lewis RV, Ramsay LE, Jackson PR, Yeo WF, Lennard MS, Tucker GT. Influence of oxidation phenotype on exercise tolerance and subjective fatigue after metoprolol and atenolol in healthy subjects. Br J Clin Pharmacol 1991;31:391-398.
27. Silas JH, Freestone S, Lennard MS, Ramsay LE. Comparison of two slow-release formulations of metoprolol with conventional metoprolol and atenolol in hypertensive patients. Br J Clin Pharmacol 1985;20:387-391.
28. Huupponen R, Kaila T, Lahdes K, Salminen L, Iisalo E. Systemic absorption of oral timolol in poor and extensive metabolizers of debrisoquine. J Ocul Pharmacol 1991;7:183-187.
29. CAST Investigators. Preliminary report: effect of encainide and flecainide on mortality in a randomized trial of arrhythmia suppression after myocardial infarction. N Engl J Med 1989;321:406-412.
30. Beckmann J, Hertrampf R, Gundert-Remy U, Mikus G, Gross AS, Eichelbaum M. Is there a genetic factor in flecainide toxicity? Br Med J 1988;297:1316.
31. Spina E, Gitto C, Avenoso A, Campo GM, Caputi AP, Perucca E. Relationship between plasma desipramine levels, CYP2D6 phenotype and clinical response to desipramine: a prospective study. Eur J Clin Pharmacol 1997;5:395-398.
32. Chen S, Chou W-H. Blouin RA, Mao Z, Humphries LL, Meek QC, Neil JR, Martin WL, Hays LR, Wedlund PJ. The cytochrome P450 2D6 (CYP2D6) enzyme polymorphism: Screening costs and influence on clinical outcomes in psychiatry. Clin Pharmacol Ther 1996;60:522-534.
33. Spina E, Martines C, Caputi AP, Obaleda J, Pinas B. Debrisoquine oxidation phenotype during neuroleptic monotherapy. Eur J Clin Pharmacol 1991;41:467-470.
34. Llerena A, Kiivet R. Fixed combination of neuroleptics with antidepressants: potential risks and estimation of use. Br J Clin. Pharmacol 1994;37:531-532.
35. Rosholm J-U *et al.* Concurrent use of more than one major psychiatric drug (polypsychopharmacy) in out-patients - a prescription database study. Br J Clin Pharmacol 1994;37:533-538.

36. Jerling M. Population pharmacokinetics and pharmacodynamics: potential use for gathering dose-concentration response. Eur J Drug Metab Pharmacokin 1996;21:113-121.
37. Linnet K, Wiborg O. Steady-state serum concentrations of the neuroleptic perphenazine in relation to CYP2D6 genetic polymorphism. Clin Pharmacol Ther 1996;60:41-47.
38. Westermeyer J. Fluoxetine-induced tricyclic toxicity: extent and duration. J Clin Pharmacol 1991;31:388-392.
39. Crewe HK, Lennard MS, Tucker GT, Woods FR, Haddock RE. The effect of selective serotonin re-uptake inhibitors on cytochrome P4502D6 (CYP2D6) activity in human liver microsomes. Br J Clin Pharmacol 1992;34:262-265.
40. Brosen K, Skjelbo E. Fluoxetine and norfluoxetine are potent inhibitors of P450IID6 the source of the sparteine/debrisoquine oxidation polymorphism. Br J Clin Pharmacol 1991;32:136-137.
41. Sindrup SH, Brosen K, Gram LF, Hallas J, Skjelbo E, Allen A, Allen GD, Cooper SM, Mellows G, Tasker TCG, Zussman BD. The relationship between paroxetine and sparteine oxidation polymorphism. Clin Pharmacol Ther 1992;51:278-287.
42. Ozdemir V, Naranjo CA, Herrmann N, Reed K, Sellers EM, Kalow W. Paroxetine potentiates the central nervous system side effects of perphenazine: Contribution of cytochrome P4502D6 inhibition *in vivo*. Clin Pharmacol Ther 1997;62:334-347.
43. Tucker GT, Lennard MS, Ellis SW, Woods HF, Cho AK, Lin LY, Hiratsuka A, Schmitz DA, Chu TYY. The demethylenation of methylenedioxymethamphetamine ("Ecstasy") by debrisoquine hydroxylase (CYP2D6). Biochem Pharmacol 1994;47:1151-1156.
44. Tucker GT. Adam and Eve make Love. Human Exp Toxicol 1996;15:455-456.
45. Kumar GN, Rodrigues AD, Buko AM, Denisson JF. Cytochrome P450-mediated metabolism of the HIV-1 protease inhibitor ritonavir (ABT-538) in human liver microsomes. J Pharmacol Exp Ther 1996;277:423-431.
46. Concar D. Deadly combination, The New Scientist, July 12,1997;20-21.
47. Eckhardt K, Li S, Ammon S, Schanzle G, Mikus G, Eichelbaum M. Same incidence of adverse drug events after codeine administration irrespective of the genetically determined differences in morphine formation. Pain 1998;76:27-33.
48. Sindrup SH, Poulsen L, Brosen K, Arendt-Nielsen L, Gram LF. Are poor metabolisers of sparteine/debrisoquine less pain tolerant than extensive metabolisers? Pain 1993;53:335-349.
49. Mikus G, Bochner F, Eichelbaum M, Horak P, Somogyi AA, Spector S. Endogenous codeine and morphine in poor and extensive metabolisers of the CYP2D6 (debrisoquine/sparteine) polymorphism. J Pharmacol Exp Ther 1994;268:546-551.
50. Caraco Y, Sheller J, Wood AJ. Pharmacogenetic determination of the effects of codeine and prediction of drug interactions. J Pharmacol Exp Ther 1996;278:1165-1174.
51. Mikus G, Trausch B, Rodewald C, Hofmann U, Richter K, Gramatte T, Eichelbaum M. Effect of codeine on gastrointestinal motility in relation to CYP2D6 phenotype. Clin Pharmacol Ther 1997;61:459-466.
52. Tyndale RF, Droll KP, Sellers EM. Genetically deficient CYP2D6 metabolism provides protection against oral opiate dependence. Pharmacogenetics 1997;7:375-379.

53. Lin LY, DiStefano EW, Scmitz DA, Hsu L, Ellis SW, Lennard MS, Tucker GT, Cho AK. Oxidation of methylamphetamine and methylenedioxymethamphetamine by CYP2D6. Drug Metab Disp 1997;25:1059-1064.
54. Wu D, Otton SV, Inaba T, Kalow W, Sellers EM. Interactions of amphetamine analogs with human liver CYP2D6. Biochem Pharmacol 1997;53:1605-1612.
55. Wilder-Smith CH, Hufschmid E, Thormann W. The visceral and somatic antinociceptive effects of dihydrocodeine and its metabolite, dihydromorphine. A cross-over study with extensive and quinidine-induced poor metabolizers. Br J Clin Pharmacol 1998;45:575-581.
56. Poulsen L, Arendt-Nielsen L, Brosen K, Sindrup SH. The hypoalgesic effect of tramadol in relation to CYP2D6. Clin Pharmacol Ther 1996;60:636-644.
57. Paar WD, Poche S, Gerloff J, Dengler HJ. Polymorphic CYP2D6 mediates O-demethylation of the opioid analgesic tramadol. Eur J Pharmacol 1997;53:235-239.
58. Capon D, Bochner F, Kerry N, Mikus G, Danz C, Somogyi AA.The influence of CYP2D6 polymorphism and quinidine on the disposition and antitussive effect of dextromethorphan in humans. Clin Pharmacol Ther 1996;60:295-307.
59. Poirier J, Roy M, Campanella G, Cloutier G, Paris S. Debrisoquine metabolism in parkinsonian patients treated with antihistamine drugs. Lancet 1987;2:386.
60. Connolly HM, Cary JL, McGoon MD, Hensrud DD, Edwards BS, Edwards WD, Schaff HV. Valvular heart disease associated with fenfluramine-phentermine. N Engl J Med 1997;337:581-588.
61. Gross AS, Phillips AC, Rieutord A, Shenfield GM. The influence of the sparteine/debrisoquine polymorphism on the disposition of dexfenfluramine. Br J Clin Pharmacol 1996;41:311-317.
62. Idle JR, Smith RL. Pharmacogenetics in the new pattern of healthcare delivery, Pharmacogenetics 1995;5:347-350.
63. Dalen P, Dahl M-L, Ruiz MLB, Nordin J, Bertilsson L. 10-hydroxylation of nortriptyline in white persons with 0,1,2,3, and 13 functional CYP2D6 genes. Clin Pharmacol Ther 1998;63:444-452.
64. Griese E-U, Zanger UM, Brudermanns U, Gaedigk A, Mikus G, Morike K, Stuven T, Eichelbaum M. Assessment of the predictive power of genotypes for the *in vivo* catalytic function of CYP2D6 in a German population. Pharmacogenetics 1998;8:15-26.
65. Tucker GT. The *in vitro* assessment of human hepatic drug metabolism. In: O'Grady J, Joubert P (eds.) Handbook of Phase I/II Clinical Drug Trials. Boca Raton: CRC Press, 1997;51-63.
66. Brynne N, Dalen P, Alvan G, Bertilsson L, Gabrielsson J. Influence of CYP2D6 polymorphism on the pharmacokinetics and pharmacodynamics of tolterodine. Clin Pharmacol Ther 1998;63:529-539.

<u>Discussion</u>: Clinical aspects of polymorphic drug metabolism

P. du Souich:

I think the problems are even greater than what you have shown, because we have not considered the patient, and his compliance, or the obsessive patient who will take everything and who will obviously notice and report every potential side-effect. We have not taken into account the time the physician needs to explain and to listen to the patient. Because the real situation is much more complicated than that we have discussed, we are very far away from reaching the right solution.

G.T. Tucker:

My concern here was to present what science has to offer, and make the point that there is also a problem of medical education.

M. Lader:

I would like to defend prescribing in psychiatry by, firstly, agreeing with what was said. There is a great problem in the large variability, but there are other factors interfering. For example, you mentioned schizophrenic patients and neuroleptics. Somewhere between 30 and 40% of schizophrenic patients are co-morbid for drug abuse. There is very little knowledge of this situation, and even less control over which particular medications they are taking. They are also, almost all of them, inveterate heavy smokers, as an additional factor. In practice, in a particular speciality like psychiatry, the practical problems are really quite immense. Not to say they cannot be resolved, but it is going to be one of the later areas of therapeutics where we can really bring in some sort of rationale.

M. Pirmohamed:

In some diseases such as cystic fibrosis, the same genotype with completely different clinical presentations exist. It is possible that there are modifier genes which modify the effect of an individual gene. It the case of CYP2D6, there may be environmental factors operating or modifier genes on completely different chromosomes, which may be affecting its activity. What is your opinion? Secondly, with regard to other drug reactions in CYP2D6, it may be possible to phenotype or genotype individuals for certain type A adverse drug reactions. But when you come to type B adverse drug reactions, the idiosyncratic ones, there may be only very specific few examples where one can genotype. When you look at the more complex type of reactions, for example hepatotoxicity and skin rashes, it seems that there may be multiple genes which are interacting together, plus the environment, to produce the phenotype or the clinical toxicity. Therefore, it becomes very difficult to be able to genotype or phenotype those individuals prospectively, and to be able to predict that they are going to get the reaction.

G.T. Tucker:

Absolutely, I agree that it is not going to be as simple as some may think in terms of genotyping. There are going to be genes that affect other genes and so on until finally we will have a whole array of genes to look at. And the more we look, the more complicated it becomes, in terms of predicting function.

A.J.J. Wood:

One way to remove the variability would be to administer an inhibitor like quinidine, but we never discuss that. Maybe the Spanish are right in having 99% of subjects with a combination therapy. If we gave everybody quinidine with their CYP2D6 substrate, they all would be poor metabolisers, as the variability would be reduced dramatically. Although the problem would not disappear, but at least the dosage would be more rational. Do you think that is reasonable?

G.T. Tucker:

If you use another drug, you might be affecting another enzyme system which affects another drug. That could introduce an additional problem, another drug interaction completely separate from the one you tried to deal with in the first place.

I.P. Hall:

I think we are being a little bit unfair on the possibilities that pharmacogenetics offer. As I understand it, there is such a large effect with the CYP2D6 that a very strong case can be made for genotyping before treating. Whether or not that is going to be effective in populations with regard to other drugs depends on two things. Firstly, it depends on whether or not there are viable alternative treatments which do not use the same metabolic pathway, and then if there is a perfectly adequate second alternative first-line treatment. The vast majority of pharmacogenetic variability in treatment response is not going to be as clear-cut as CYP2D6. There has to be some threshold to determine when it is worthwhile genotyping. The idea that you might have a chip where you identify a hundred common treatment response genes, genotype your population and then say, if you are going to get hypertension, you get drug X, if you get diabetes, you get drug Y is fine, but the effects have to be large enough. I do not think there are good examples at the moment of other targets where there is such a large big effect as for CYP2D6.

G.T. Tucker:

I guess that is exactly why the chip technology is concentrating initially on polymorphic CYPs. But still the technology has to be shown to have clinical relevance.

E.M. Sellers:

I would like to make a comment concerning the impact of environmental and other factors as possible gene regulators. It is probably important to remember that gene-regulation is organ-specific, and that there is now increasing evidence that the expression of cytochrome P450 in the brain is cell-type specific, and the regulation of those cell types in the brain is also very specific. It is quite easy to demonstrate that you can have cell-specific, cytochrome-specific induction in the brain with absolutely no effect whatsoever on hepatic expression of the cytochromes. So the extent that the central cytochromes are playing a role, either in endogenous-like answered response or whether they actually have a drug-metabolising role, is something that is essentially invisible to us. Therefore, studying clearance is a poor model for this situation.

M.M. Reidenberg:

A lot of us have been proposing for a while the idea that we need to identify which of these sources of variability that we have been discovering are clinically important. We have seen with classic examples, such as the tricyclic antidepressants and the CYP2D6 polymorphism, that people who do know about it and do understand it, do not seem to use this information in their clinical practice. In my opinion, rather than trying to prove the clinical importance of each of these sources of variability that we are identifying, we have to concentrate more on discovering the situations in which knowledge of the existence of a specific source of variability is clinically important. As clinical pharmacologists, we need to discover a lot more of when this variability is important, rather than assume that every one is equally important.

D.C. Brater:

I would like to comment on the example of mibefradil, where it was absolutely predictable that drug interactions were going to be problematic. It is surprising that a highly respected pharmaceutical company did not realize this beforehand and modify their studies and marketing accordingly, instead of having a disaster on their hands. Education about relevance of drug reactions goes beyond demonstrating the clinical relevance to our clinician colleagues.

M. Lader:

Related to all these drug interactions, I would like to consider a simple drug like lithium. With lithium, if you are looking for correlations with clinical response, there is only a broad spectrum of levels that you can look at. And even if you look at the toxicology, when you reach the high levels, you may have somebody who is perfectly comfortable at 1 mM concentration and another person who is going into toxicity at this level. The intra-cellular mechanisms are so important here, even with a simple drug like lithium, that they probably swamp the individual disposition of the compound and the variability in that. Until we know a lot more about what these drugs are actually doing at the cellular level, the concentrations are really a secondary issue.

M.M. Reidenberg:

Your point is well-taken because we do not differentiate drugs that move throughout the body and to the site of action by passive diffusion, from those that are involved in active transport. A basic theory that was developed in the 1940s essentially presupposes that drugs move by passive diffusion. For many organic molecules, this is a reasonable assumption. But when we consider other classes of molecules, then this assumption often breaks down.

T. Salmonson:

Firstly, I want to point out that mibefradil was not approved in Sweden. The problem is we are not today where we may be in the future. The health care system is under severe time and financial pressures and the industry acts accordingly. The drug industry therefore dislikes any type of labelling restriction which makes the drug more difficult to prescribe and/or handle, even if it means only avoiding taking the drug with food. This problem is partly due to lack of easily accessible information at the time of prescribing, and perhaps a lot can be done with modern technology to improve this. Although we should continue to focus on all the sources of variability, we also have to focus on why we are not considering even the most obvious sources of variability that do not need sophisticated measurements, such as gender or weight.

When we have problems correcting for such simple factors, how can we imagine that we will be successful in correcting for genotypes? The challenge is to show that there is a consequence for all these variabilities. We have also to be better at predicting the clinically relevant sources of variability. We are extremely good at detecting potential interactions with today's technology and we at the regulatory side can be blamed for including pharmacokinetically significant interactions on the labelling without considering the clinical relevance. This makes it impossible for the prescriber to consider all of these issues. So we need to be better at identifying clinically relevant interactions and sources of variability. And the challenge for us is how we can stimulate this development and reward knowledge and penalise lack of knowledge, instead of the opposite, which is the present situation.

J. Benítez:
Regarding the mibefradil case, it seems unbelievable and it is surprising that one of the biggest drug companies in the world has made such a mistake, and the FDA allowed it to occur, after removing from the market terfenadine for similar reasons. In about 100 psychiatric patients we studied the importance of CYP2D6 from a clinical point of view. We found that whether the patients were actually smokers or not was the most important factor. When we studied the possible interaction between fluvoxamine and thioridazine, a tremendous inhibition through CYP1A2 was observed, leading us to advise about the possible danger in giving these two drugs together. But apparently most clinical pharmacologists, including myself, did not think of this. A too simplistic view was taken and people were studying their favourite cytochrome, for example, 2D6, 1A2, 3A4. This reminds me of the frustrations related to therapeutic drug monitoring, about which we were very optimistic some years ago but I think it was oversold. If the results have not been as good as expected, it is because we took a too simplistic view, and I think we are making the same mistake again. Much more studies are needed, about how cytochromes interact with each other, how dietary components like caffeine and juice interact together. Too frequently results are not published because there is no clear clinical correlation.

J. Urquhart:
One of the places that might be useful to look at is therapeutic failure. Everything indicates a drug ought to work, but when it does not work then there is some kind of pharmacoescalation, either in drug, in dose or both. Considering this from a logical point of view, three possibilities exist: 1. Clinically unrecognised non-complier; 2. Clinically unrecognised non-absorption or some kind of absorption barrier problem; and 3. Non-responder. The clinical failure situation focuses attention on the resolution of these 3 possibilities, and when the problem is resolved, it should be clear what is happening. However, this does not deal with toxicity, but it at least deals with therapeutic failure.

M.M. Reidenberg:
The same approach can be used for toxicity, and the example I would use is digoxin, where you make the digoxin toxicity diagnosis clinically, looking at the digoxin level. If the digoxin level is very high, you have made a mistake on the renal function. If it is normal, then you look at serum potassium, serum calcium and so on, and it is a very different list. This way of thinking, we do clinically with at least digoxin, so that conceptually I think this process is understood.

A.J.J. Wood:

Anticoagulants could be a good example of our failure to having good end-points with other drugs, because there is certainly a good relationship between the extent of anticoagulation and the risk of haemorrhage, which is a devastating adverse effect but it is pretty easy for people to define. On the contrary, it is a lot harder to define an end-point in psychiatry for distinguishing between efficacy and toxicity. If you feel bad, it could be because you have not had your depression improved, or because your depression might have improved but the drug's toxicity has made you feel worse. Sometimes, the complexity makes it really hard to separate out efficacy from toxicity.

P. du Souich:

Probably we need to improve our pharmacodynamic tools to assess the effects of drugs. If we were able to speak to the physicians on pharmacodynamic grounds, they would understand us much better than when we talk to them about half-lives and clearances.

P.B. Watkins:

I patented the erythromycin breath test and for the last decade have been proposing use of the test to individualize dosing of CYP3A4 substrates with narrow therapeutic indices. My experiences point out some of the problems with gaining acceptance for phenotyping tests. The first drug we targeted was cyclosporin A. This seemed to be a good candidate as it has a narrow therapeutic index and its pharmacokinetics vary substantially among patients. Moreover, the physician must place the patient on a sufficient but nontoxic dose as soon as possible after transplantation. It is therefore not possible to start at a low dose and slowly increase it, which is often the strategy used for dosing other drugs with narrow therapeutic indices. Both clinicians and members of pharmaceutical industry found our studies scientifically appealing. However, one seemed interested in funding or participating in studies that might show the true utility of the test; no once even seemed interested in the concept of reducing the need for blood level monitoring. I have been told that blood level monitoring is more lucrative than the sale of the drug, which may account for this reluctance.

The second category of drugs we are examining are chemotherapies which are CYP3A4 substrates and where pharmacokinetics predict clinical response. Again, it is not desirable to start with a low dose and escalate, as the tumor can develop drug resistance. Alternatively, these drugs are very toxic in high doses. I have participated in several discussions within industry were scientists and clinicians have argued for phenotyping studies, but marketing executives have viewed bundling any sort of special test testing to their drug as a competitive disadvantage. To date, marketing has won these discussions.

U. Klotz:

It would be interesting to know whether all the clinical pharmacologists working in the area of pharmacogenetics and CYP2D6 and in units capable of phenotyping, routinely carry out this analysis. If it is not done by clinical pharmacologists in their own units, you cannot expect it from practitioners or other physicians. For instance, in my hospital we have patients on certain drugs who were not routinely phenotyped. If we do not consider such an important factor for individualisation of dosage, we place ourselves in a weak position.

J. Benítez:
Obviously phenotyping is not done routinely but when there exist special problems with some patients. Phenotyping is not routinely done anywhere as far as I know.

G.T. Tucker:
I mentioned a study, in a major centre of therapeutic drug monitoring showing that the levels of nortriptiline were significantly higher in the presence of neuroleptics. However, physicians using this drug did not lower the dose. If this is true in a leading TDM centre, then it is unlikely that phenotyping will catch on as a routine procedure.

M.M. Reidenberg:
The question I would raise is whether there is any clinical need to act on the situation for these drugs when there was a difference in mean levels but there was not a very steep concentration-effect relationship. At least, the psychiatrists at my university and at the University of Pittsburgh, with whom I have discussed this matter and who are well aware of this clinical pharmacology issue, find that, in practice, it is of little importance. Among all the reasons for variability in the response of depressed patients to treatment, the pharmacokinetic degree of variability in tricyclics is such a small part of the total that it can be ignored without perceiving any detriment.

G.T. Tucker:
That could be true of the desired response, but it may not be true of adverse response, whether overt toxicity or impaired quality of life.

Variability in Human Drug Response
G.T. Tucker, Editor

Enzyme Inhibition and Induction - PK/PD Impact

Ulrich Klotz[a] and Kari T. Kivistö[b]

[a]Dr. Margarete Fischer-Bosch-Institute of Clinical Pharmacology, Stuttgart, Germany

[b]Department of Clinical Pharmacology, University of Helsinki, Finland

ABSTRACT

Disposition and action of many drugs depend on their (extra-) hepatic metabolism which is accomplished by several cytochrome P450 (CYP) enzymes and/or conjugating activities. The CYP3a subfamily is the most abundant in the liver and in the small intestine.At these metabolic sites high clearance drugs sustain presystemic elimination. Ingredients of grapefruit juice have no influence on the systemic clearance of various drugs whereas intestinal drug metabolism may be decreased and consequently oral bioavailability increases. Midazolam represents a probe of CYP3A4. Its oral availability is higher during treatment with fluconazole, itraconazole, ketoconazole, diltiazem, verapamil, erythromycin or grapefruit juice ingestion. On the other side midazolam metabolism is induced by rifampicin. Thus, switching from inhibition to induction causes an about 400 fold change in the AUC of oral midazolam which has a significant impact on the sedative action of this benzodiazepine. Using verapamil as a model drug it was shown that rifampicin will induce, not only hepatic but also intestinal drug metabolism. During oral coadministration of both drugs, steady state concentrations of verapamil decreased more than 30 fold and the response was nearly abolished. These examples show that inhibition or induction of drug metabolizing enzymes will have an impact on PK and both contribute to variability in drug response.

Key words: inhibition, induction, drug metabolism, pharmacokinetics, pharmacodynamics

Correspondence: Prof. Dr. Ulrich Klotz, Dr. Margarete Fischer-Bosch-Institut für Klinische Pharmacologie, Auerbachstrasse 112, D-70376 Stuttgart, Germany, Tel: +49-711-81-01-37-02, Fax: +49-711-85-92-95, Email: ulrich.klotz@ikp-stuttgart.de

Funding acknowledgement: This work was supported by the Robert Bosch Foundation Stuttgart and Helsinki University Central Hospital Research Fund.

INTRODUCTION

Most drugs undergo biotransformation before excretion by renal, biliary or other routes. The liver, which contains a number of drug metabolising systems, is the major site of metabolism. Among those enzymes the cytochrome (CYP) P450 superfamily enzymes represent the most important class [1,2]. More recently it has been revealed that these enzymes are also present at extrahepatic sites, especially in the small intestine [3].

During the past numerous *in vitro* and *in vivo* studies have been performed indicating that the activity of the various CYP can be modified, i.e. drugs, environmental factors or food constituents can inhibit or induce these enzymes. Impairment or acceleration of drug metabolism will lead to pharmacokinetic (PK) changes which may have also pharmacodynamic (PD) consequences [4,5].

This article will concentrate on *in vivo* studies in man where interactions between different compounds have been investigated. In these interaction studies often probe drugs have been used to characterize indirectly the *in vitro* activity of certain CYP [6,7]. The pharmacokinetic modifications due to inhibiting or inducing agents can be best visualized by changes in the plasma level-time profiles (AUC measurements) or by the calculation of systemic (CL) and oral (CL_0) clearance of the affected drugs [8].

We will present some recent examples from literature and our own work to illustrate the clinical impact of the observed PK- and/or PD-changes, rather than provide a comprehensive overview of the involved problems.

GRAPEFRUIT JUICE AS INHIBITOR

The inhibitory potential of grapefruit juice was serendipitously discovered during an interaction study with ethanol (EtOH) and Ca-channel blockers to mask the typical flavor of EtOH [9]. Since then, with an increasing number of drugs, such as felodipine, nifedipine, nitrendipine, nisoldipine, terfenadine, cyclosporine and midazolam, elevated plasma concentrations following oral administration have been observed when grapefruit juice was concomitantly ingested. Most studies focused on drugs that are CYP3A substrates, since this subfamily is particularly inhibited, especially in the intestinal epithelium. Consequently, the affected drugs showed a substantial increase in their relative oral bioavailability (F) ranging from a mean value of about 40% to over 250% [10, 11]. In the case of terfenadine [12,13] and midazolam [14] these PK-changes were associated with more pronounced PD-effects. Recently, it was suggested that 6',7'-dihydroxybergamottin is the putative inhibiting agent in the grapefruit juice [15]. The unpredictability of the magnitude of the individual increase in F would suggest to reduce the oral dosage of the affected CYP3A-substrates.

EtOH AS INDUCER

EtOH is consumed worldwide in tremendous amounts and it is an effective inducer of hepatic drug metabolism, especially involving pathways mediated by CYP2E1. Therefore individuals consuming chronically EtOH have an accelerated metabolism of CYP2E1 substrates, such as chlorzoxazone (CZX), paracetamol, halothane, enflurane, methoxyflurane, sevoflurane and many organic solvents [16]. The metabolic ratio of CZX, a probe of CYP2E1, increased significantly from 0.43 in non-induced subjects to 1.2 in EtOH-induced patients and it normalized within 1 week after withdrawal of EtOH (17].

The hepatotoxic potential of paracetamol resides in its reactive metabolite N-acetyl-p-benzo-chinonimine which is formed by CYP2E1 [18]. In two recent reviews, 67 and 94 cases of paracetamol-induced hepatotoxicity associated with regular intake of EtOH were presented indicating the risk of combined use of both agents [19,20]. Likewise, the hepato- and nephrotoxic potential of fluorinated volatile anaesthetics depends on the CYP2E1-mediated formation of reactive metabolites and inorganic fluoride. Therefore it is conceivable that induction of CYP2E1 by EtOH may increase the toxicity of these drugs [16].

INHIBITION OF DRUG METABOLISM BY CIMETIDINE

Due to its imidazole ring structure cimetidine binds to the heme part of several CYP [21]. Therefore it is not surprising that this H_2-receptor antagonist inhibits the metabolism of many drugs (Table 1) which are substrates of different CYP. CL of these substances is decreased on average by 20 to 50% by cimetidine [22,23]. With some drugs (e.g. diazepam, theophylline, carbamazepine, phenytoin, lidocaine, warfarin), the increased plasma concentrations were associated with a more pronounced PD response [22-24]. Therefore it appears prudent to reduce the dose of these drugs or to use ranitidine which does not inhibit drug metabolism.

Table 1.
Drugs, whose hepatic elimination is impaired by cimetidine

acenocoumarole	cyclosporine	5-fluorouracil	moricizine	propranolol
alprazolam	dapsone	flurazepam	nicardipine	quinidine
amitriptyline	debrisoquine	flurbiprofen	nicotine	quinine
amoxicillin	desipramine	glibenclamide	nifedipine	sparteine
antipyrine	desmethyldiazepam	glipizide	nimodipine	sulindac
bromazepam	diazepam	imipramine	nitrazepam	tacrine
bupivacaine	digitoxin	indomethacin	nitrendipine	theobromine
caffeine	diltiazem	labetalol	nortriptyline	theophylline
carbamazepine	doxepine	lidocaine	paroxetine	tolbutamide
carbocysteine	encainide	mebendazole	pentoxifylline	triamteren
chlordiazepoxide	enoxacin	metformine	pethidine	triazolam
chlormethiazole	estradiol	methadone	phenytoin	valproic acid
chloroquine	ethanol	metoprolol	pindolol	verapamil
chlorpromazine	felodipine	metronidazole	piroxicam	warfarin
clobazam	flecainide	midazolam	prednisone	

RIFAMPICIN AND VERAPAMIL

Drug metabolism in the liver and gut wall can be induced by rifampicin and especially substrates of CYP3A4 (e.g. cyclosporine, midazolam) are cleared much faster during coadministration of rifampicin and consequently F of these drugs is dramatically reduced [25,26].

In other studies verapamil was chosen as a model drug, because several CYP (CYP3A4, CYP1A2, CYP2C) are involved in its metabolism and stereoselective aspects can be investigated with this racemic drug. In young [27] and elderly [28] subjects it was found that 12 days' co-treatment with rifampicin (600 mg once daily) and verapamil (120 mg twice daily) resulted in a more than 30-fold increase ($p < 0.001$) in the oral CL of the cardioactive S-verapamil, whereas systemic CL following an iv-dose of 10 mg was increased only about 1.3-fold. F of both enantiomers was dropped almost to zero and consequently the effect of oral verapamil on atrioventricular conduction was nearly abolished ($p < 0.01$). Induction by rifampicin caused a considerable reduction of stereoselectivity after both iv- and po-administration. As rifampicin altered the PK and PD of verapamil in both populations to a much greater extent after po-dosing compared with iv-administration, it was concluded that - independent of the age - prehepatic (gut wall) metabolism of verapamil was preferentially induced by rifampicin [27,28].

INHIBITION AND INDUCTION OF THE METABOLISM OF MIDAZOLAM

Midazolam represents a well-established probe for CYP3A4 [6,7] and its PK/PD-properties and relationships have been described thoroughly [29]. There is a marked interindividual variation in both CYP3A4 activity in the liver and pharmacokinetics of CYP3A4 substrates. Furthermore, CYP3A4 is readily inhibited or induced by a number of drugs, resulting in many clinically significant drug interactions. The erythromycin breath test is currently the best validated measure of CYP3A4 activity in the liver *in vivo*. The results of this test have been shown to correlate with the clearance of intravenously administered midazolam [30], and the clearance of intravenous midazolam seems to provide a good estimate of the activity of CYP3A4 in the liver. It should be noted that assays of CYP3A4 activity in the liver are not suitable for accurate assessment of intestinal CYP3A4 activity. This is an important issue because many CYP3A4 substrates undergo significant first-pass metabolism not only in the liver but also in the gut. The first-pass metabolism of CYP3A4 substrates, i.e. the combined CYP3A4 activity in the liver and gut, can, however, be predicted by administering the probe orally.

After oral administration, midazolam undergoes extensive first-pass metabolism in the intestinal wall and the liver and, therefore, its concentrations in plasma are markedly altered by inhibition and induction of CYP3A4. The effects of various drugs on the AUC of oral midazolam are illustrated in Figure 1 [31-36]. In these studies, a single dose of midazolam was given orally after a 2- to 6-day pretreatment with the inhibitor. Most of these interactions are clinically significant, that is, the sedative effect of midazolam is greater and lasts longer during co-administration of a potent CYP3A4 inhibitor. This holds also true for triazolam, the pharmacokinetics of which are also very susceptible to inhibition (and induction) of CYP3A4.

Plasma concentrations of numerous drugs are reduced to a clinically significant extent by co-administration of rifampicin. In a recent study, in which a single dose (15 mg) of midazolam was given orally after a 5-day pretreatment with rifampicin (600 mg once daily) or placebo, rifampicin decreased the AUC of midazolam by 96% compared with placebo [37]. As a result, the pharmacodynamic effects of midazolam, measured by several psychomotor tests, were practically abolished. It is therefore reasonable to assume that orally administered midazolam (and triazolam) are ineffective as hypnotic agents during concomitant treatment with rifampicin and other potent CYP3A4 inducers such as phenytoin and carbamazepine.

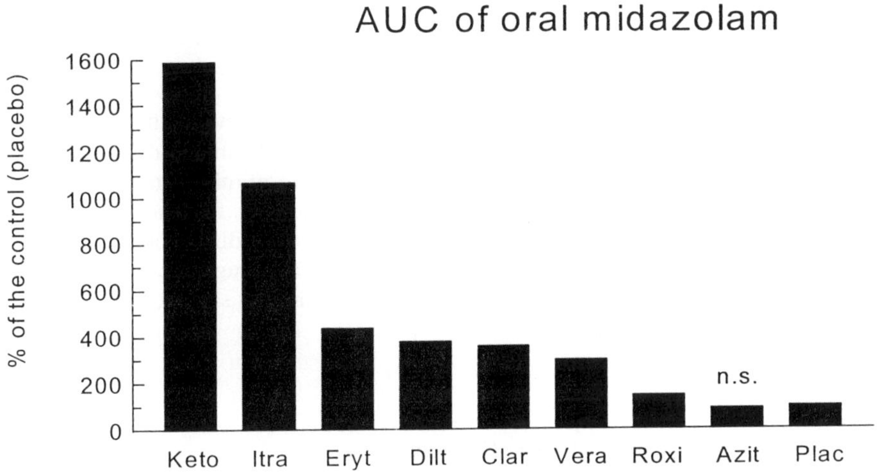

Figure 1: The effect of various drugs on the AUC of oral midazolam compared with placebo. Keto, ketoconazole; Itra, itraconazole; Eryt, erythromycin; Dilt, diltiazem; Clar, clarithromycin; Vera, verapamil; Roxi, roxithromycin; Azit, azithromycin; Plac, placebo. N.S., not significantly different from placebo. Data from references [31-36].

To summarise, midazolam is a sensitive probe of CYP3A4 activity *in vivo*, since its pharmacokinetics are very susceptible to inhibition and induction of CYP3A4. By using orally administered midazolam (or triazolam) as a probe, the potential of drugs to affect CYP3A4 activity *in vivo* can be assessed. For example, the pharmacokinetics of midazolam were unaffected by azithromycin [35], strongly suggesting that azithromycin does not cause clinically significant interactions with CYP3A4 substrates.

PROTON PUMP INHIBITORS (PPI) AS INHIBITORS OR INDUCERS

Omeprazole can induce (CYP1A subfamily) and inhibit (CYP2C19) drug metabolism [38,39]. It is controversial whether this is of clinical significance and whether other PPI, such as pantoprazole or lansoprazole share the same interaction potential [22,40]. Therefore we recently tested in a randomized, placebo-controlled, 4-way cross-over study in 20 healthy, non-smoking and drug-free volunteers (extensive metabolizers of CYP2C19, *H. pylori* negative) whether 10 days' treatment with omeprazole (40mg/day), pantoprazole (80mg/day) or lansoprazole (60mg/day) affected the steady state disposition of theophylline (350 mg bid given as a slow release preparation), a common probe of CYP1A2. During all 4 parts of the study plasma concentration time profiles following the last theophylline dose were nearly identical and the 90% C.I. for the ratios for bioequivalence criteria (e.g. AUC; peak; mean and trough C_{ss}; % PTF) fluctuated around unity. Therefore it appears very unlikely that the 3 PPI, tested at a sufficiently high dosage, have a significant effect on the CYP1A2 activity [41].

CONCLUSIONS

According to the examples given drug metabolizing enzymes can be more or less specifically inhibited or induced by a variety of compounds ingested in form of food constituents or drugs (Table 2). The affected (pre-)systemic elimination will influence the disposition (PK) of many therapeutic agents and consequently their action (PD) can be affected as well. The interactions may necessitate dosage modifications, and sometimes selection of alternative drugs with a lower potential for drug interactions should be considered. In summary, enzyme inhibition and induction can significantly contribute to variability in human drug response.

Table 2.
Typical inhibitors and inducers of some CYP-enzymes

Enzyme	**Inhibitory reference compounds**	**Inducers**
CYP1A1	α-naphtoflavone	methylcholanthrene
CYP1A2	furafylline, fluvoxamine	smoking, omeprazole
CYP2A6	methoxsalen, pilocarpine	phenobarbital
CYP2C8/9/18	sulfaphenazole	phenobarbital, rifampicin
CYP2C19	fluconazole, omeprazole	phenobarbital, rifampicin
CYP2D6	quinidine	not inducible
CYP2E1	diethyldithiocarbamate	ethanol, INH
CYP3A(4)	ketoconazole, itraconazole	rifampicin, dexamethasone, anticonvulsants

ACKNOWLEDGEMENT: The valuable secretarial help of Mrs. H. Köhler and Mrs. G. Wilder is highly appreciated.

REFERENCES

1. Gonzalez FJ. Human cytochromes P450 : problems and prospects. Trends Pharmacol Sci 1992;13:346-352.
2. Guengerich FP. Human cytochrome P450 enzymes. Life Sci 1992;50:1471-1478.
3. Krishna DR, Klotz U. Extrahepatic metabolism of drugs in humans. Clin Pharmacokinet 1994;26:144-160.
4. Pelkonen O, Breimer DD. Role of environmental factors in the pharmacokinetics of drugs: considerations with respect to animal models, P-450 enzymes, and probe drugs. In: Welling PG, Balant LP (eds.) Handbook of Experimental Pharmacology 110. Berlin: Springer, 1994;289-332.
5. Lin JH, Lu AYH. Role of pharmacokinetics and metabolism in drug discovery and development. Pharmacol Rev 1997;49:403-449.
6. Vesell ES. The model drug approach in clinical pharmacology. Clin Pharmacol Ther 1991;50:239-248
7. Kivistö KT, Kroemer HK. Use of probe drugs as predictors of drug metabolism in humans. J Clin Pharmacol 1997;37:40S-48S.
8. Wilkinson GR. Clearance approaches in pharmacology. Pharmacol Rev 1987; 39:1-47.
9. Bailey DB, Spence JD, Munoz C, Arnold JMO. Interaction of citrus juices with felodipine and nifedipine. Lancet 1991;1:268-269.
10. Walter-Sack I, Klotz U. Influence of diet and nutritional status on drug metabolism. Clin Pharmacokinet 1996;31:47-64.
11. Wilkinson GR. The effects of diet, aging and disease-states on presystemic elimination and oral drug bioavailability in humans. Adv Drug Deliv Rev 1997;27:129-159.
12. Benton RE, Honig PK, Zamani K, Cantilena LR, Woosley RL. Grapefruit juice alters terfenadine pharmacokinetics, resulting in prolongation of repolarization on the electrocardiogram. Clin Pharmacol Ther 1996;59:383-388.
13. Honig PK, Wortham DC, Lazarev A, Cantilena LR. Grapefruit juice alters the systemic bioavailability and cardiac repolarization of terfenadine in poor metabolizers of terfenadine. J Clin Pharmacol 1996;36:345-351.
14. Kupferschmidt HHT, Ha HR, Ziegler WH, Meier PJ, Krähenbühl S. Interaction between grapefruit juice and midazolam in humans. Clin Pharmacol Ther 1995;58:20-28.
15. Edwards DJ, Bellevue III FH, Woster PM. Identification of 6', 7'-dihydroxybergamottin, a cytochrome P450 inhibitor, in grapefruit juice. Drug Metab Disp 1996;24:1287-1290.

16. Klotz U, Ammon E. Clinical and toxicological consequences of the inductive potential of ethanol. Eur J Clin Pharmacol 1998;54:7-12.
17. Dilger K, Metzler J, Bode JC, Klotz U. CYP2E1 activity in patients with alcoholic liver disease. J Hepatol 1997;27:1009-1014.
18. Park BK, Kitteringham NR, Pirmohamed M, Tucker GT. Relevance of induction of human drug-metabolizing enzymes: pharmacological and toxicological implications. Br J Clin Pharmacol 1996;41:477-491.
19. Zimmerman HJ, Maddrey WC. Acetaminophen (paracetamol) hepatotoxicity with regular intake of alcohol: analysis of instances of therapeutic misadventure. Hepatology 1995;22:767-773.
20. Collins C, Starmer GA. A review of the hepatotoxicity of paracetamol at therapeutic or near therapeutic dose levels, with particular reference to alcohol users. Drug Alcohol Rev 1995;14:63-79.
21. Klotz U, Reimann I. Drug interactions through binding to cytochrome P450: The experience with H_2-receptor blocking agents. Pharm Res 1984;2:59-62.
22. Guengerich FP. Role of cytochrome P450 enzymes in drug-drug interactions. Adv Pharmacol 1997;43:7-35.
23. Gerber MC, Tejwani GA, Gerber N, Bianchine JR. Drug interactions with cimetidine. An update. Pharmacol Ther 1985;27:353-370
24. Klotz U, Kroemer HK. The drug interaction potential of ranitidine: an update. Pharmacol Ther 1991;50:233-244.
25. Hebert MF, Roberts JP, Prueksaritanont T, Benet LZ. Bioavailability of cyclosporine with concomitant rifampin administration is markedly less than predicted by hepatic enzyme induction. Clin Pharmacol Ther 1992;52:453-457.
26. Backman JT, Kivistö KT, Olkkola KT, Neuvonen PJ. The area under the plasma concentration-time curve for oral midazolam is 400-fold larger during treatment with itraconazole than with rifampicin. Eur J Clin Pharmacol 1998;54:53-58.
27. Fromm MF, Busse D, Kroemer HK, Eichelbaum M. Differential induction of prehepatic and hepatic metabolism of verapamil by rifampin. Hepatology 1996;24:796-801.
28. Fromm MF, Dilger K, Busse D, Kroemer HK, Eichelbaum M, Klotz U. Gut wall metabolism of verapamil in older people: effect of rifampicin-mediated enzyme induction. Br J Clin Pharmacol 1998;45:247-255.
29. Allonen H, Ziegler G, Klotz U. Midazolam kinetics. Clin Pharmacol Ther 1981; 30:653-661.
30. Lown KS, Thummel KE, Benedict PE, Shen DD, Turgeon DK, Berent S, Watkins PB. The erythromycin breath test predicts the clearance of midazolam. Clin Pharmacol Ther 1995;57:16-24.
31. Olkkola KT, Aranko K, Luurila H, Hiller A, Saarnivaara L, Himberg J-J, Neuvonen PJ. A potentially hazardous interaction between erythromycin and midazolam. Clin Pharmacol Ther 1993;53:298-305.
32. Backman JT, Aranko K, Himberg J-J, Olkkola KT. A pharmacokinetic interaction between roxithromycin and midazolam. Eur J Clin Pharmacol 1994;46:551-555.

33. Backman JT, Olkkola KT, Aranko K, Himberg J-J, Neuvonen PJ. Dose of midazolam should be reduced during diltiazem and verapamil treatments. Br J Clin Pharmacol 1994;37:221-225.
34. Olkkola KT, Backman JT, Neuvonen PJ. Midazolam should be avoided in patients receiving the systemic antimycotics ketoconazole or itraconazole. Clin Pharmacol Ther 1994;55:481-485.
35. Backman JT, Olkkola KT, Neuvonen PJ. Azithromycin does not increase plasma concentrations of oral midazolam. Int J Clin Pharmacol Ther 1995;33:356-359.
36. Yeates RA, Laufen H, Zimmermann T. Interaction between midazolam and clarithromycin: comparison with azithromycin. Int J Clin Pharmacol Ther 1996;34:400-405.
37. Backman JT, Olkkola KT, Neuvonen PJ. Rifampin drastically reduces plasma concentrations and effects of oral midazolam. Clin Pharmacol Ther 1996;59:7-13.
38. Diaz D, Fabre I, Daujat M, Saint Aubert B, Bories P, Michel H., Maurel P. Omeprazole is an aryl hydrocarbon-like inducer of human hepatic cytochrome P-450. Gastroenterology 1990;99:737-747.
39. Andersson T, Cederberg C, Edvardsson G, Heggelund A, Lundborg P. Effect of omeprazole treatment on diazepam plasma levels in slow versus normal rapid metabolizers of omeprazole. Clin Pharmacol Ther 1990;47:79-85.
40. Andersson T. Pharmacokinetics, metabolism and interactions of acid pump inhibitors. Focus on omeprazole, lansoprazole and pantoprazole. Clin Pharmacokinet 1996;31:9-28.
41. Dilger K, Templin S, Kadus W, Klotz U. Do proton pump inhibitors (PPI) affect the disposition of theophylline? Naunyn Schmiedeberg's Arch Pharmacol 1998;358(suppl 3)R-770.

Discussion: Enzyme inhibition of polymorphic drug metabolism

E.M. Sellers:

Perhaps we need to give a little bit more attention to how we characterise variations in activity. We tend to use ratios of parent drug to metabolite, which from a psychometric point of view are very unsatisfactory. We should probably be focusing much more on fractional clearances and absolute recoveries by particular pathways, because these give a much more accurate estimate of what is the real activity of the enzyme.

U. Klotz:

We discovered in this interaction study that there were quite dramatic differences by comparing the ratio technique with using area under the curves. But it is much more tedious to measure a whole time profile during the dosing intervals than just a single measurement. For routine use the ratio technique is much more convenient, but it is much more variable.

P. Rolan:

The extent of the variability of the caffeine metabolic ratio is surprising, because that test has been suggested as a screening tool and if its variability is that large, it means that you could fail to find an effect just due to the variability. I wonder whether part of the problem was again selecting the ratio, because there are at least five metabolic caffeine ratios.

U. Klotz:

We used the ratio (MR) which, according also to Geoffrey Tucker and other experts, is independent of the renal excretion [MR = (AFMU+1X+1U)/1,7U]

G.T. Tucker:

The issue of what index of enzyme activity you use is really quite important. From a theoretical point of view certainly I would defend the metabolic ratio over urine metabolite recovery as an index, because the latter depends not just on the pathway you are interested in but on parallel pathways also. Theoretically, the urinary drug to metabolite ratio for a simple system is a function of the partial clearance by the enzyme you are interested in, in the denominator, and in the numerator you have the renal clearance of the parent drug. Thus, renal clearance is the potential source of noise in using these ratios as markers of enzyme activity. The kinetic bases of the indices that we use should be considered more carefully.

N.L. Benowitz:

In the verapamil studies when you look at inhibition, is there a general relationship between hepatic CYP3A4 activity and intestinal activity, or are these regulated separately?

U. Klotz:

For a long time it was thought that CYP3A4 in the intestinal wall and in the liver were using the same substrates. The same inhibitors and the same inducers could affect both sites, and there might be some kind of co-regulation. But more recently, some evidence has appeared showing that both enzymes are probably regulated in a slightly different way.

P. du Souich:

I would like to reiterate again that it is very difficult to interpret the effect of a drug on theophylline kinetics, because at least four enzymes are contributing to its clearance. When you modify one of these enzymes you do not know exactly how the alternative pathways will respond. We do not know if they will remain exactly the same, and follow predictable first-order kinetics or not. Another practical point I would like to make from the examples you have shown, should we think about developing drugs for alternative routes of administration, for example, sublingual, transcutaneous or even inhaled drugs, to try to avoid these effects of intestinal and liver variability?

U. Klotz:

This could be one alternative to get round intestinal metabolism, although comparative studies with different routes of administration are required.

A.J.J. Wood:

We need to be careful just extrapolating from studies done with one route to another route and assuming that the effects will be exactly the same. I suspect that the effects are not identical.

J. Urquhart:

If you are going to use other routes, you need more potent drugs and there are not very many of them.

U. Klotz:

Bioavailability then becomes an issue, because to develop a new formulation you have to complete new studies in terms of efficacy and toxicity. Then, it is probably much easier to perform 2 or 3 interaction studies, instead.

Variability in Human Drug Response
G.T. Tucker, Editor

Adverse drug reactions: role of enzyme inhibition and induction

Munir Pirmohamed and Brian Kevin Park

Department of Pharmacology and Therapeutics, The University of Liverpool, Ashton Street, Liverpool, U.K.

ABSTRACT

Human drug metabolising enzymes can be induced or inhibited by drugs, foodstuffs, and alcohol. which can predispose to toxicity from both endogenous and exogenous substrates. For endogenous substrates, enzyme inhibition can lead to a deficiency of an essential metabolite or accumulation of an otherwise non-toxic compound. Enzyme induction by increasing metabolism of endogenous compounds can lead to a deficiency state, e.g. vitamin D deficiency with phenytoin. With drugs, perturbation of enzyme activity can lead to both type A and type B adverse drug reactions (ADRs) depending on whether phase I or phase II pathways are affected. Thus type A ADRs can result from inhibition or induction of phase I pathways, the toxicity being due to the parent drug or active metabolite, respectively. Type B ADRs result form induction of phase I, or inhibition of phase II pathways, with a resultant imbalance between bioactivation and detoxication. Knowledge of drug effects on metabolic pathways is important so that their potential to cause toxicity can be anticipated. In the long-term, it is important to develop "cleaner" compounds so that the problem of enzyme inhibition and enzyme induction can be eliminated, and together with it, the potential of such drugs to cause ADRs.

Key words: hypersensitivity, idiosyncratic, interaction, toxicity, chemically reactive metabolites.

Correspondence: Dr. M. Pirmohamed, Department of Pharmacology and Therapeutics, University of Liverpool, Ashton Street, Liverpool L69 3GE, U.K., Tel: +44-151-794-5549, Fax: +44-151-794-5540, Email: munirp@liv.ac.uk

INTRODUCTION

An adverse drug reaction (ADR) may be defined as any undersirable effect of a drug beyond its anticipated therapeutic effects occurring during clinical use [1]. ADRs are common and account for 2-6% of all hospital admissions [2]. A recent meta-analysis has suggested that ADRs are the fourth commonest cause of death in the USA [3].

In general, ADRs can be divided into two types, type A and type B [1]. Type A reactions represent an augmentation of the pharmacological actions of a drug, are dose-dependent and therefore readily reversible on drug withdrawal, or after dose-reduction. In contrast, type B, or idiosyncratic adverse reactions, are bizarre, and cannot be predicted from the known pharmacology of the drug. Type A reactions account for over 80% of all ADRs.

There are many factors which predispose to ADRs: these have been considered in more detail elsewhere [4,5]. The purpose of this chapter is to evaluate the role of inhibition and induction of enzymes in predisposing to ADRs. When considering the role of either enzyme inhibition or enzyme induction in ADRs, it is important to note that (a) the toxicity may arise as a result of an alteration in the metabolism of either endogenous or exogenous substances (Table 1), and (b) both type A and type B reactions may arise as a result of modulation of enzyme activity.

Table 1
Mechanisms of adverse drug reactions resulting from effects of changes in enzyme activity for endogenous and exogenous substrates

	Endogenous substrates	Exogenous substrates
Enzyme inhibition	· Deficiency of essential metabolite, production of abnormal and biologically inactive metabolites, or accumulation of intermediary products which become toxic when present in excess	· Increased levels of parent drug resulting in dose-dependent toxicity · Decreased bioinactivation of an active metabolite resulting in idiosyncratic toxicity
Enzyme induction	· Increased metabolism of an endogenous substrate resulting in a deficiency state	· Increased production of a toxic metabolite resulting in either dose-dependent (idiosyncratic) toxicity

PHARMACOKINETIC CONSIDERATIONS

The toxiclogical impact of enzyme inhibiton is dependent on

(i) the degree and duration of enzyme inhibition (as determined by the potency of the inhibitor, the nature of inhibition and the pharmacokinetics of the inhibitor), and

(ii) the biological importance of the enzyme and its ability to overcome inhibition by either synthesis of more enzyme or utilization of alternative biochemical pathways.

The impact of enzyme inhibition on drug half-life is very sensitive to the fraction of the dose normally metabolised via the inhibited pathway [6]. Thus, if drug clearance is dependent on one pathway, then inhibition of that pathway, will lead to supra-pharmacological concentrations of the inhibited drug, and possible toxicity. When drug clearance is dependent on more than one pathway, inhibition of one of the pathways may have little effect on plasma drug concentrations, and thus is unlikely to cause toxicity. The exception to this are drugs with a narrow therapeutic index, such as warfarin and phenytoin, where a relatively modest change in plasma levels may result in a shift from a therapeutic response to a toxic effect [6].

Enzyme induction by increasing drug clearance will lead to a reduction in parent drug concentration, and thus loss of efficacy [7]. Loss of efficacy is not considered as an adverse drug reaction in the context of this chapter, but nevertheless is important, since it can result in re-emergence of the underlying disease process, for example, thrombosis in a patient administered an enzyme inducer while anticoagulated on warfarin. Clearly, the effect of enzyme induction can be overcome by increasing the dose of the drug. Whether the dose needs to be increased and by how much depends on whether drug clearance is dependent on one or more than one metabolic pathway. This has been considered in detail in a recent review [7]. With particular respect to this chapter, more important is a consideration of toxic metabolite formation via the induced pathway. The rate of reactive metabolite formation will increase as a function of the change in the maximal velocity of the reaction (V_{max}). If the reactive metabolite is normally only a minor metabolite (<5%), then the total dose of the toxic metabolite will increase substantially. Such an increase in reactive metabolite formation may be adequate to overcome the detoxication processes, unless these are also induced, resulting in toxicity.

DRUGS AND THE METABOLISM OF ENDOGENOUS SUBSTRATES

Inhibition of the metabolism of endogenous substrates

Various drugs designed as enzyme inhibitors to achieve their therapeutic actions may also result in the interruption of the metabolism of other closely related endogenous compounds or the same endogenous compound but at a different site in the body, resulting in an adverse drug reactions [6]. Examples of enzymes inhibited, the endogenous substrates affected, and the toxicity which results because of the inhibition, are listed in table 2

Prevention of ADRs with some drugs may be possible by developing more selective enzyme inhibitors [1]. Non-steroidal anti-inflammatory drugs best exemplify this. Inhibition of cyclo-oxygenase in the joints is responsible for their therapeutic action, while inhibition of cyclo-oxygenase in extra-articular tissues such as the stomach and kidney, can result in peptic ulceration and renal insufficiency, respectively. The recent discoveries that there are two isoforms of COX (COX-1 and COX-2), and that COX-2 expression is enhanced in inflammatory conditions, has led to the development of selective COX-2 inhibitors based on the hypothesis that sparing of COX-1 activity may prevent toxicity. Preliminary clinical experience has suggested that selective COX-2 inhibitors have both anti-inflammatory and gastrointestinal sparing properties, but whether this is translated into long-term safety will only become evident with clinical experience [8].

Table 2.
Examples of adverse drug reactions produced as a result of inhibition of the metabolism of endogenous substrates

Enzyme	Enzyme inhibitor	Endogenous substrate	Adverse reaction
Angiotensin converting enzyme	ACE inhibitors, e.g. captopril	Bradykinin	Angio-oedema
Cholinesterase	Anti-cholinesterases, e.g. neostigmine	Acetylcholine	Abdominal cramps, salivation and diarrhoea
Cyclo-oxygenase	Non-steroidal anti-inflammatory drugs, e.g. diclofenac	Prostaglandins	Peptic ulceration, nephrotoxicity
Cytochrome P450 enzymes	Ketoconazole	Corticosteroids, testosterone	Adrenal suppression, impotence
Dihydrofolate reductase	Methotrexate	Folic acid	Megaloblastic anaemia
Monoamine oxidase	Iproniazid	Catecholamines	Hypertensive crises

Induction of the metabolism of endogenous substrates

Induction of the metabolism of endogenous substrates such as thyroid hormones and vitamin D may lead to clinically significant deficiency of such substrates. For example, use of phenobarbitone in rats leads to increased glucuronidation of the thyroid hormones, which is followed by functional adaptation of the thyroid gland, with respect to size and activity. Subclinical depression of thyroid hormone concentrations has been reported in epileptics and in patients taking rifampicin, although the incidence of clinical hypothyroidism in such patients is low [7,9]. Enzyme inducers can also perturb the metabolism of steroids and fat-soluble vitamins. Induction of vitamin D metabolism by drugs such as phenytoin can lead to osteomalacia [10].

DRUGS AND THE METABOLISM OF EXOGENOUS SUBSTRATES

The rate of elimination of a lipophilic drug is governed largely by its rate of metabolism. Metabolism via either the phase I oxidation pathways and/or the phase II conjugation pathways is usually associated with an increase in the water solubility of the compound and thus enhanced clearance. Metabolism can also lead to the formation of toxic, chemically reactive metabolites from drugs (a process termed bioactivation), which if not detoxified by detoxication mechanisms in body, can bind to cellular macromolecules and lead to various forms of idiosyncratic toxicity (such as tissue necrosis, hypersensitivity reactions and teratogenicity) [4,5,11].

Modulation of any of these pathways by either enzyme inhibitors or enzyme inducers can increase the risk of toxicity (table 1). Therefore, an enzyme inhibitor may (a) reduce elimination of the drug leading to dose-dependent toxicity, or (b) by inhibiting the detoxication pathways, decrease inactivation of a toxic metabolite and predispose to idiosyncratic toxicity. Conversely, enzyme induction (of the phase I metabolic pathways) may increase chemically reactive metabolite formation.

Table 3.
Cytochrome P450 isozymes involved in the metabolism of drugs and xenobiotics in man

P450 isoform	Substrates	Inducers	Inhibitors
CYP1A2	Clozapine Theophylline	Cigarette smoke Omeprazole	Ciprofloxacin Furafylline
CYP2A6	Halothane Methoxyflurane	Phenytoin Rifampicin	Tranylcypromine
CYP2C9	Diclofenac Tolbutamide Warfarin	Barbiturates Rifampicin	Sulphaphenazole
CYP2C19	Citalopram Diazepam Omeprazole	Rifampicin	Tranylcypromine
CYP2D6	Codeine Haloperidol Metoprolol Nortriptyline	Not inducible	Quinidine
CYP2E1	Enflurane Halothane Paracetamol	Alcohol (chronic use)	Disulfiram
CYP3A4	Amiodarone Carbamazepine Cyclosporin Terfenadine	Carbamazepine Glucocorticoids Phenytoin Rifampicin	Ketoconazole Erythromycin
CYP4A1	Testosterone	Clofibrate	-

Only few substrates, inhibitors and inducers have been mentioned for each P450 isoform.

The enzymes most liable to undergo inhibition and induction and thereby be involved in ADRs are the cytochrome P450 enzymes. There are many different P450 isoforms, and many of these can be induced and inhibited in a selective fashion, resulting in different forms of drug toxicity [12]. Table 3 provides a summary of the different P450 isoforms together with their inducers and inhibitors.

Enzyme inhibition and dose-dependent adverse drug reactions

The concomitant administration of a drug with a narrow therapeutic index together with an enzyme inhibitor can lead to adverse drug interactions, which can be severe and occasionally fatal. Many such interactions have been reported, and the drugs with a narrow therapeutic index most likely to be involved are the aromatic anticonvulsants, theophylline, cyclosporin, warfarin, terfenadine and cisapride [13]. In all cases, inhibition of the relevant P450 isoform needed for metabolism of these drugs is involved in the pathogenesis of the ADR. The reader is referred elsewhere for a more detailed discussion of such adverse drug reactions [13].

An area which has generated a lot of media interest and has resulted in drug regulatory action is the interaction between non-sedating antihistamines and CYP3A4 inhibitors. Astemizole and terfenadine, both non-sedating antihistamines, have been reported to cause life-threatening cardiac arrhythmias [14]. Attention has primarily focused on terfenadine, which is the most widely used. Terfenadine is a pro-drug that is converted to a carboxylic acid metabolite by CYP3A4 [5]. Terfenadine cannot normally be detected in the plasma, unless taken in overdosage or when its metabolism is inhibited. The latter has been reported to occur by various drugs including ketoconazole, itraconazole, erythromycin and clarithromycin [15]. Grapefruit juice also inhibits the metabolism of terfenadine [16]. When any of these drugs are given together with terfenadine, the elevated plasma terfenadine concentration leads to prolongation of the QT-interval, which in turn, may lead to a polymorphic ventricular tachycardia termed "torsades de pointes" [14]. Both terfenadine and astemizole block the ventricular potassium channels, particularly the rapidly activating component of the delayed rectifier, which increases the duration of the action potential and the QT-interval [17]. In order to reduce the risk of arrhythmias with terfenadine, the legal status of the drug has recently been changed, so that it is now only available as a prescription-only medicine [14]. In addition, its active metabolite (fexofenadine), which does not affect potassium [18], has recently been marketed as a drug in its own right.

Enzyme inhibition and idiosyncratic toxicity

Inhibition of P450 enzymes can actually lead to a reduction in the formation of a toxic or chemically reactive metabolite, and may thereby protect against idiosyncratic toxicity (discussed below). Conversely, inhibition of detoxication enzymes can decrease bioinactivation of the toxic metabolite, and increase the propensity of a drug to cause idiosyncratic toxicity. Given the wide and overlapping substrate specificities of most of the detoxication enzymes, such situations fortunately are uncommon. An area that has caused concern however is the increase in frequency of teratogenicity in patients on combination anti-epileptic therapy which includes valpromide and valproic acid. Both these drugs are inhibitors of microsomal epoxide hydrolase, which catalyses the hydrolysis of various epoxides, including arene oxides. Lindhout *et al.* [19] reported a 58% rate of foetal malformations associated with combination therapy (which included valproic acid); inhibition of foetal microsomal epoxide hydrolase by valproic acid, thus increasing foetal exposure to reactive epoxides has been suggested to be the mechanism [20].

Enzyme induction and dose-dependent toxicity

Enzyme induction increases the clearance of a drug and therefore should protect against dose-dependent toxicity. However, if the toxicity is due to an active metabolite, then enzyme induction will increase the risk of toxicity. The clearest example of this is paracetamol which causes hepatotoxicity when taken in overdosage, and still causes about 160 deaths per year in the UK [21]. According to the definition of adverse drug reactions given above, paracetamol hepatotoxicity should not be classified as an adverse drug reaction, since the hepatic injury occurs when the drug is used inappropriately. However, it is important to note that the occurrence of liver damage with paracetamol and its severity is a function not only of the dose but also of various host factors [5]. Indeed, paracetamol hepatotoxicity has been reported with therapeutic drug use. For example, a recent study in 67 alcoholics who had sustained liver injury after paracetamol ingestion, showed that 40% had taken less than 4g/day (the maximum recommended therapeutic dose) while another 20% had taken between 4-6g/day (which is also regarded as a non-toxic dose) [22]. In therapeutic dosage, paracetamol is largely metabolised by phase II processes (glucuronidation and sulphation) to stable metabolites, but between 5-10% also undergoes P450 metabolism to the toxic quinoneimine metabolite [23]. This is detoxified by cellular glutathione. In overdosage, saturation of the phase II metabolic pathways results in a greater proportion of the drug undergoing bioactivation. This ultimately leads to depletion of cellular glutathione, and allows the toxic metabolite to bind to hepatic proteins resulting in hepatocellular damage [23]. The use of N-acetylcysteine in the treatment of paracetamol overdosage illustrates the important point that elucidation of the mechanism of drug toxicity can lead to the development of rational therapies which will prevent the toxicity. Alcoholics show increased susceptibility to paracetamol overdosage because excess alcohol consumption results in depletion of glutathione [24] and induction of the P450 isoform CYP2E1 [25]. Recent studies in knockout mice have shown that CYP2E1 is the primary isoform involved in the bioactivation of paracetamol [26]. Patients on enzyme-inducing anticonvulsants (which leads to induction of CYP3A4) are also more susceptible to paracetamol hepatotoxicity, and require treatment with N-acetylcysteine at lower plasma paracetamol concentrations [27].

Dapsone, a drug used in the treatment of leprosy, is associated with dose-dependent methaemoglobinaemia [28]. This is thought to be due to P450-mediated (CYP3A4, CYP2C9 and CYP2E1) activation of dapsone to the hydroxylamine metabolite [29]. The hydroxylamine is taken up by red cells where it is co-oxidised with haemoglobin to form nitroso-dapsone and methaemoglobin. Dapsone is usually co-administered with the potent enzyme inducer rifampicin in the treatment of leprosy. In these patients, it has been shown that rifampicin significantly increases the formation clearance of dapsone hydroxylamine by fourfold and methaemoglobinaemia by 1.7-fold [30].

Enzyme induction and idiosyncratic toxicity

Enzyme induction by increasing drug bioactivation (and hence chemically reactive metabolite formation) may overcome the detoxication processes and lead to idiosyncratic toxicity. However, it is important to note that there is very little direct data to support this. This is partly due to the fact that predisposition to idiosyncratic toxicity is multi-factorial, and the presence one predisposing factor, i.e. enzyme induction, may be compensated for by the lack of other predisposing factors [1]. The important examples of enzyme induction predisposing to idiosyncratic ADRs include the following:

- Isoniazid by itself causes hepatotoxicity in 1% of patients. Co-administration with rifampicin increases the frequency of hepatitis to 7%; this is thought to be secondary to induction of bioactivation of isoniazid to reactive hydrazine intermediates [31].
- Alcohol is metabolised by alcohol dehydrogenase (80%) and CYP2E1 (20%). Chronic alcoholics have induction of CYP2E1 and thus a higher proportion of alcohol undergoing metabolism via CYP2E1. Metabolism of alcohol by CYP2E1 causes the formation of toxic hydroxyethyl radicals, which have been implicated in the pathogenesis of alcoholic liver disease. Thus, autoinduction of its own metabolism by alcohol may increase the risk of liver injury [5].
- Carbamazepine causes generalised hypersensitivity in small number (1:1000-5000) of patients taking the drug. Bioactivation of carbamazepine by CYP3A4 to a toxic arene oxide metabolite is thought to be the initial step in the pathogenesis of toxicity [32]. Carbamazepine induces CYP3A4, and therefore bioactivation to the arene oxide metabolite [33]. However, there is varaibility in induction at the same dose levels, which may serve as a factor in predisposing to this form of idiosyncratic toxicity [34].

PREVENTION OF ADVERSE DRUG REACTIONS BY MODULATION OF ENZYME ACTIVITY

If induction of P450 enzymes predisposes to drug toxicity, then it would seem logical to suppose that therapeutic use of an enzyme inhibitor may prevent toxicity. Using this rationale, and dapsone-induced methaemoglobinaemia as the paradigm, we were able to show that its conversion to dapsone hydroxylamine, and thus methaemoglobinaemia, could be prevented *in vitro* [35], *in vivo* in volunteers [36] and in patients with dermatitis herpetiformis [37], by cimetidine, a P450 inhibitor. The use of disulfiram, a CYP2E1 inhibitor, before halothane anaesthesia has also been suggested (but not yet proven) as a way of preventing halothane hepatitis [38].

Induction of detoxication enzymes may also protect against toxicity, although this has not been used therapeutically. Vegetables such as broccoli contain potent inducers of quinone reductase and glutathione transferase; this has been put forward as the explanation why consumption of vegetables reduces the risk of cancer [39]. Oltipraz, which is an inducer of phase II enzymes (quinone reductase, glutathione transferase and glucuronyl transferase), has been shown to protect against the acute toxicities of many xenobiotics, and inhibits experimental carcinogenesis [40].

CONCLUSION

Human drug metabolising enzymes can be induced or inhibited by a variety of xenobiotics. This contributes to the intra-individual and inter-individual variation in the rate and route of metabolism of xenobiotics, which in some instances, predisposes to an ADR. Any type of

ADR (i.e. type A or type B) can result from a change in enzyme activity. Through knowledge of the metabolic pathways, and the properties of any co-administered drug, it may be possible to anticipate and avoid type A ADRs. For type B ADRs, this is more difficult, since even knowledge of the pathway affected by a concomitantly administered drug does not necessarily allow accurate prediction of the toxicity. The ultimate aim in the future must be to develop pharmacologically "cleaner" drugs so that the problem of enzyme inhibition and enzyme induction can be prevented, and at least some of the factors causing ADRs avoided.

REFERENCES

1. Pirmohamed M, Breckenridge AM, Kitteringham NR, Park BK. Adverse drug reactions: current status. Br Med J 1998;316:1295-1298.
2. Einarson TR. Drug-related hospital admissions. Ann Pharmacother 1993;27:832-840.
3. Lazarou J, Pomeranz BH, Corey PN. Incidence of adverse drug reactions in hospitalized patients - A meta-analysis of prospective studies. JAMA 1998;279:1200-1205.
4. Park BK, Pirmohamed M, Kitteringham NR. Idiosyncratic drug reactions: a mechanistic evaluation of risk factors. Br J Clin Pharmacol 1992;34:377-395.
5. Pirmohamed M, Kitteringham NR, Park BK. The role of active metabolites in drug toxicity. Drug Saf 1994;11:114-144.
6. Pirmohamed M, Park BK. Enzyme inhibition-mediated toxic effects of drugs. In: Sandler M, Smith J (eds.) Design of enzyme inhibitors as drugs. Oxford: OUP, 1994:800-818.
7. Park BK, Kitteringham NR, Pirmohamed M, Tucker GT. Relevance of induction of human drug-metabolizing enzymes: pharmacological and toxicological implications. Br J Clin Pharmacol 1996;41:477-491.
8. Yeomans ND, Cook GA, Giraud AS. Selective COX-2 inhibitors: Are they safe for the stomach? Gastroenterology 1998;115:227-229.
9. Larkin JG, Macphee GJA, Beastall GH, Brodie MJ. Thyroid hormone concentrations in epileptic patients. Eur J Clin Pharmacol 1989;36:213-216.
10. Park BK, Kitteringham NR. Assessment of enzyme induction and enzyme inhibition in humans: toxicological implications. Xenobiotica 1990;20:1171-1185.
11. Pirmohamed M, Madden S, Park BK. Idiosyncratic drug reactions: metabolic bioactivation as a pathogenic mechanism. Clin Pharmacokin 1996;31:215-230.
12. Kitteringham NR, Pirmohamed M, Park BK. The pharmacology of the cytochrome P450 enzyme system. Baill Clin Anaesthesiol 1998;in press.
13. Pirmohamed M, Orme ML'E. Drug interactions of clinical importance. In: Davies DM, Ferner RE, de Glanville H (eds.) Textbook of Adverse Drug Reactions. London: Chapman & Hall, 1998:888-912.
14. Rankin AC. Non-sedating antihistamines and cardiac arrhythmia. Lancet 1997;350:1115-1116.
15. Ament PW, Paterson A. Drug interactions with the nonsedating antihistamines. American Family Physician 1997;56:223.
16. Benton RE, Honig PK, Zamani K, Cantilena LR, Woosley RL. Grapefruit juice alters terfenadine pharmacokinetics resulting in prolongation of repolarization on the electrocardiogram. Clin Pharmacol Ther 1996;59:383-388.

17. Salata JJ, Jurkiewicz NK, Wallace AA, Stupienski RF, Guinosso PJ, Lynch JJ. Cardiac electrophysiological actions of the histamine h-1-receptor antagonists astemizole and terfenadine compared with chlorpheniramine and pyrilamine. Circ Res 1995;76:110-119.
18. Woosley RL, Chen YW, Freiman JP, Gillis RA. Mechanism of the cardiotoxic actions of terfenadine. JAMA 1993;269:1532-1536.
19. Lindhout D, Hoppener RJEA, Meinardi H. Teratogenecity of anti-epileptic drug combinations with special emphasis on epoxidation (of carbamazepine). Epilepsia 1984;25:77-83.
20. Kerr BM, Rettie AE, Eddy C, *et al.* Inhibition of human liver microsomal epoxide hydrolase by valproate and valpromide: *in vitro/in vivo* correlation. Clin Pharmacol Ther 1989;46:82-93.
21. Bray GP. Liver failure induced by paracetamol. Br Med J 1993;306:157-158.
22. Zimmerman HJ, Maddrey WC. Acetaminophen (paracetamol) hepatotoxicity with regular intake of alcohol: analysis of instances of therapeutic misadventure. Hepatology 1995;22:767-773.
23. Nelson SD. Molecular mechanisms of the hepatotoxicity caused by acetaminophen. Semin Liver Dis 1990;10:267-278.
24. Lauterburg BH, Velez ME. Glutathione deficiency in alcoholics: Risk factor for paracetamol hepatotoxicity. Gut 1988;29:1153-1157.
25. Raucy JL, Lasker JM, Lieber CS, Black M. Acetaminophen activation by human liver cytochromes P-450IIE1 and P-450IA2. Arch Biochem Biophys 1989;271:270-283.
26. Lee SST, Buters JTM, Pineau T, Fernandezsalguero P, Gonzalez FJ. Role of cyp2e1 in the hepatotoxicity of acetaminophen. J Biol Chem 1996;271:12063-12067.
27. Bray GP, Harrison PM, O'Grady JG, Tredger JM, Williams R. Long-term anticonvulsant therapy worsens outcome in paracetamol-induced fulminant hepatic failure. Hum Exp Toxicol 1992;11:265-270.
28. Park BK, Pirmohamed M, Tingle MD, Madden S, Kitteringham NR. Bioactivation and bioinactivation of drugs and drug metabolites: relevance to adverse drug reactions. Tox in vitro 1994;8:613-621.
29. Gill HJ, Tingle MD, Park BK. N-hydroxylation of dapsone by multiple enzymes of cytochrome P450: implications for inhibition of haemotoxicity. Br J Clin Pharmacol 1995;40:531-539.
30. Occhipinti DJ, Choi A, Deyo K, Danziger LH, Fischer JH. Influence of rifampicin and clarithromycin on dapsone disposition and methemoglobin concentrations. Clin Pharmacol Ther 1995;57:163.
31. Pirmohamed M, Park BK. Mechanisms of hypertransaminemia. In: Cameron RG, Feuer G, de la Iglesia FA (eds.) Drug-Induced Hepatotoxicity. Berlin: Springer-Verlag, 1996:341-366.
32. Madden S, Maggs JL, Park BK. Bioactivation of carbamazepine in the rat in-vivo - evidence for the formation of reactive arene oxide(s). Drug Metab Dispos 1996;24:469-479.
33. Pirmohamed M, Kitteringham NR, Breckenridge AM, Park BK. The effect of enzyme induction on the cytochrome P450-mediated bioactivation of carbamazepine by mouse liver microsomes. Biochem Pharmacol 1992;44:2307-2314.

34. Pirmohamed M, Allott R, Kitteringham NR, Choonara I, Breckenridge AM, Park BK. Lymphocyte microsomal epoxide hydrolase activity in patients on chronic anticonvulsant therapy. Br J Clin Pharmacol 1993;36:159P.
35. Tingle MD, Coleman MD, Park BK. The effect of preincubation with cimetidine on the N-hydroxylation of dapsone by human liver microsomes. Br J Clin Pharmacol 1991;32:120-123.
36. Coleman MD, Scott AK, Breckenridge AM, Park BK. The use of cimetidine as a selective inhibitor of dapsone N-hydroxylation in man. Br J Clin Pharmacol 1990;30:761-767.
37. Rhodes LE, Tingle MD, Park BK, Chu P, Verbov JL, Friedmann PS. Cimetidine improves the therapeutic toxic ratio of dapsone in patients on chronic dapsone therapy. Br J Dermatol 1995;132:257-262.
38. Kharasch ED, Hankins D, Mautz D, Thummel KE. Identification of the enzyme responsible for oxidative halothane metabolism - implications for prevention of halothane hepatitis. Lancet 1996;347:1367-1371.
39. Zhang H, Zdolsek JM, Brunk UT. Alloxan cytotoxicity involves lysosomal damage. Apmis 1992;100:309-316.
40. Egner PA, Kensler TW, Prestera T, *et al.* Regulation of phase 2 enzyme-induction by oltipraz and other dithiolethiones. Carcinogenesis 1994;15:177-181.

Discussion: Adverse drug reactions: Role of enzyme inhibition and induction

H.K. Kroemer:
Terfenadine interaction is a good example, because its metabolism could be explained from the *in vitro* data. But it would not have occurred to anyone that this parent compound, which is basically inactive in terms of H_1 blockade, would block specifically the potassium channel in the heart. The current problem is to predict how relevant the QT prolongation is. A lot of studies have shown that there is an inhibition of the metabolism of some drugs by ketoconazole leading to QT_C prolongation at a specific percentage but it would be difficult to set the threshold. Secondly, from my point of view, it is time to discard the term idiosyncrasy. Maybe 10 years ago we would have attached this term, for example, to many of these CYP2D6-dependent reactions, which we understand nowadays. Idiosyncrasy should define a type of adverse drug reaction which we cannot explain based on our current knowledge.

M. Pirmohamed:
An idiosyncratic reaction is a functional term which does not imply any specific aetiology and for which we do not understand the mechanism. With regard to your first comment, there is a pharmacodynamic variance for these effects and a lot of drug companies are screening for drug actions on potassium channels. Through the knowledge basis we are obtaining of the metabolic and pharmacodynamic profile, hopefully in the future, it will be possible to prevent these kinds of severe interactions from occurring in clinical practice.

L. Aarons:
To actually describe idiosyncratic reactions as dose-independent seems to deny causality, and I suspect the real reason is that, as you just said, you do not have the information to describe the dose-response relationship.

M. Pirmohamed:
It is apparently dose-independent, but what we are looking at is the external dose. The internal dose is unknown as is the dose of the reactive metabolite formed in the body. If one was able to measure the reactive metabolite being formed accurately, then one may be able to say they are dose-independent in terms of the reactive metabolite itself, but dose-independent in terms of the parent drug.

A.J.J. Wood:
The term idiopathic might be better than idiosyncratic which is a moving target. It reflects our lack of knowledge now or in the past but it is not necessarily applicable to the present. Cough following ACE-inhibitors would have been idiosyncratic, I guess, in the absence of an explanation. In the presence of an explanation, it is not. I suspect the dose-effect depends on the concentration of bradykinin. It is knowledge of what the compound is that produces the effect, that presumably is dose-related, not necessarily the dose of the parent drug. For this reason I am not even sure that that is a very helpful definition any more, either.

M.M. Reidenberg:

These definitions are really contingent upon present knowledge. I think, as much as we dislike the term idiosyncratic, it is so well-established throughout medicine that it would be difficult to abolish the term now. We might gain more by defining it clearly in the way we have done: an adverse reaction that, based on present knowledge, is both not predictable and not understood.

M. Pirmohamed:

The term hypersensitivity also causes a lot of problems and is often misused. There needs to be some kind of definition which everybody uses, because different people tend to use the term hypersensitivity or idiosyncrasy differently in different contexts.

D.A. Smith:

The comment I wanted to make was about the specificity of the toxicity, and in particular when teratogenicity exists. Some toxic reactions, for example, a skin rash, some sort of blood dyscrasia, etc., are often associated for the sort of compounds you were describing. But considering teratogenicity, it always seems to me a very specific target because always the same sort of malformations are present. It is a specific set of syndromes which must occur by an interaction at a specific time in the growth of the foetus. I think this is difficult to relate this to the reactive metabolite theory because this theory holds that there is a specific target, one particular receptor or one particular gene.

M. Pirmohamed:

Not necessarily, because what one could hypothesise also is that it depends when, during foetal development, you actually take the drug, or what is the concentration of the drug or its reactive metabolite at that particular point because different organs are developed at different times. If one can interfere with the development of a particular organ, then one can develop a specific form of toxicity. If you examine different forms for teratogenicity, they do have similar features. The exact nature of the teratogenicity will depend on when that particular drug was taken during pregnancy and what particular target was hit at the time. That does not go against the reactive metabolite theory but clearly what one needs to do is to identify which particular target proteins, or target DNA system or target receptors are being hit by that particular reactive metabolite or parent drug.

Variability in Human Drug Response
G.T. Tucker, Editor

Approaches to studying the role of transporters in drug interactions in man

Paul B. Watkins

General Clinical Research Center, The University of Michigan Medical Center, Ann Arbor, MI, USA

ABSTRACT

It has been suggested that some drug interactions occur due to changes in the activities of xenobiotic transport proteins, such as P-glycoprotein, a "counter transport" protein present in the epithelial cells (enterocytes) lining the small intestine. It has been difficult to study the role of P-glycoprotein in drug interactions in man in part because most substrates of P-glycoprotein are also substrates for a drug metabolizing enzyme (CYP3A4) present in hepatocytes and enterocytes. We have developed techniques to safely quantitate liver CYP3A4 activity and enterocyte CYP3A4 and P-glycoprotein concentrations in humans. The large interpatient variation in each of these three variables makes it possible to use multiple regression to estimate the contribution of each parameter to the apparent oral clearance of specific drugs. This approach has shown the role of P-glycoprotein in drug interactions involving cyclosporin A and may be readily applicable to the study of other enterocyte transport proteins. A complimentary approach would be to develop safe and selective inhibitors of transporters to "knock out" the variable. The potential value of this approach has been demonstrated with Seville orange juice, which contains inhibitors of CYP3A4 but does not appear to contain inhibitors of P-glycoprotein.

Key words: CYP3A4, p-glycoprotein, cyclosporin A, grapefruit juice, Seville orange juice, drug interactions.

Correspondence: Prof. Paul B. Watkins, General Clinical Research Center, The University of Michigan Medical Center, A7119 UH, 1500 E. Medical Center, Ann Arbor, Michigan 48109-0108, USA, Tel: +1-734-936-8083, Fax: +1-734-647-9554, Email: pwatkins@umich.edu

INTRODUCTION

In the last decade, there has been great progress in understanding the regulation of human drug metabolizing enzymes, particularly the cytochromes P450. In some instances, this information has provided attractive explanations for known drug interactions, and successfully predicted drug interactions not yet observed in the clinic. However, it now appears likely that some drug interactions believed to have a metabolic basis may at least in part result from changes in the activity of transport proteins. An example of this appears to be drug interactions attributed to induction or inhibition of CYP3A4.

CYP3A4 is the most abundant cytochrome P450 present in the liver [1] and small intestine [2,3]. CYP3A4 has been shown to be the major enzyme involved in the metabolism of many important drugs in several classes, including immunosuppressants, calcium channel blockers, cancer chemotherapies antihistaminics, sedatives, synthetic estrogens, and HIV protease inhibitors [4]. Indeed, it has been estimated that up to one-half of all drugs in clinical use, or under development, are capable of being metabolized by CYP3A4 [5]. Treatment with some drugs causes inhibition or induction of CYP3A4, and this has appeared to account for many drug interactions [4]. For example, ketoconazole is a potent inhibitor of CYP3A4, and this appears to account for why blood levels of CYP3A4 substrates tend to rise during therapy with ketoconazole. Conversely, rifampin is a potent inducer of CYP3A4 in both liver and intestine [3], and this provides an attractive explanation for why blood levels of CYP3A4 substrates tend to fall during treatment with rifampin. However, it is now clear that drug interactions involving CYP3A4 substrates can not always be explained by induction or inhibition of CYP3A4. For example, all but 5% of administered fexofenadine (Allegra®) is excreted from the body unmetabolized, yet ketoconazole treatment results in a 2.6 fold increase in the plasma AUC of parent drug [6].

NEW APPROACHES

A potential additional explanation for CYP3A4 substrate/drug interactions has been provided by the discovery of p-glycoprotein (MDR1 gene product). This versatile xenobiotic transport protein is present in the brush border of the small intestine epithelial cell (enterocyte) [7], and functions to pump substrates against the absorption gradient [8]. Most substrates for CYP3A4 are also substrates for Pgp [9,10] and some CYP3A4 inhibitors (eg. ketoconazole [11]) and inducers (rifampin [12,13]) also appear to inhibit and induce Pgp. Hence, drug interactions involving CYP3A4 substrates could result from induction of inhibition of p-glycoprotein. Current pharmacokinetic approaches, such as the simultaneous administration of unlabelled drug intravenously and labelled drug orally, are useful in distinguishing liver and intestinal contributions to "first pass" effects, but are not capable of distinguishing the roles of CYP3A4 and p-glycoprotein at the level of the small intestine [14,15]. This is because metabolites generated by CYP3A4 in the enterocyte are often pumped by p-glycoprotein back into the intestinal lumen, and therefore would not be detected in blood [14].

To assess the relative contributions of CYP3A4 and p-glycoprotein in the oral availability of drugs, we have pursued a strategy that is based on the observation that there exist large interindividual differences in the activity of CYP3A4 in the liver and intestine, and in the intestinal levels of p-glycoprotein that can not be attributed to induction or inhibition by drugs [1,16-19]. In addition, there appears to be no correlation between the levels or either of these three parameters within an individual (i.e. they behave as independent variables) [18,19]. We reasoned that if **intra**individual changes in any of these three parameters caused by induction or inhibition produce corresponding changes in the clearance and dosing requirements of a CYP3A4 substrate, it logically follows that **inter**individual differences in activity of CYP3A4 should account, at least in part, for **inter**individual differences in the oral kinetics that drug.

Moreover, we reasoned that the relative strengths of the correlations between each of these three parameters and variation in the pharmacokinetics (PK) of the CYP3A4 substrate would estimate the relative importance of variable. To test this hypothesis, it would have been desirable to be able to perform liver biopsies to directly measure CYP3A4 activity. However, since the risks of liver biopsy are substantial, we developed the intravenous [14C N-methyl] erythromycin breath test (ERMBT) as an alternate means of quantitating liver CYP3A4 activity in living people [20]. This test is based on the observations that CYP3A4 catalyzes N-demethylation of erythromycin and that the carbon in the cleaved methyl group is rapidly converted to exhaled CO2 which can be easily trapped. Although there was initially some controversy [21], the ERMBT is now generally regarded as a "gold standard" probe based test for hepatic CYP3A4 activity [22,23]. In human studies we, and others, have used the ERMBT to demonstrate that variation in liver CYP3A4 activity accounts in part for interpatient differences in pharmacokinetics of several orally or intravenously administered CYP3A4 substrates [24-28], including CsA [18,28-32].We have also developed methods to quantitate CYP3A4 and p-glycoprotein in mucosal "pinch" biopsies that can be rapidly and safely obtained in people using a standard endoscopic instrument [18,33].

THE MULTIPLE REGRESSION APPROACH

To perform a study, 20 subjects not receiving known inducers of inhibitors of CYP3A4 or p-glycoprotein receive the ERMBT and intestinal biopsies. A standard pharmacokinetic study is then performed with a drug of interest. The apparent oral clearance (CL/F) is used as the dependent variable, and the ERMBT and enterocyte concentrations of CYP3A4 and Pgp are used as independent variables in multiple regression analyses. Using this approach ([18,26] we have found that variation in enterocyte concentration of CYP3A4 (but not Pgp) correlates significantly with CL/F of felodipine ([26] supporting a substantial role of the intestinal enzyme in the disposition of this drug. However, in a similar study examining CL/F of cyclosporin A, enterocyte concentrations of Pgp (and not of CYP3A4) was a significant predictor [18]. This suggests that Pgp (and not CYP3A4) is the relevant enterocyte factor for CL/F of CsA, and the probable locus for the intestinal component of CsA drug interactions involving inducers or inhibitors. However, these observations alone do not exclude the possibility that significant CsA metabolism by CYP3A4 occurs in the intestine. As recently reviewed [15,34], Pgp may actually influence the extent of metabolism by CYP3A4 in the intestine by controlling the intraenterocyte concentrations of substrate, limiting product inhibition, or controlling the duration of absorption (i.e. total amount of metabolism occurring in the intestine would be proportional to the duration of the absorptive phase if enzyme saturation occurs). Hence, our multiple regression approach does not allow unequivocal conclusions about the role of enterocyte CYP3A4 in drug disposition.

THE KNOCKOUT APPROACH

A novel approach for distinguishing the roles of enterocyte CYP3A4 and p-glycoprotein became apparent during our examination of the effects of grapefruit juice on enterocyte CYP3A4 and felodipine kinetics. Grapefruit juice has been shown to substantially increase the oral availability of many CYP3A4 substrates [35-43], including felodipine [35,44,45] and cyclosporin A [46-50] We noted that after grapefruit juice treatment, variation in enterocyte concentration of CYP3A4 no longer significantly predicted CL/F of felodipine, which became chiefly a function of liver CYP3A4 activity as measured by the ERMBT([26]. Grapefruit juice had in effect eliminated or "knocked out" enterocyte CYP3A4 as a relevant variable, presumably by shifting the bulk of metabolism to the liver. We reasoned that this approach could potentially represent a useful and fairly direct strategy for assessing the role of enterocyte CYP3A4 in the disposition of drugs.

We and others [51-53] now believe that furanocoumarins (FCs) are the major active agents present in grapefruit juice accounting for the irreversible inhibition of CYP3A4 in enterocytes. We have shown that a major FC in grapefruit juice 6',7'-dihydroxybergamottin, or DHB, is a mechanism-based inactivator of CYP3A4 [51]. Mechanism-based inactivation is an attractive property for our "knock out" agent, as it is likely to be more P450-specific than reversible inhibition [54]. In addition, because it is irreversible, its duration of action will depend on the synthesis of new enzyme.

If the sole effect of grapefruit juice is to decrease enterocyte CYP3A4 activity, we might predict, based on our inability to identify a contribution of enterocyte CYP3A4 to the CL/F of cyclosporin A [18], that grapefruit juice would have no effect on the oral kinetics of cyclosporin A. However, grapefruit juice does significantly increases the oral availability of cyclosporin A [46-50]. To address the effects of DHB on cyclosporin A disposition, we used the fact that DHB is present in fruit other than grapefruit, including the Seville orange. In collaboration with David Edwards (at Wayne State University), a 2-way cross over study was performed in healthy volunteers to determine whether Seville orange juice would improve the oral availability of cyclosporin A [55]. We found that Seville orange juice (containing ~40 ·M DHB) did not at all increase mean AUC values for cyclosporin A, although whole grapefruit juice (containing ~40 ·M DHB) produced a significant increase in AUC in these same subjects [56]. To determine if Seville orange juice causes an in vivo fall in CYP3A4 protein, we performed small bowel biopsies in 2 of the subjects who participated in the trial, before and after they received Seville orange juice. An unequivocal fall in enterocyte CYP3A4 concentration was observed in each subject [56]. Hence, substantial decreases in enterocyte CYP3A4 level had no effect on the apparent oral clearance of cyclosporin A. This supports the conclusion from our multiple regression approach [18] that enterocyte CYP3A4 is unlikely to be the locus for drug interactions involving cyclosporin A. In addition, the observations suggest that the effects of grapefruit juice on CsA oral availability can not be attributed to DHB, and presumably reflect inhibitors of Pgp present in the juice.

CONCLUSION

In summary, the multiple regression approach has appeared to provide insight into the role p-glycoprotein may play in the oral availability of cyclosporin A, and this approach should be applicable to other substrates and intestinal transporters. The "knock out" approach also appears to show promise if safe selective inhibitors of transport proteins can be developed.

Combining these approaches with traditional pharmacokinetic strategies should improve our understanding of relative contributions of liver and intestine to the oral availability of drugs.

REFERENCES

1. Shimada T, Yamazaki H, Mimura M, Inui Y, Guengerich FP. Interindividual variations in human liver cytochrome P-450 enzymes involved in the oxidation of drugs, carcinogens and toxic chemicals: studies with liver microsomes of 30 Japanese and 30 Caucasians. J Pharmacol Exp Ther 1994;270:414-423.
2. Watkins PB, Wrighton SA, Schuetz EG, Molowa DT, Guzelian PS. Identification of glucocorticoid-inducible cytochromes P-450 in the intestinal mucosa of rats and man. J Clin Invest 1987;80:1029-1036.
3. Kolars JC, Schmiedlin-Ren P, Schuetz JD, Fang C, Watkins PB. Identification of rifampin-inducible P450IIIA4 (CYP3A4) in human small bowel enterocytes. J Clin Invest 1992;90:1871-1878.
4. Bertz RJ, Grannerman GR. Use of *In Vitro* and *In Vivo* Data to Estimate the Likelihood of Metabolic Pharmacokinetic Interactions. Clin Pharmacokinet 1997;32:210-258.
5. Benet LZ, Kroetz DL, Sheiner LB. Pharmacokinetics of drug absorption, distribution and elimination, In: Hardman JG, Limbird LeMolinoff PB, eds. Goodman and Gilman's the pharmacological basis of therapeutics. New York: McGraw-Hill, 1996:3-29.
6. Kaye WH, Sitaram N, Weingartner H, Ebert MH, Smallberg S, Gillin JC. Modest facilitation of memory in dementia with combined lecithin and anticholinesterase treatment. Biol Psychiatry 1982;17:275-280.
7. Thiebaut F, Tsuruo T, Hamada H, Gottesman MM, Pastan I, Willingham MC. Cellular localization of the multidrug-resistance gene product P-glycoprotein in normal human tissues. Proc Natl Acad Sci USA 1987;84:7735-7738.
8. Hsing S, Gatmaitan Z, Arias IM. The function of Gp170, the multidrug-resistance gene product, in the brush border of rat intestinal mucosa. Gastroenterology 1992;102:879-885.
9. Wacher VJ, Wu C-Y, Benet LZ. Overlapping substrate specificities and tissue distribution of cytochrome P450 3A and P-glycoprotein: implications for drug delivery and activity in cancer chemotherapy. Mol Carcinog 1995;13:129-134.
10. Schuetz EG, Furuya KN, Schuetz JD. Interindividual variation in expression of P-glycoprotein in normal human liver and secondary hepatic neoplasms. J Pharmacol Exp Ther 1995;275:1011-1018.
11. Siegsmund MJ, Cardarelli C, Aksentijevich I, Sugimoto Y, Pastan I, Gottesman MM. Ketoconazole effectively reverses multidrug resistance in highly resistant KB cells. J Urol 1994;151:485-491.
12. Lown KS, Kolars JC, Ghosh M, Schmiedlin-Ren P, Watkins PB. Induction of MDR1 expression in normal rat and human intestine in vivo. Gastroenterology 1996;110:A344 (Abstract).
13. Fricker G, Drewe J, Huwyler J, Gutmann H, Beglinger C. Relevance of p-glycoprotein for the enteral absorption of cyclosporin A: In vitro in vivo correlation. Br J Pharm 1996;118:1841-1847.

14. Watkins PB. The barrier function of CYP3A4 and P-glycoprotein in the small bowel. Adv Drug Deliv Rev 1997;27:161-170.
15. Benet LZ, Wu C-Y, Hebert MF, Wacher VJ. Intestinal drug metabolism and antitransport processes: a potential paradigm shift in oral drug delivery. J Cont Release 1996;39:139-143.
16. Schmucker DL, Woodhouse KW, Wang RK, et al. Effects of age and gender on in vitro properties of human liver microsomal monooxygenases. Clin Pharmacol Ther 1990;48:365-374.
17. Forrester LM, Henderson CJ, Glancey MJ, et al. Relative expression of cytochrome P450 isoenzymes in human liver and association with the metabolism of drug and xenobiotics. Biochemistry 1992;281:359-368.
18. Lown KS, Mayo RR, Leichtman AB, et al. Role of intestinal P-glycoprotein (*mdr1*) in interpatient variation in the oral bioavailability of cyclosporin A. Clin Pharmacol Ther 1997;62:248-60.
19. Turgeon DK, Leichtman AB, Blake DS, et al. Prediction of interpatient and intrapatient variation in OG 37-325 dosing requirements by the erythromycin breath test. A prospective study in renal transplant recipients. Transplantation 1994;57:1736-1741.
20. Watkins PB, Murray SA, Winkelman LG, Heuman DM, Wrighton SA, Guzelian PS. Erythromycin breath test as an assay of glucocorticoid-inducible liver cytochromes P-450. Studies in rats and patients. J Clin Invest 1989;83:688-697.
21. Kinirons MT, O'Shea D, Downing TE, et al. Absence of correlations among three putative in vivo probes of human cytochrome P4503A activity in young healthy men. Clin Pharmacol Ther 1993;54:621-629.
22. Watkins PB. Noninvasive tests of CYP3A enzymes. Pharmacogenetics 1994;4:171-184.
23. Kivisto KT, Kroemer HK. Use of probe drugs as predictors of drug metabolism in humans. J Clin Pharmacol 1997;37:40S-48S.
24. Cheng CL, Smith DE, Carver PL, et al. Steady state pharmacokinetics of delavirdine in HIV-positive patients: Effect on erythromycin breath test. Clin Pharmacol Ther 1997;61:531-543.
25. Lown KS, Thummel KE, Benedict PE, et al. The erythromycin breath test predicts the clearance of midazolam. Clin Pharmacol Ther 1995;57:16-24.
26. Lown KS, Bailey DG, Fontana RJ, et al. Grapefruit juice increases felodipine oral availability in humans by decreasing intestinal CYP3A protein expression. J Clin Invest 1997;99:2545-2553.
27. Darbar D, Dell'Orto S, Morike K, Wilkinson GR, Roden DM. Dietary salt increases first-pass elimination of oral quinidine. Clin Pharmacol Ther 1997;61:292-300.
28. Cakaloglu Y, Tredger JM, Devlin J, Williams R. Importance of cytochrome P450IIIA activity in determining dosage and blood levels of FK 506 and cyclosporine in liver transplant recipients. Hepatology 1994;20:309-316.
29. Watkins PB, Hamilton TA, Annesley TM, Ellis CN, Kolars JC, Voorhees JJ. The erythromycin breath test as a predictor of cyclosporine blood levels. Clin Pharmacol Ther 1990;48:120-129.
30. Turgeon DK, Normolle DP, Leichtman AB, Annesley TM, Smith DE, Watkins PB. Erythromycin breath test predicts oral clearance of cyclosporine in kidney transplant recipients. Clin Pharmacol Ther 1992;52:471-478.

31. Turgeon DK, Leichtman AB, Lown KS, et al. P450 3A activity and cyclosporine dosing in kidney and heart transplant recipients. Clin Pharmacol Ther 1994;56:253-260.
32. Stein CM, Kinirons MT, Pincus M, Wilkinson GR, Wood AJJ. Comparison of the dapsone recovery ratio and the erythromycin breath test as in vivo probes of CYP3A4 activity in patients with rheumatoid arthritis receiving cyclosporine. Clin Pharmacol Ther 1996;59:47-51.
33. Lown KS, Kolars JC, Thummel KE, et al. Interpatient heterogeneity in expression of CYP3A4 and CYP3A5 in small bowel. Lack of prediction by the erythromycin breath test. Drug Metab Dispos 1994;22:947-955.
34. Watkins PB. The role of p-glycoprotein in limiting the oral availability of drugs. Pharmacol Rev 1997;(In Press).
35. Bailey DG, Spence JD, Munoz C, Arnold JMO. Interaction of citrus juices with felodipine and nifedipine. Lancet 1991;337:268-269.
36. Bailey DG, Arnold MO, Strong A, Munoz C, Spence JD. Effect of grapefruit juice and naringin on nisoldipine pharmacokinetics. Clin Pharmacol Ther 1993;54:589-594.
37. Soons PA, Vogel BA, Roosemalen MC, et al. Grapefruit juice and cimetidine inhibit stereoselective metabolism of nitrendipine in humans. Clin Pharmacol Ther 1991;50:394-403.
38. Fuhr U, Harder S, Lopez-Rojas P, Muller-Peltzer H, Kern R, Staib AH. Increase of verapamil concentrations in steady state by coadministration of grapefruit juice. Naunyn-Schmiedeberg's Arch Pharmacol 1994;349:R134.
39. Benton RE, Honig PK, Zamani K, Cantilena LR, Woosley RL. Grapefruit juice alters terfenadine pharmacokinetics, resulting in prolongation of repolarization on the electrocardiogram. Clin Pharmacol Ther 1996;59:383-388.
40. Weber A, Jager R, Borner A, et al. Can grapefruit juice influence ethinylestradiol bioavailability? Contraception 1996;53:41-47.
41. Kupferschmidt HHT, Ha HR, Ziegler WH, Meier PJ, Krahenbuhl S. Interaction between grapefruit juice and midazolam in humans. Clin Pharmacol Ther 1995;58:20-28.
42. Hukkinen SK, Varhe AV, Olkkola KT, Neuvonen PJ. Plasma concentrations of triazolam are increased by concomitant ingestion of grapefruit juice. Clin Pharmacol Ther 1995;58:127-131.
43. Saquinavir with grapefruit juice. Posit Aware 1996;7:5.
44. Bailey DG, Arnold JMO, Munoz C, Spence JD. Grapefruit juice-felodipine interaction: Mechanism, predictability, and effect of naringin. Clin Pharmacol Ther 1993;53:637-642.
45. Bailey DG, Arnold JMO, Bend JR, Tran LT, Spence JD. Grapefruit juice-felodipine interaction: reproducibility and characterization with the extended release drug formulation. Br J Clin Pharmacol 1995;40:135-140.
46. Ducharme MP, Provenzano R, Dehoorne-Smith M, Edwards DJ. Trough concentrations of cyclosporine in blood following administration with grapefruit juice. Br J Clin Pharmacol 1993;36:457-459.
47. Ducharme MP, Warbasse LH, Edwards DJ. Disposition of intravenous and oral cyclosporine after administration with grapefruit juice. Clin Pharmacol Ther 1995;57:485-491.

48. Hollander A, van Rooij JMD, Lentjes E, et al. The effect of grapefruit juice on cyclosporine and prednisone metabolism in transplant patients. Clin Pharmacol Ther 1995;57:318-324.

49. Yee GC, Stanley DL, Pessa LJ, et al. Effect of grapefruit juice on blood cyclosporin concentration. Lancet 1995;345:955-956.

50. Min DI, Ku YM, Perry PJ, et al. Effect of grapefruit juice on cyclosporine pharmacokinetics in renal transplant patients. Transplantation 1996;62:123-125.

51. Schmiedlin-Ren P, Edwards DJ, Fitzsimmons ME, et al. Mechanisms of enhanced oral availability of CYP3A4 substrates by grapefruit constituents: Decreased enterocyte CYP3A4 concentration and mechanism-based inactivation by furanocoumarins. Drug Metab Dispos 1997;25:1228-1233.

52. Fukuda K, Ohta T, Oshima Y, Ohashi N, Yoshikawa M, Yamazoe Y. Specific CYP3A4 inhibitors in grapefruit juice: furocoumarin dimers as components of drug interaction. Pharmacogenetics 1997;7:391-396.

53. Edwards DJ, Bellevue FH, Woster PM. Identification of 6',7'-dihydroxybergamottin, a cytochrome P450 inhibitor, in grapefruit juice. Drug Metab Dispos 1996;24:1287-1290.

54. Halpert JR, Guengerich FP, Bend JR, Correia MA. Selective inhibitors of cytochromes P450. Toxicol Appl Pharmacol 1994;125:163-175.

55. Summers WK, Viesselman JO, Marsh GM, Candelora K. Use of THA in treatment of Alzheimer-like dementia: Pilot study in twelve patients. Biol Psychiatry 1981;16:145-153.

56. Edwards DJ, Fitzsimmons MF, Schuetz EG, et al. 6'7'-dihydroxybergamottin in grapefruit juice and Seville orange juice: Effects on cyclosporine disposition, enterocyte CYP3A4, and p-glycoprotein. Clin Pharmacol Ther 1999;(In Press).

Discussion: Approaches to studying the role of enzyme inhibition and induction

J. Urquhart:
What role does the CYP3A4 at the brush border have in systemic metabolism?

P.B. Watkins:
I have assumed that the enzyme would only act on xenobiotics during the process of absorption, but there is some evidence that it may also be involved in systemic elimination. Ken Thummell in Seattle performed some studies during the phase of a liver transplant operation when the liver is removed from the body. Giving midazolam intravenously, a very good probe for CYP3A4, the mean extraction across the intestinal bed was 8% but there was one individual whose metabolic extraction was 25%. This suggests that the intestine may be a major organ of systemic extraction for some drugs in some people. Additionally, it has been known for a long time that certain drugs, particularly erythromycin, are actively transported into the gut lumen presumably by a p-glycoprotein (P-GP).

N. Benowitz:
You make the assumption that you can translate your data from intestinal biopsy enzyme activity to total intestinal enzyme activity. But, obviously, there are a lot of complexities in regulation, and local regulation could occur to a different degree in different parts of the small intestine. With respect to the CPY3A4 or P-GP activity, how sure are you that you can extrapolate from a single biopsy to the whole intestinal mass?

P.B. Watkins:
Our endoscope can only reach the first part of the small intestine. Nevertheless, we have obtained excellent correlations between the proximal and distal "phenotypes" in human intestine biopsies. Even though the level of expression falls as you proceed down the small bowel towards the colon, it appears to fall in parallel for individuals.

D.C. Brater:
Referring back to the differential regulation of hepatic and intestinal metabolism, if you bathe the liver in the same kind of environment that you bathe the intestinal mucosa, is there still differential regulation?

P.B. Watkins:
We have treated normal volunteers with known inducers of liver CYP3A4. With rifampicin we have seen induction in both liver and intestine within 24 h. However, after 48 h we have seen no evidence of induction in intestine with high therapeutic doses of phenobarbital, dexamethasone or clotrimazole. Now we plan to begin studies to treat for up to 2 weeks. These observations suggest that the actual molecular mechanisms of induction may be fundamentally different in the intestine and liver. On the other hand, the recently cloned pregnene-X receptor is expressed in the intestine as well as the liver. Therefore, at least the major receptor involved in xenobiotic induction of CYP3A4 appears to be present for xenobiotic induction in both intestine and liver.

U. Klotz:

You mentioned that another mechanism is the down-regulation of CYP3A4 by grapefruit juice ingredients, but you did not see a change in the mRNA of CYP3A4. Do you know a little bit more about the mechanism of this down-regulation?

P.B. Watkins:

We are testing at the moment in cells that express CYP3A4 whether mechanism based inactivation by furanocoumarins in the juice is followed by accelerated degradation of the protein, as has been shown with other P450s following mechanism-based inhibition.

P. du Souich:

The enterocyte is perfused from the mesenteric capillary through a short-cut which goes straight to the portal flow. The vasodilation of this mesenteric capillary will obviously be present during the absorption of food. But under fasting conditions, when the perfusion of the enterocyte is minimal, the access of some drugs to this enterocyte after intravenous administration will also be minimal. If you give it orally, the product needs to come from the mesenteric artery, and then reach the mesenteric capillaries in the enterocyte, which are closed when you are fasting. That is why I think the contribution of the intestine to the systemic clearance is very low and it is very difficult to interpret the exact role of the intestine in the systemic clearance of a drug. It may change significantly during the day, depending on its own perfusion.

P.B. Watkins:

It is the free fraction of the drug that is relevant and accessible for intestinal metabolism and the availability of this free faction is another factor, in theory, that could explain why intestinal metabolism can be low.

D.A. Smith:

The work that has been done on the role of P-GP in drug disposition of drugs has been very valuable. Although it is thought to be important for macrolides, at least, there is more and more data emerging that it is also just as important for small molecules. This is the case for the beta-blocker talinolol, a very small and metabolically stable compound, which is definitely secreted in the gastrointestinal tract by P-GP, and shows a marked verapamil interaction.

P. Rolan:

Atovaquone is a very lipophilic compound of intermediate bioavailability, that is not metabolised and reaches the bile unchanged. A population analysis showed that people on rifampin had an approximately double apparent oral clearance of this compound. At the time we did not understand this result. We thought that rifampin increases the clearance of some metabolised compounds, and this might due to an effect on transporters either in the gut or in the liver.

P.B. Watkins:

The other example is the follow-up compound to terfenadine in the United States, fexofenadine, which is excreted 85% unchanged from the body. Nonetheless there is an interaction between fexofenadine and ketaconazole or erythromycin which may be explained again by modulation of P-GP activity.

H.K. Kroemer:
It has been published that P-GP does not have much of a role in the initial verapamil-rifampin interaction, because the amount excreted in urine does not fall significantly following rifampin administration. About the linear regression approach you mentioned, in one part of the regression you use a functional assay, the erythromycin breath test, and in the other part of the lineal regression you use a non-functional test of the expression of P-GP using Western blots. Considering the problems that exist with blotting P-GP, is there a direct relationship between the expression of P-GP and the function of transport in the intestine?

P.B. Watkins:
We know that we get the same answer from the immunoblot and enzymatic assays for CYP3A4. But you are right, especially when you are talking about an energy-dependent pump, it is not at all clear that the amount of protein would correlate with the actual activity, at least under all circumstances. However, in cancer cell lines the level of the P-GP protein does generally correlate with the amount of activity of the enzyme. In addition, the correlation of the P-GP protein measurements with cyclosporin oral availability also supports a close relationship between expression and function.

A.J.J. Wood:
Another non-metabolised substrate for P-GP is digoxin, which could probably explain the digoxin-quinidine, the digoxin-verapamil and the digoxin-ketoconazole interactions that we never really understood very well. Related to the cyclosporin studies, did you use the micro-emulsion cyclosporin?

P.B. Watkins:
The question refers to the fact that the older cyclosporine formulation Sandimmune®) has been replaced by a newer formulation (Neoral®) which is micro-emulsified and is absorbed much quicker and shows less inter-individual variations in kinetics. We used the Sandimmune® formulation, but in some studies with Neoral® we found that the correlations with the erythromycin breath test results were dramatically improved, presumably because of the removal of the P-GP and perhaps other variables from the regression.

A.J.J. Wood:
It might be because the new formulation, although it has been sold as a micro-emulsion preparation, actually contains inhibitors of CYP3A and potentially of P-GP as well, improving the bioavailability.

S. Erill:
The issue of the intracellular concentration of drugs was mentioned. In the case of cancer cells, P-GP plays a role in the intracellular concentration of anti-cancer drugs. Are there data on P-GP in cells other than enterocytes?

P.B. Watkins:

The majority of work on P-GP has been done on cancer, looking at it as a mechanism for resistance to chemotherapy. The higher levels of expression of P-GP, the lower the intracellular concentration. However, considering the presence of P-GP in the blood-brain barrier, it may be that inter-individual differences in the level of expression could account for differences between people in the CNS concentration of some drugs. The pharmacokinetic concepts are not simple ones that most of us know of, and importantly, there are not a lot of studies in progress, or even ways to study it that I know of.

A.J.J. Wood:

We have shown that P-GP is an important, perhaps the most important, determinant of HIV-protease inhibitors' entry into the CNS. We have recently looked at the effects of loperamide, an antidiarrhoeal agent, which is a very potent opiate. Since loperamide is a P-GP substrate it does not enter the CNS, and does not produce CNS opiate effects as other opiates do. If you inhibit P-GP with quinidine you can get respiratory depression with loperamide, but there are no respiratory effects in the absence of quinidine. So it is obvious that some of the drugs that are thought to have local effects, are actually producing them because of their ability to be pumped out of certain tissues by P-GP.

E.M. Sellers:

In my opinion, it is unlikely that the notions of individualisation are going to be widely accepted soon. Drug regulations and drug reimbursement policy, and socio-economic differences, along with social values and prejudice around issues of gender and race, all favor studying large groups and group differences. Practically, it is very difficult for the pharmaceutical industry to develop individualized dose approaches because of cost and labelling implications. It is very unlikely that the pharmaceutical industry is going to change, without regulatory change. I doubt whether physician education is going to have much of an impact.

H.K. Kroemer:

Before looking at individualisation, I think it should be made clear at some point to what extent the need for individualisation exists. The P-GP issue in cancer is a very good example. *In vitro* P-GP was a major determinant of resistance of cancer cells, yet all the clinical studies have been a complete disaster. This is because we now understand that the response of a given cancer to drug therapy is extremely complex. We should consider how far we take this individualisation, because obviously a cancer is as individual as the patient who carries this cancer.

A.J.J. Wood:

One of the reasons why the P-GP inhibitors did not work in cancer was that they were all potent CYP3A inhibitors as well. Part of the problem is that we need to individualise not only drugs and people, but need to have more selective probes for targeting CYP3A selectively from P-GP or vice versa. If you inhibit CYP3A, then you will get effects that are quite different from what you might have predicted from just targeting P-GP.

P. Rolan:

Convincing people of the importance of individualisation, and proving the clinical relevance of needing to assess it is difficult because, overall, we are so poor with most of our drugs at measuring any effect whatsoever. There is a major debate about whether the drugs of most of the major therapeutic classes do anything at all. There has been, for example, this recent issue in the popular press that all anti-depressants are placebos. There are other drugs we would expect to need to individualise because of their underlying heterogeneity, such as the treatment for Alzheimer's disease in the elderly. Since we cannot measure the effect on the population with these drugs, let alone on individuals, it is not surprising we cannot see the clinical relevance. Under these circumstances, the argument the clinical pharmacologists could put forward is best called the precautionary principle. If we have an unidentified source of variability that increases plasma concentrations four-fold, it would be very difficult to show that this is clinically relevant, because adverse event frequencies could be already low in the population, and you might not be able to detect a different principle. If you believe the drug is working through the circulation, and there are some people who have much higher concentrations, it is a reasonable starting-point to reduce the dose and then see if there are any changes. In conditions where the effect is very easy to measure, migraine for example, patients are very happy to individually titrate and use quite a lot of variability in individual response. In contrast, the pharmaceutical industry advocates one dose for everybody, because they do parallel groups studies with no individual titration therefore their recommendations are not useful and patients titrate themselves successfully anyway. We should propose the precautionary principle and the regulators should take it on board again. If we cannot see any difference in adverse drug reaction nor in efficacy it is probably because we cannot detect a difference rather than because one does not really exist. Under those circumstances it is prudent to take advance action to avoid problems, if a drug obtains a reputation for poor safety this can cause market resistance and poor sales. Since it is unlikely to have been detected in the clinical data base, I think we should be trying to propose individualisation when the size of variability is very large.

Variability in Human Drug Response
G.T. Tucker, Editor

Genetic polymorphisms in cardiovascular disease: focus on renin angiotensin system

Gershan K. Davis[a] and Naseer H. Naqvi[b]

[a]Consulting Physician/Cardiologist, Chorley and South Ribble District General Hospital, Chorley, Lancashire, UK

[b]Department of Medicine, Chorley and South Ribble District General Hospital, Chroley, Lancashire, UK

ABSTRACT

Cardiovascular Disease is an important cause of morbidity and mortality in Western Communities. The conditions of coronary artery disease, hypertension and heart failure predominate as the main types of cardiovascular disease. The renin angiotensin system (RAS) is one of the main systems responsible for cardiovascular homeostasis and the effect of genetic polymorphisms of components of this system may be important as it may affect the circulating or local concentrations of these components and thus predispose to the development of cardiovascular disease.

In addition, the possibility of these genetic polymorphisms affecting the response to treatment in patients with cardiovascular diseases needs further investigation, particularly in relation to pharmacological agents which target this system such as angiotensin converting enzyme inhibitors and more recently angiotensin II receptor antagonists.

This presentation describes the common RAS gene polymorphisms and discusses their associations with the common cardiovascular conditions as well as describes the rapid PCR based assays used in their detection. Information on the effect of these polymorphisms on treatment is presented. Examples of non RAS gene mutations are also highlighted.

Key words: angiotensin converting enzyme, hypertension, heart failure.

Correspondence: Dr. Greshan K. Davis, Chorley and South Ribble District General Hospital, Euxton Lane, Chorley, Lancashire PR7 1PP, United Kingdom, Tel: +44-1257-26-1222 Fax: +44-1257-24-5575, Email: GERSHAN@classic.msn.com

INTRODUCTION

The Renin Angiotensin System is one of the major systems involved in maintaining cardiovascular homeostasis and as such polymorphisms in genes coding for components of this system may have an impact on cardiovascular disease. Other systems that may also impact on cardiovascular disease include the fibrinolytic system and lipid metabolism.

THE RENIN ANGIOTENSIN SYSTEM

The renin angiotensin system (RAS) is one of the body's most powerful regulators of arterial pressure and body fluid volumes. Traditionally the RAS has been thought of as an endocrine system with circulating renin originating largely from the kidney where it is synthesised and stored in the juxtaglomerular cells of the kidney. The concept of the existence of tissue renin angiotensin systems proposes a paracrine mode of operation for the RAS with angiotensin II being produced in target organs via local RAS biochemical cascades. To support this RAS components have all been demonstrated at various tissue sites including the heart [1]. Enzymatic pathways however independent of renin and ACE also contribute to the development of angiotensin II in tissues, blood vessels and the heart. Chymase is an efficient angiotensin II forming enzyme and has been found in the human cardiac interstitium, endothelial cells and mast cells.

Renin

Renin was first discovered in 1898 [2]. It is synthesised as a pre-prorenin molecule within renin synthesizing cells. Human renin secreting cells have been identified in the juxtaglomerular apparatus (JGA) of the kidney with the aid of histochemical stains. The human renin gene is located on the short arm of chromosome 1 q32, [3] and contains ten exons (coding sequences) and nine introns (non-coding sequences) and spans 12.5 kilobases (kb) [4]. Various restriction fragment length polymorphisms are known to occur. These include the *Taq* I and *Bgl* I polymorphisms which are located in the 5' region, the *Hind*III in the 3' region and the *Hinf* I in the first intron. No significant associations have been found so far between human essential hypertension and the renin gene alleles [5].

Angiotensinogen

The angiotensinogen gene is located near the renin gene on chromosome 1q 42-3 [6]. It encompasses five exons and four introns and spans approximately 13 kilobases [7]. The first exon is short (37 nucleotides) and corresponds to the 5'untranslated sequence of the mRNA. The second exon codes for 59 percent of the protein and contains the nucleotide sequences coding for the signal peptide and ANG1. Exons 3 and 4 code for 48 and 62 amino acids of the protein and the last exon codes for the C terminal part of the protein and the 3' untranslated sequence of the mRNA. Mutations have been discovered within the 5' end of the gene as well as within exons and intron 3.

The potential role of the AGT gene in human essential hypertension has been investigated in two large series of hypertensive sibships. Evidence was obtained of genetic linkage between the AGT gene and hypertension. In particular a strong linkage was found in patients characterised by a diastolic blood pressure greater than 100mmHg or the prescription of two or more antihypertensive drugs. One common variant has been shown to be linked to the determination of circulating angiotensinogen levels and hypertension. This variant is found within exon 2 and is the result of a single DNA base dimorphism (T or C). This produces a substitution of methionine (ATG) for threonine (ACG) at position 235 of the angiotensinogen amino acid sequence. Possession of alleles specifying threonine at this position is associated with high plasma angiotensinogen concentrations with 10 and 20 percent increases in heterozygotes (MT) and homozygotes (TT) respectively compared with wild type homozygotes. This AGT variant was found more frequently in hypertensive probands in some populations of White European ancestry [8] especially in the more severe index cases than in controls. The association of this variant with hypertension has been confirmed in Caucasians [9] and Japanese hypertensive patients [10] but not in African Caribbeans [11].

Angiotensin Converting Enzyme

ACE is a carboxypeptidase which hydrolyzes di- and tripeptides from the C terminus of peptides. The majority of the human ACE molecule projects into the extracellular space and is bound to the plasma membrane via a C-terminal region which spans across the membrane and is linked to a short cytoplasmic tail. ACE converts angiotensin I (Ang I) to angiotensin II (Ang II) by removal of the C terminal peptide His-Leu. ACE also cleaves the C-terminal dipeptide (Phe-Arg) from bradykinin, thus giving it the ability to activate a pressor agent and inactivate a vasodilator. ACE is homogenously distributed throughout the human heart with only low levels in the valves.

ACE GENE AND ACE I/D POLYMORPHISM

The Nancy study [12] showed a familial resemblance in plasma ACE levels between genetically related adult subjects. This was consistent with a major genetic contribution to the determination of plasma ACE levels. Two ACE alleles were discovered [13] which differed in size due to the insertion of a 287 base pair (bp) DNA sequence in intron 16 of the ACE gene. The larger allele was assigned the symbol I (insertion) and the shorter allele the symbol D (deletion).

Population Variations in ACE I/D genotypes

There are important population differences in the frequency of genetic markers including those of the renin angiotensin system. The ACE DD genotype shows a wide variation in frequency between populations. It is found in only 2% of Samoans but up to 42% in Caucasians [14]. Ishigami *et al.* [15] have reported significant differences in genotype frequences between Japanese population and Caucasians. DD genotype frequency in their normal control population was 18%. In Lee's [16] normal subjects, the D allele frequency was 0.3. The D allele frequency is higher in Black Nigerians [17] and the Afro Caribbean population compared to Europeans [18].

Effect of ACE gene I/D polymorphism on ACE levels

The effect of ACE genotype on tissue and plasma ACE levels is co-dominant with mean plasma ACE levels in DD subjects approximately twice those of II caucasian subjects. The ID genotype individuals have intermediate ACE levels [13,19]. The I allele is a marker for the major gene effect on serum ACE which is due to an as yet unidentified variant of the ACE gene. There is tight linkage of this ACE polymorphic marker site to a locus that regulates gene expression (site of major gene effect). This major gene has co-dominant effects and accounts for 44% of the total variability of ACE levels while the marker I/D polymorphism accounts for 28% of the variation [20].

Population variations in the effect of the ACE I/D genotype on serum ACE levels

Genetic studies in African-Caribbean families from Jamaica have shown that the ACE I/D polymorphism is in moderate linkage disequilibrium with an ACE linked quantitative trait locus. In this population two quantitative trait loci jointly influence serum ACE levels with one locus located close to or within the ACE locus and accounting for 27% of the total variability [21]. In a black healthy population no variation in serum ACE activity was found with ACE genotype [22]. The effect of ACE genotype on serum ACE levels also applies in the Caucasian hypertensive population [23]. No variation has been found in plasma angiotensin II levels and aldosterone with ACE genotype [24].

ACE gene I/D polymorphism and myocardial infarction

The deletion polymorphism in the ACE gene (DD genotype) was reported to show an increased frequency in patients with myocardial infarction who were recruited between three and nine months after the event in a retrospective multicenter, case-control study [25]. The overall increase in risk was modest with an odds ratio of 1.34 for patients with the DD genotype (an increase in risk of MI with the DD genotype of 34%). This varied between 1.1 and 2.1 in the four populations studied. A sub-group analysis in patients who had sustained an MI despite being at low risk on established criteria (low body mass index and low apolipoprotein B) showed that the DD genotype assumed much greater importance with an odds ratio of 3.2. The DD genotype thus seemed to act independently and in a non-additive fashion to other known risk factors. At least 15 other studies have been published. They support or question this association. Samani *et al.* [26], performed a meta-analysis of the available studies and found support for the proposition that the D allele confers an increased risk of MI with a pooled estimate odds ratio of 1.26 (increased risk of 26%). The studies however were conducted in different ethnic groups and as recruitment was at variable intervals post MI, there is the possibility of selection by mortality affecting the results. The mechanism by which the D allele influences the risk of MI is unclear with published studies reporting different effects on coronary atheroma [27, 28]. Ludwig *et al.* [28] suggests that the polymorphism confer significant risk of infarction by influencing the conversion to MI with no apparent effect on the development of atherosclerotic coronary artery disease.

Effect of ACE I/D on Left Ventricular dilatation after Myocardial Infarction

There is evidence that the ACE genotype may affect ventricular remodelling presumably through its effects on circulating and tissue renin angiotensin systems. Ohmichi *et al.* [29] assessed 79 post myocardial infarction patients (4-7 months post MI) and found that patients with the ACE DD genotype had lower left ventricular ejection fractions and greater end systolic volume indices as determined by left ventriculography compared to II patients. Schunkert *et al.* [30], in a study of 96 patients, found DD patients to have significant LV dilatation at 1 year post MI compared to ID and II patients using echocardiographic assessment. Raynolds *et al.* [31] showed a higher frequency of the DD genotype in-patients with ischaemic cardiomyopathy. Sakuramoto *et al.* [32], showed that patients with idiopathic dilated cardiomyopathy and the DD genotype had a worse clinical response to ACE inhibitor therapy. These initial reports suggest a role for the ACE polymorphism in ischaemic heart failure and LV dilatation after myocardial infarction.

ACE gene I/D polymorphism and hypertension

The ACE gene has been shown not to be associated with a genetic predisposition to high blood pressure in a Caucasian population [24, 33, 34]. Other studies have shown associations with the I allele [35] and the D allele [36]. No significant differences have been found between the I/D allele frequency in the Japanese population with and without essential hypertension [37] or in the Chinese population [38]. In the African-American population however, Duru *et al.* [39] found a significant difference in genotype frequency with a higher prevalence of the D allele in patients with hypertension compared with normotensives. This finding was confirmed in this ethnic group by Rutledge *et al.* [40]. Also, in the Afro Caribbean population Barley *et al.* [41] found a positive association between the frequency of the D allele and increasing blood pressure.

ACE gene I/D polymorphism and Left Ventricular Mass and function

The DD genotype is known to be over represented in diseases characterised by left ventricular hypertrophy and dysfunction. Kupari *et al.* [42] have shown that in the absence of cardiac disease the ACE polymorphism has no effect on LV mass to body height ratio or indices of LV systolic or diastolic function detectable by echocardiography. The results of studies in which the study population is unselected are inconclusive. A large study on subjects from the Framingham Heart Study, Lindpaintner *et al.* [43] did not find an association between the D allele and LV mass using echocardiography while in the Japanese population, Iwai *et al.* [44] found an association between the D allele and LV mass.

ACE gene I/D polymorphism in Hypertensive Left Ventricular Hypertrophy

There is evidence that the ACE genotype is an independent predictor of the development of LVH in normotensive men [30] and hypertensives [44]. It has been suggested that the effect of blood pressure on left ventricular mass index (LVMI) in essential hypertension is expressed only in the presence of the ACE gene deletion allele [45]. Conversely, it can be hypothesised that for an equal reduction of blood pressure, DD patients may have less reduction in LV mass index. It is tempting to speculate that the cause of the association of the DD genotype with LVH is that subjects with the DD genotype have increased cardiac ACE activity and angiotensin II concentrations locally.

ACE I/D Polymorphism and Antihypertensive Treatment

In a normal healthy population enalapril 10 mg reduced serum ACE activity in DD genotype subjects more than II subjects at 2, 4, and 6 hours post dose but the fall in ACE activity was greater in II subjects at 24 hours [46]. The expression of the AT_1 receptor in mononuclear cells of healthy subjects and patients with hypertension has been shown to vary with ACE genotype. The levels of expression decreased significantly with ACE inhibitor treatment in subjects with the DD genotype [47]. No association between the ACE I/D polymorphism and BP reduction has been documented in essential hypertensives treated with lisinopril 10 mg daily [48].

ANGIOTENSIN II RECEPTORS AND THE AT1 RECEPTOR POLYMORPHISM

Two subtypes (AT_1 and AT_2) of angiotensin binding receptors are known to exist in humans. The AT1 subtype mediates the physiological actions of Ang II such as vasoconstriction and salt and water retention. Two structurally distinct AT_1 receptor isoforms however have been demonstrated in animal species (AT_{1a} and $AT_{1b.}$The AT_2 receptor is highly expressed in animal embryonic tissues such as the brain and kidney but is expressed at low levels in normal adult tissues [49]. There is evidence that the AT_2 receptor mediates an antigrowth effect and apoptosis and hence may exhibit functional antagonism to the AT_1 receptor. Both the AT receptors belong to the group of seven transmembrane receptors. The gene for the human angiotensin type 1 (AT_1) receptor is located on chromosome 3 while the X chromosome contains the gene for the angiotensin type 2 (AT_2) receptor. The angiotensin II type 1 receptor gene is polymorphic with the (A1166C) polymorphism located at the 5' end of the 3' un-translated region of the gene. This is the most relevant variant of this receptor's polymorphism to cardiovascular disease. It has been found to be associated with aortic stiffness in hypertensive but not normotensive subjects and it has been suggested that this may be due to a potentiation of angiotensin II effects in the presence of hypertension [50].

EXAMPLE OF RAPID METHODS FOR DETERMINING GENOTYPES

ACE

It is possible to genotype for the ACE gene polymorphism using molecular biological methods such as the polymerase chain reaction (PCR) based assay which was first described by Rigat *et al.* [51] and is an established rapid technique. This method requires the use of genomic DNA usually from blood samples. PCR is an *in vitro* method for selectively replicating a discreet DNA fragment using an enzyme. Two oligonucleotide primers (usually 18-25bp) which have complimentary sequences to the sense and antisense strands in the target DNA are used to define the fragment to be amplified. Amplification takes place via a repetitive series of thermocycles. The thermocycles correspond to the process of template denaturation (90-95°C), annealing of primers to the separated DNA strands (40-65°C), and extension of the annealed primers by a heat stable enzyme *Taq* DNA polymerase. The newly synthesised products can act as a template in the following cycles thus resulting in exponential increase in the desired product. The PCR based assay uses two primers which flank the insertion sequence and thus allows discrimination among three genotypes: II, ID, DD. Occasionally, amplification of the I allele is suppressed leading to mistyping of an ID heterozygote as DD [52].

Angiotensinogen M235T polymorphism

The T235 allele of the angiotensinogen gene can be detected by a modification of the method of Russ *et al.* [53]. PCR products are digested with 1U of the restriction enzyme *Tth*111 I at 65^{0}C for 6 hours.

AT1 Receptor Polymorphism

This can also be performed using a PCR based assay and by using a restriction enzyme to digest the PCR product. Genotyping for the A1166C AT_1R gene variant can thus be performed by using the sense primer: 5'ATAATGTAAGCTCATCCACC-3' and the antisense primer: 5'GAGATTGCATTTCTGTCAGT-3'.

The PCR reaction is cycled and the PCR product can be digested overnight with 5U of the

restriction enzyme *Dde*I at 37^{0}C.
PCR products or digested products are electrophoresed on 2.0% agarose gels and visualised via ethidium bromide mediated fluorescence using ultraviolet transillumination.

NON RAS POLYMORPHISMS

Lipoprotein lipase

Genetic variation helps to determine in part the levels of lipids in the blood. Lipoprotein lipase is a cofactor involved in the hydrolysis of triglycerides in chylomicrons and very low density lipoproteins. Over 50 deletions and point mutations have been reported in the gene for LPL. Two common mutations cause a substitution of aspartic acid at position 9 to asparagine and asparagine at position 291 to serine. These common mutations tend to cause an elevation in plasma triglyceride levels and or low high density lipoprotein levels. This effect is particularly associated with body mass index.

Fibrinogen genes

The three fibrinogen genes are together in approximately 50kb on the long arm of chromosome 4. Each chain is manufactured as a separate RNA with the levels of all three being coordinated. The promoter region for the beta fibrinogen gene is of the order of 150base pairs and sequence changes in this region of the gene may have a direct effect on the rate of transcription and plasma fibrinogen levels. One such change is a G/A variation at position –455 with the A allele in healthy individuals showing higher fibrinogen levels [54].

Homocysteine

Evidence is accumulating that an increased blood level of homocysteine is a risk factor for premature atherosclerosis and an independent risk factor for coronary artery disease. 5, 10 methylenetetrahydrofolate reductase (MTHFR) is a key enzyme catalyzing homocysteine. Recently an alanine/valine polymorphism of the MTHFR gene has been reported with the VV genotype correlating with increased plasma levels of homocysteine. Pharmacological doses of folate can reduce plasma homocysteine levels.

REFERENCES

1. Paul M, Wagner J, Dzau VJ. Gene expression of the renin-angiotensin system in human tissues. Quantitative analysis by the polymerase chain reaction. J Clin Invest 1993;91:2058-2064.
2. Tigerstedt R, Bergman PG. Niere und Kreislauf. Skandinavishes Archiv fur Physiologie 1898;8:223-271.
3. Cohen-Haguenauer O, Soubrier F, Van Cong N, Serero S, Turleau C, Jegou C, Gross MS, Corvol P, Frezat J. Regional mapping of the human renin gene to 1q32 by in situ hybridisation. Ann Genet 1989;32:16-20.
4. Hadman JA, Mort YJ, Catanzaro DF, Tallam JT, Baxter JD, Morris BJ, Shine J. Primary structure of human renin gene. DNA 1984;3:457-468.
5. Naftilan AJ, Williams R, Burt D, Paul M, Pratt RE, Hobart P, Chirgwin J, Dzau VJ. A

lack of genetic linkage of renin gene restriction length polymorphisms with human hypertension. Hypertension 1989;14:614-618.
6. Gaillard-Sanchez I, Mattei MG, Clauser E, Corvol P. Assignment by insitu hybridisation of the angiotensinogen gene to chromosome band 1q4, the same region as the human renin gene. Hum Genet 1990;84:341-343.
7. Gaillard I, Clauser E, Corvol P. Structure of human angiotensinogen gene. DNA 1989;8:87-99.
8. Jeunemaitre X, Soubrier F, Kotelevstev YV, Lifton RP, Williams CS, Charru A, Hunt SC, Hopkins PN, Williams RR, Lalouel JM, Corvol P. Molecular basis of human hypertension:role of angiotensinogen. Cell 1992;71:169-180.
9. Jeunemaitre X, Charru A, Chatellier G, *et al.* M235T variant of the human angiotensinogen gene in unselected hypertensive patients. J Hypertens 1993;11[Suppl:5];580-581.
10. Hata A, Namikawa C, Sasaki M, *et al.* Angiotensinogen as a risk factor for essential hypertension in Japan. J Clin Invest 1994;93:1285-1287.
11. Caulfield M, Lavender P, Newell-Price J, Farrall M, Kamdar S, Daniel H, Lawson M, DeFreitas P, Fogarty P, Clark AJ. Linkage of the angiotensinogen gene locus to human essential hypertension in African Caribbeans. J. Clin. Invest. 1995;96:687-692.
12. Cambien F, Alhnec-Gelas F, Herbeth B, Andre JL, Rakotovao R, Gonzales MF, Allegrine J, Bloch C. Familial resemblance of plasma angiotensin-converting enzyme level: the Nancy study. Am J Hum Genet 1988;43:774-780.
13. Rigat B, Hubert C, Alhenc-Gelas F, Cambien F *et al.* An insertion/deletion polymorphism in the Angiotensin I-converting Enzyme Gene Accounting for half of the variance of serum enzyme levels. J. Clin Invest. 1990; 86:1343-1346.
14. Johanning GL, Johnston KE, Tamura T, Goldenburg RL. Ethnic differences in angiotensin converting enzyme polymorphism [letter]. J Hypertens 1995;13:710-711.
15. Ishigami T, Iwamoto T, Tamura K, Yamaguchi S, Iwasawa K, Uchino K, Umemura S, Ishii M: Angiotensin I converting enzyme (ACE) gene polymorphism and essential hypertension in Japan. Ethnic difference of ACE genotype. Am J Hypertension 1995;8:95-97.
16. Lee EJ: Population genetics of the angiotensin converting enzyme gene in Chinese. Br J Clin Pharmacol 1994;37:212-214.
17. Barley J, Blackwood A, Carter ND, Crewes DE, Cruckshank JK, Jeffrey S, Ogienlesi AO, Seagnill GA: Angiotensin converting enzyme insertion/deletion polymorphism: association with ethnic origin. J Hypertens 1994;12:955-957.
18. Barley J, Blackwood A, Miller M, Markandu ND, Carter ND, Jeffrey S, Cappuccio FB, MacGregor GA, Sagnella GA: Angiotensin converting enzyme gene I/D polymorphism, blood pressure and the renin angiotensin system in Caucasian and Afro-Caribbean peoples. J Hypertens 1996;10:31-35.
19. Costerousse O, Allegrini J, Lopez M, Alhenc-Gelas F. Angiotensin 1-converting enzyme in human circulating mononuclear cells: genetic polymorphism of expression in T-lymphocytes. Biochem J 1993;290:33-40.
20. Tiret L, Rigat B, Visvikis S, Breda C, Corvol P, Cambien F, Soubrier F. Evidence from combined segregation and linkage analysis, that a variant of the angiotensin I-converting enzyme gene controls plasma ACE levels. Am J Hum Genet 1992;51:197-205.
21. McKenzie CA, Julier C, Forrester T, McFarlane-Anderson N, Keavney B, Lathrop GM,

Ratcliffe PJ, Farall M: Segregation and linkage analysis of serum angiotensin I - converting enzyme levels evidence for two quantitative-trait loci. Am J Hum Genet 1995;57:1426-1435.
22. Bloem LJ, Manatunga AK, Pratt JH. Racial differences in the relationship of an angiotensin I converting enzyme gene polymorphism to serum angiotensin I converting enzyme activity. Hypertension 1996;27:62-66.
23. Morris BJ, Monaghan TC, Perich R, Stokes GS, Jackson B, Schrader AP: Genotypic influence on plasma dipeptidyl carboxypeptidase - 1 activity in hypertensives. Clin Exp Pharmacol Physiol 1994;21:343-346.
24. Harrap SB, Davidson HR, Connor JH, Soubrier F, Corvol P, Fraser R, Foy CJ, Watt GC: The angiotensin I converting enzyme gene and predisposition to high blood pressure: Hypertension 1993;21:455-460.
25. Cambien F, Poirier O, Lecerf L, Evans A, Cambou JP, Arveiler D, Luc G, Bord JM, Bora Richard S, Tiret L, Amouyel P, Alhenc-Gelas F, Scubrier F. Deletion polymorphism in the gene for angiotensin converting enzyme is a potent risk factor for myocardial infarction. Nature 1992;359:641-644.
26. Samani NJ, Thompson JR, O'Toole L, Channer K, Woods KL. A meta analysis of the association of the deletion allele of the angiotensin-converting enzyme gene with myocardial infarction. Circulation 1996;94:708-712.
27. Mattu RK, Needham EW, Galton DJ, Frangos E, Clark AJ, Caulfield M. A DNA variant of the angiotensin converting enzyme gene locus associates with coronary artery disease in the Caerphilly Heart Study. Circulation 1995;91:270-274.
28. Ludwig E, Corneli PS, Anderson JL, Marshall HW, Lalouel JM, Ward RH. Angiotensin converting enzyme gene polymorphism is associated with myocardial infarction but not with the development of coronary stenosis. Circulation 1995;91:2120-2124.
29. Ohmichi N, Iwa N, Nakamura Y, Kinoshita M. The genotype of the angiotensin converting enzyme gene and global left ventricular dysfunction after myocardial infarction. Am J Cardiol 1995;76:326-329.
30. Schunkert H, Hense HW, H, Holmer SR, Stender M, Perz S, Keil U, Lorell BH, Riegger G. Association between a deletion polymorphism of the angiotensin-converting enzyme gene and left ventricular hypertrophy. N Engl J Med 1994;330:1634-1638.
31. Raynolds MV, Bristow MR, Bush EW, Abraham WT, Lowes BD, Zisman LS, Taft CS, Perryman MB. Angiotensin converting enzyme DD genotype in patients with ischaemic or idiopathic dilated cardiomyopathy. Lancet 1993;342:1073-1075.
32. Sakuramoto H, Shimizu M, Yokota Y, Terashima M, Yokoyama M. Angiotensin Converting enzyme genotype DD showed poor response to angiotensin converting enzyme inhibitors in patients with idiopathic dilated cardiomyopathy [abstract]. Circulation 1994;Vol 90 No 4:I-452.
33. Schmidt S, Van Hooft IMS, Grobbee DE, Ganten D, Ritz E. Polymorphism of the angiotensin I converting enzyme gene is apparently not related to high blood pressure: Dutch Hypertension and Offspring Study. J Hypertension 1993;11:345-348.
34. Higashimori K, Zhao Y, Higaki J, Kamitani A, Katsuya T, Nakura J, Miki T, Mixami H, Ogihara T. Association analysis of a polymorphism of the angiotensin converting enzyme gene with essential hypertension in the Japanese population. Biochem Biophys Res Comm 1993;2:399-404.
35. Zee RYL, Lou YK, Griffiths LR, Morris BJ. Association of a polymorphism of the

angiotensin I converting enzyme gene with essential hypertension. Biochem Biophys Res Commun 1992;184:9-15.
36. Morise T, Takeuchi Y, Takeda R. Angiotensin converting enzyme polymorphism and essential hypertension. Lancet 1994;343:125.
37. Ishigami T, Iwamoto T, Tamura K, Yamaguchi S, Iwasawa K, Uchino K, Umemura S, Ishii M: Angiotensin I converting enzyme (ACE) gene polymorphism and essential hypertension in Japan. Ethnic difference of ACE genotype. Am J Hypertension 1995;8:95-97.
38. Chiang FT, Lai ZP, Chern TH, Tseng CD, Hsu KL, Lo HM, Tseng YZ: Lack of association of the angiotensin converting enzyme polymorphism with essential hypertension in a Chinese Population. Am J Hypertension 1997;10:197-201.
39. Duru K, Farrow S, Wang JM, Lockette W, Kurtz T: Frequency of a deletion polymorphism in the gene for angiotensin converting enzyme is increased in African-Americans with Hypertension. Am J Hypertens 1994;9:759-762.
40. Rutledge DR, Kubilis P, Browe CS, Ross EA: Polymorphism of the angiotensin I converting enzyme gene in essential hypertensive patients. Biochem Mol Biol Int 1995;35:661-668.
41. Barley J, Blackwood A, Miller M, Markandu ND, Carter ND, Jeffrey S, Cappuccio FB, MacGregor GA, Sagnella GA: Angiotensin converting enzyme gene I/D polymorphism, blood pressure and the renin angiotensin system in Caucasian and Afro-Caribbean peoples. J Hypertens 1996;10:31-35.
42. Kupari M, Perola M, Koskinen P, Virolainen J, Karhunen P. Left ventricular size, mass, and function in relation to angiotensin-converting enzyme gene polymorphism in humans. Am J Physiol 1994;267:H1107-H1111.
43. Lindpaintner K, Lee M, Larson MG, Rao VS, Pfeffer MA, Ordovas JM, Schaefer EJ, Wilson AF, Wilson PWF, Vasan RS, Myers RH, Levy D. Absence of association or genetic linkage between the angiotensin-converting enzyme gene and left ventricular mass. N Engl J Med 1996;334:1023-1028.
44. Iwai N, Ohmichi N, Nakamura Y, Kinoshita M. DD Genotype of the Angiotensin Converting Enzyme Gene is a risk factor for Left Ventricular Hypertrophy. Circulation 1994;90:2622-2628.
45. Prasad N, O'Kane K P, Johnstone H A *et al.* The relationship between blood pressure and left ventricular mass in essential hypertension is observed only in the presence of the angiotensin converting enzyme gene deletion allele. QJM 1994;87:659-662.
46. Todd GP, Chadwick IG, Higgins KS, Yeo WW, Jackson PR, Ramsay LE: Relation between changes in blood pressure and serum ACE activity after single dose of enalapril and ACE genotype in healthy subjects. Br J Clin Pharm 1995;39:131-134.
47. Dieguez-Lucena JL, Aranda-Lara P, Ruiz-Galdon M, Villanova-Garcia J, Morell-Ocana M, Engel-Reyes A. Angiotensin I-converting enzyme genotypes and angiotensin II receptors Response to therapy. Hypertension 1996;28:98-103.
48. Dudley C, Keavney B, Casadei B, Conway J, Bird R, Ratcliffe P. Prediction of patient responses to antihypertensive drugs using genetic polymorphisms:investigation of renin-angiotensin system genes. J Hypertens 1996;14:259-262.
49. Aguilera G, Kapur S, Feuillan P. Developmental changes in angiotensin II receptor subtypes and AT_1 receptor mRNA in rat kidney. Kidney Int 1994;46:973-979.
50. Benetos A, Gautier S, Ricard S, Topouchian J, Asmar R, Poirier O, Larosa E, Guize L,

Safar M, Soubrier F, Cambien F. Influence of angiotensin-converting enzyme and angiotensin II type 1 receptor gene polymorphisms on aortic stiffness in normotensive and hypertensive patients. Circulation 1996;94:698-703.

51. Rigat B,Hubert C, Corvol P, Soubrier F. PCR detection of the insertion/deletion polymorphism of the human angiotensin converting enzyme gene (DCP1) dipeptidyl carboxypeptidase 1. Nucleic Acids Res 1992;20:1433.
52. Shanmugan V, Sell KW, Saha BK. Mistyping ACE heterozygotes. PCR Methods Appl 1993;2:120-121.
53. Russ AP, Maerz W, Ruzicka V, Stein U, Gross U. Rapid detection of the hypertension associated Met235-Thr allele of the human angiotensinogen gene. Hum Mol Genet 1993;2:609-610.
54. Thomas A, Kelleher C, Green F *et al.* Variation in the promoter region of the beta fibrinogen gene is associated with plasma fibrinogen levels in smokers and non-smokers. Thromb Haemost 1991;65:487-490.

Discussion: Genetic polymorphisms in cardiovascular disease: focus on renin angiotensin system

M.M. Reidenberg:

You mentioned that the ACE/ID polymorphism was in an intron. Is there any evidence that this is actually pathophysiologically important, or is it still possible that this could be a marker for something close to it on the chromosome?

G.K. Davis:

The current thinking is that it is possibly a marker for something close to it on the chromosome. It has not yet been identified exactly where the locus affecting ACE levels is located.

A. Breckenridge:

Does the level of ACE, whether or not determined by the polymorphism you have described, affect the expression of AII receptors? If so, this would be a very convenient homeostatic mechanism for the body and this might account for the diversity of the results of the studies that you have described. You said quite clearly that there is not a very strong or clear clinical correlate for the impressive genetic work you have described. Possibly, there is this kind of feed-back loop with respect to expression of AII receptor.

G.K. Davis:

I think there is some specific work in terms of either ACE and AT1 receptors, that we may have to look at. The expression of the AT1 receptor in mononuclear cells has been shown to vary with ACE genotype (Dieguez-Lucena *et al.*, Hypertension, 1996).

M. Pirmohamed:

Firstly, since tissue levels of ACE may be much more important pathophysiologically than serum levels of ACE, how closely do serum levels relate to tissue levels of ACE? And secondly, there was initially evidence that the ACE gene polymorphism could be associated with myocardial infarction, particularly in low-risk patients, although it was refuted through a prospective study.

G.K. Davis:

There is a relationship between the ACE I/D polymorphism and tissue levels of ACE for normal hearts, (Jan Danser *et al.*, Circulation, 1995). The overall result in the meta-analysis done by (Samani *et al.*, Circulation, 1996) was a positive effect of the D allele on the risk of MI. The large negative prospective study (by Lindpainter *et al.*, N Engl J Med, 1995) could be due to differences in genetic backgrounds.

P. du Souich:

A study about the effect of growth hormone on dilated cardiomyopathy was published two years ago (Fazio *et al.*, N Engl J Med, 1996) but it has not been reproduced. How could the polymorphism you have described affect the effect of growth hormone?

G.K. Davis:

I cannot comment specifically on how ACE may interact with growth hormone. A point of interest I probably should mention is the fact that angiotensin II type 2 receptors exist in the heart as well as in other tissues. Whether or not the angiotensin II type 2 receptor is thought to have some form of anti-proliferative effect itself is another feature of the inter-relationship which has yet to be clarified.

A.J.J. Wood:

What should be our standard for reporting positive associations? Should we demand a pathophysiological hypothesis first, or should we view these as data-dredging exercises?

G.K. Davis:

I think the way cardiovascular medicine has developed is that we did the studies and found that some of the treatments were effective, for example, ACE inhibitors in heart failure and hypertension, although we did not actually have pathophysiological explanations at the time. We used the treatment based on the results we had at the time. Now, there is a lot of work on amongst different genes, and there is quite a list of different genes that may be related to coronary artery disease or hypertension. The information is forthcoming, but we should also look for some form of unifying mechanism, some pathophysiological reason to explain any effect.

A.J.J. Wood:

If you were a journal editor, for example, would you be more reluctant to accept an article that did not have a therapeutic basis to it? If you did not have a positive ACE inhibitor trial in post-myocardial infarction, should you not be less willing to accept a gene association?

G.K. Davis:

I would not say I would be less willing to accept a gene association, but I think that a positive trial result would give an association a lot more strength, at least in terms of the pathophysiology of the condition.

D.C. Brater:

There is an experiment of nature with high ACE levels in sarcoidosis where there is no increase in cardiovascular disease or hypertension. This seems to contradict hypotheses about the importance of these phenotypes?

G.K. Davis:

The fact is that the experiments done so far have shown that aside from hypertension, heart failure and hypertrophic cardiomyopathy, high ACE levels also seem to be a poor prognostic marker for quite a lot of independent cardiovascular conditions. To some extent, the question at the moment is whether or not it is all related to angiotensin-II, the main effector hormone and whether this is related to increased ACE levels. I think angiotensin-II is the effector hormone, and there is a lot of independent information as regards different cardiovascular conditions supporting this. Although I can not recall any increased cardiovascular events in patients with sarcoidosis, there is strong data with regard to a lot of the other conditions and increased ACE levels.

I.P. Hall:

Two issues should be considered. There is a high rate of polymorphic variation in the human genome, and therefore it is critical we do not do endless association studies. Therefore you need to have some functional evidence to indicate something is relevant. With respect to the ID polymorphism, I think it is problematic that it is intronic. One could argue that there is something else which is controlling ACE levels. This brings me to the second point: a lot of association studies have problems with drifting phenotypes. The difficulty is that, if you go after enough end-points, you will see associations, and looking at the ID story, some studies detect association with left ventricular change, some with risk of myocardial infarction and some have reported changes in blood pressure in some populations, but these are not the same pathophysiological processes. The danger is that one will assume that this is a meaningful polymorphism, because the body of evidence related to all the associations even if, on careful examination, the associations do not seem so valid.

E.M. Sellers:

In other fields, the explanation for varying reported results very often turns out to be inadequate control of ethno-racial origin. To what extent, can we be sure with these reports that in fact there is clear evidence that the ethno-racial groups have been homogeneous?

G.K. Davis:

From some of the study data actually presented, we can see that there is ethnic variation in the frequency of polymorphism. Therefore the interpretation has to be within the groups that are studied. There is certainly no firm explanation as to the actual pathophysiology, and studies have been carried out in different ethnic groups. We do have that sort of scepticism about intronic polymorphisms, and that has certainly been the feeling throughout the analysis of the data and accounts for the number of studies that have been performed looking at it in different ways.

M.M. Reidenberg:

I suspect this is an area where the risk of publication bias is very high, in that the positive studies get reported, and not the negative ones. At this stage, if there were some way to develop a registry of studies, such as has been attempted for clinical trials, it would be very fruitful in keeping people from making erroneous conclusions about the one positive study out of a series that looked at the same thing.

G.K. Davis:

Another area that we are studying is whether these polymorphisms themselves have any clinical relevance in terms of patient management and predicting patient response.

Variability in Human Drug Response
G.T. Tucker, Editor

Pharmacogenetics of respiratory system drugs

Ian P. Hall

Division of Therapeutics, University Hospital, Nottingham, UK.

ABSTRACT

Genetic factors can affect the pharmacokinetics of respiratory drugs in a number of ways. Defects in drug metabolising enzymes are the best characterised genetic factors: approximately 10% of Caucasians are slow acetylators (ie have a low affinity N-acetyltransferase isozyme) and will therefore (for example) metabolise isoniazid less rapidly and are more susceptible to peripheral neuropathy. Common polymorphisms in drug targets may also affect treatment response.

Of these polymorphisms the treatment modifying effects of the β_2 adrenoceptor polymorphism and 5-LO promoter polymorphism are best described. Individuals homozygous for the Gly 16 β_2 adrenoceptor polymorphism demonstrate bronchodilator tachyphylaxis (Tam *et al.* 1997). This polymorphism has a high allelic frequency in the Caucasian population (Gly 16 homozygotes 37 %, n = 626). 5-LO promoter polymorphisms modify promoter activity and hence can potentially alter the response to 5-LO inhibition (In *et al.* 1997). Thus common genetic variants of genes whose products are targets of respiratory system drugs may alter treatment response in individuals.

Polymorphism are known to exist in the β_2 adrenoceptor (cpdpm 16,27, 164), the H_1 receptor (degenerate polymorphism at codon 356) and the 5-lipoxygenase (5-LO) promoter (alleles 11-5).

Key words: Drug metabolism, polymorphism, pharmacogenetics, β_2 adrenoceptor, 5-lipoxygenase.

Correspondence: Dr. I.P. Hall, Division of Therapeutics, University Hospital, Nottingham, NG7 2UH, United Kingdom, Tel: +44-(0)115-970-9905 Fax: +44-(0)115-942-22-323, Email: ian.hall@nottingham.ac.uk

Funding acknowledgement: National Asthma Campaign; Medical Research Council.

INTRODUCTION

The role of genetic factors in determining variability in treatment response to drugs used in the management of respiratory disease has only recently attracted attention. This is perhaps surprising given that it has been clear for many years that there is marked inter-individual variability in treatment response to given drugs. In this review I will discuss the evidence for genetic polymorphism in the target proteins of respiratory drugs used in the management of asthma and chronic obstructive pulmonary disease (COPD). It must however be remembered that genetic variability can be important in treatment response for drugs used in the treatment of other respiratory disease. Perhaps the best example is the contribution of hepatic metabolising enzyme polymorphisms to the risk of developing peripheral nerve toxicity in individuals treated with isoniazid: slow acetylators (10 % of the population) are at increased risk of neurotoxicity due to the reduced hepatic metabolism of isoniazid.

The major target proteins of drugs used in the treatment of airflow obstruction are G-protein coupled receptors, steroid receptors, the phosphodiesterase family of isoenzymes and metabolising enzymes involved in leukotriene metabolism. These will be systematically reviewed below.

β_2 ADRENOCEPTORS

By far the largest literature on the influence of genetic polymorphisms to disease susceptibility and treatment response concerns β_2 adrenoceptor polymorphism. The β_2 adrenoceptor is situated on chromosome 5q.31 and following initial work by Liggett and co-workers [1] which identified 4 single base substitutions which resulted in amino acid changes in the receptor as well as 5 degenerate single base substitutions (ie polymorphism which do not alter the amino acid code of the receptor) extensive studies have been performed to address the potential functionality of the nondegenerative polymorphisms.

The 4 polymorphisms which alter the amino acid code of the receptor are situated at codons 16, 27, 34 and 164. Of these the valine to methionine 34 substitution appears to be of no functional significance and is also rare and hence has not been studied in human populations. However the other 3 polymorphisms all occur in the Caucasian population two being common. All 3 appear to be functionally relevant.

Perhaps the most interesting from the pharmacogenetic point of view is the polymorphism at codon 164 (threonine to isoleucine). This polymorphism is relatively uncommon with an allelic frequency of 3 % in the Caucasian population. Because each individual has 2 genes for the β_2 adrenoceptor homozygous individuals would be expected to be rare: to date none have been studied formally. When the isoleucine 164 version of the receptor was expressed in recombinant cell lines there was a reduction in agonist induced activation of adenylyl cyclase and also altered receptor sequestration following long term agonist stimulation [2]. Interestingly the amino acid 164 sits deep in transmembrane domain IV and is very close to the proposed "exosite" where the hydrophobic tail of the long acting β_2 agonist salmeterol is believed to bind. Because the threonine - isoleucine 164 polymorphism is non conservative one would predict charge alteration in this region of the 4th transmembrane spanning domain and it seems likely therefore that individuals carrying this polymorphism may display an altered response to salmeterol. Because no individual homozygous for this polymorphism has yet been studied the response of such individuals to salmeterol (or other β agonists) remains unknown.

In contrast to the amino acid 164 polymorphism the polymorphisms at amino acid 16 (arginine-glycine) and 27 (glutamine-glutamate) are common in Caucasian populations. Neither amino acid substitution confers altered agonist binding efficiency: this is hardly surprising given that both polymorphisms are in the N terminal extra cellular part of the receptor. However these polymorphisms have effects on receptor downregulation in both transformed cell systems and in primary cell cultures of known genotype. The glycine 16 variant of the receptor confers increased receptor downregulation following agonist exposure, whereas the glutamate 27 variant is protected in part from receptor downregulation [3,4]. Two published studies have suggested that individuals with asthma carrying the glycine 16 variant (which downregulates to a greater extent than the arginine 16 version of the receptor) have altered bronchodilator responses following treatment with β agonists. In a single blind placebo controlled cross over trial with formoterol bronchodilator subsensitivity was observed following 2 weeks treatment with formoterol 24 g b.d. in those individuals homozygous for the glycine 16 variant, whereas individuals with the arginine 16 variant of the receptor had maintained bronchodilator responses [5]. In the second study asthmatic children were more likely to have significant reversibility to inhaled β_2 agonist if they did not have the glycine 16 variant of the receptor [6]. However, a third study, examining the potential contribution of this polymorphism to adverse asthma control in asthmatics taking fenoterol failed to demonstrate any contribution from Glycine 16 [7].

In contrast to the codon 16 polymorphism, polymorphism at codon 27 does not appear to dictate response to β_2 agonist drugs, although in one study both allelic association and linkage was observed between the aminoacid 27 polymorphism and IgE levels in asthmatic families [8]. These data may possibly be explained by linkage disequilibrium with other potential candidate genes on chromosome 5q including the Th_2 cytokine cluster.

Finally it is important to note that the amino acid 16 and 27 polymorphisms are in strong linkage disequilibrium in the Caucasian population and that there are racial differences in the distribution of these polymorphisms [9]. In particular the glutamate 27 polymorphism is rare in both the Japanese and Black Afro-Caribbean population (unpublished data).

HISTAMINE H_1 RECEPTORS

Although antagonists at histamine H_1 receptors are relatively poor bronchodilators there is marked variability in the response of individuals in their response to inhaled histamine. Because there is a good correlation between PD20 values obtained with both methacholine and histamine within individuals this would suggest that inter-individual variability of the bronchoconstrictor response to inhaled histamine is a feature of non specific bronchial hyperreactivity rather than due to genetic variability of the response to histamine alone. Nonetheless, we have recently screened the coding region for the histamine H_1 receptor for variants by single stranded confirmational polymorphism analysis (SSCP): this method is around 95 % sensitive for detecting single base substitutions or other polymorphisms. In marked contrast to the β_2 adrenoceptor we were unable to find any single base substitutions or other polymorphisms which altered the amino acid code of the histamine H_1 receptor, although we did find 1 degenerate polymorphism at codon 356 (A-G, allelic frequency 3.8 %) [10]. Hence it appears that genetic variation in the coding region of the H_1 receptor gene is unlikely to contribute to variability in individual responses to histamine.

MUSCARINIC RECEPTORS

Both muscarinic M_2 and M_3 receptors are expressed on airway smooth muscle. The muscarinic M_3 receptor is likely to be important in the contractile response of airway smooth muscle to muscarinic agonists such as acetylcholine released following vagal stimulation. The exact function of the muscarinic M_2 receptors present on these cells remains unclear: the M_2 receptor is negatively coupled to adenylyl cyclase and hence stimulation of these receptors can partially prevent the relaxant action of drugs such as β_2 agonists working through receptors positively coupled to adenylyl cyclase.

There are no described polymorphisms in either the M_2 or the M_3 receptor in the current literature. Whilst we have not screened the coding region (or regulator regions) of the M_3 receptor for polymorphism we have performed a limited screen of the coding region for the M_2 receptor and to date have not found evidence for polymorphism. There is a known polymorphic marker approximately 3 kilobases upstream of the M_2 gene however which could be used for linkage studies.

5-LIPOXYGENASE

The 5-lipoxygenase pathway is important in generation of the bronchoconstrictor leukotrienes, of which the most potent is leukotriene (LT) D4. Whilst the receptor for LTD4 has not been cloned the metabolising enzyme 5-lipoxygenase has been screened for polymorphic variants. Drazen and co-workers have described a number of variants in the promoter for this gene (called alleles 1-5) which interfere with potential Spl/Egr-1 transcriptional factor binding sites. Using reporter gene approaches this group has been able to show that these promoter polymorphisms alter the transcriptional activity of a surrogate reporter gene implying that individuals carrying the different alleles for this promoter polymorphism may have altered transcriptional activity of the 5-LO gene *in vivo* [11]. There are at present no published data on the potential for these polymorphisms to alter response to 5-lipoxygenase inhibitors in asthmatic populations. In addition to known polymorphisms in the 5-lipoxygenase promoter gene there is also a known polymorphism in the LT C4 synthase gene which in one study was shown to be associated with aspirin induced asthma.

GLUCOCORTICOID RECEPTORS

Whilst it is clear that there is a wide spectrum in steroid responsiveness in asthma with some individuals appearing to be essentially steroid resistant and other individuals having a good clinical response to steroids the biochemical basis for this variability remains unclear. In one study the glucocorticoid receptor from steroid sensitive and steroid resistant asthmatics was sequenced and no genetic basis for the variability in treatment response was found [12]. However there are many potential downstream targets for the glucocorticoid receptor which to date have not been examined for genetic polymorphism.

PHOSPHODIESTERASE ISOENZYMES

It is now clear that there are many different phosphodiesterase isoenzymes [13]. On the basis of sequence homology these have been divided into a number of families: however the genes for phosphodiesterase isoenzymes are somewhat complex often with several exons leading to potential splice variants. In the airways it appears that members of the Type 3 and Type 4 isoenzyme families are likely to be the most important in both airway smooth muscle and in inflammatory cells. At present the only respiratory drugs targeted at this system and in widespread use are theophylline and its derivatives: these act as non-selective phosphodiesterase isoenzymes. Whether or not polymorphisms alter activity of individual phosphodiesterase isoenzymes has not been explored, although this would be a difficult topic for research give the multiplicity of phosphodiesterase isoforms.

CONCLUSIONS

It is estimated that approximately 1 in 1000 bases in coding region DNA and 1 in 500 bases in non-coding region DNA are polymorphic within the human genome. This however is clearly an oversimplification in that some genes show marked variability (eg the β_2 adrenoceptor, with a frequency of polymorphisms of >1 in 200) at one extreme and genes such as the histamine H_1 receptor of similar length but with a rate of polymorphism of 1 in 1500 at the other extreme. Given this high rate of genetic variability many polymorphisms will be identified which can potentially alter the function of a gene. In addition to coding region polymorphisms many regulatory sequences can potentially also be polymorphic and may alter transcriptional activity of that gene. Given this high rate of genetic variability it is critical to assess the functional relevance of identified polymorphisms before performing pharmacogenetic studies. Many genetic variants are likely to be clinically silent, producing no functional effects. However it is likely that genetic polymorphism within specific genes plays a major role in determining the inter-individual variability in treatment response to drugs used in the treatment of respiratory (and other) disease.

REFERENCES

1. Reishaus E, Innis M, MacIntyre N, Liggett SB. Mutations in the gene encoding for the β_2 adrenergic receptor in normal and asthmatic subjects. Am J Resp Cell Mol Biol 1993;8:334-9.
2. Green SA, Cole G, Jacinto M, Innis M, Liggett SB. A polymorphism of the human β_2-receptor within the fourth transmembrane domain alters ligand binding and functional properties of the receptor. J Biological Chemistry 1993;268:23116-21.
3. Green SA, Turki J, Innis M, Liggett SB. Amino-terminal polymorphisms of the human β_2-adrenergic receptor impart distinct agonist-promoted regulatory properties. Biochem (USA) 1994;33:9414-9.
4. Green SA, Turki J, Bejarano P, Hall IP, Liggett SB. Influence of β_2 adrenergic receptor genotypes on signal transduction in human airway smooth muscle cells. Am J Resp Cell Mol Biol 1995;13:25-33.

5. Tan KS, Hall IP, Dewar JC, Dow E, Lipworth BJ. β_2 adrenoceptor (β_2-AR) polymorphism determines susceptibility to bronchodilator desensitisation in asthmatics. Lancet 1997;4;350:995-999.
6. Martinez FD, Graves PE, Baldini M *et al.* Association between genetic polymorphisms of the β_2 adrenoceptor and response to albuterol in children with and without a history of wheezing. J Clin Invest 1997;100:3184.
7. Hancox RJ, Sears MR, Taylor DR. Polymorphism of the β_2 adrenoceptor and the response to long-term β_2 agonist therapy in asthma. Euro Resp J 1998;11:589-593.
8. Dewar JC, Wheatley A, Wilkinson J, Thomas NS, Doull I, Morton N, Lio P, Harvey J, Liggett SB, Holgate ST, Hall IP. The glutamine 27 β_2 adrenoceptor polymorphism is associated with elevated IgE levels in asthmatic families. J All Clin Immunol 1997;100:261-265.
9. Dewar JC, Wheatley AP, Venn A, Morrison JFJ, Britton J, Hall IP. β_2 adrenoceptor polymorphisms are in linkage disequilibrium, but are not associated with asthma in an adult population. Clin Exp All 1998;28:442-448.
10. Dewar JC, Hall IP. A novel degenerate polymorphism in the human histamine H_1 receptor gene. Am J Resp & Crit Care Med 1998 (in press) (abstract).
11. In KH, Asano K, Beler D, Grosholz J, Finn PW, Silverman EK *et al.* Naturally occurring mutations in the human 5-lipoxygenase gene promoter that modify transcription factor binding and reporter gene transcription. J Clin Invest 1997;99:1130-1137.
12. Lane SJ, Arm JP, Staynov DZ, Lee TH. Chemical mutational analysis of the human glucocorticoid receptor cDNA in glucocorticoid-resistant bronchial asthma. Am J Respir Cell Mol Biol 1994;11:42-48.
13. Beavo JA: Cyclic nucleotide phosphodiesterases: functional implications of multiple isoforms. Physiol Rev 1995;75:725-748.

<u>Discussion</u>: Pharmacogenetics of respiratory system drugs

M.T. Kinirons:

Has anybody looked at the relationship of some of these polymorphisms with sudden death?

I.P. Hall:

The β_2 adrenoceptor has been studied. There have been a number of epidemiological studies suggesting that giving asthmatic individuals high doses of β-agonists may predispose to sudden death. This was initially noted with isoprenaline inhalers, back in the late 1960s and resulted in them being removed from the market in many countries. Subsequently an epidemic of asthma deaths in New Zealand in the 1970s suggested fenoterol to be the clue. A couple of retrospective studies, (Hancox RJ *et al.*, Eur Resp J, 1998), (Weir TD *et al.* Am J Respir Crit Cared Med, 1998), have been done on this issue but they suggested that there is no association between genotype and sudden death.

N.L. Benowitz:

It is interesting to speculate about what the lack of tolerance related to agonism might mean for the cardiovascular system. The development of tolerance could be an important homeostatic mechanism. Do people who have the mutation for this β_2 gene have any cardiovascular physiological abnormalities?

I.P. Hall:

We have been working with John Cockcroft, who is a cardiovascular pharmacologist, and we did studies where we infused isoprenaline into the forearm vasculature of individuals. Then we looked at vasodilator responses to isoprenaline by plethysmography. The data, published in abstract form, show an association, which is actually more striking for venodilation than for arteriodilation, between a preserved response and a non-down-regulating genotype. There is also quite a marked racial difference in these polymorphisms. For example, the black South African population, which is known to have blunted vasodilator responses to isoprenaline, has got a markedly reduced frequency of the non-down-regulating, glutamate 27 genotype.

P. Rolan:

Treating patients some years ago, I noticed some who were very poorly controlled with oral doses of steroids of 30 mg or more. These patients did not seem to get better, but they became cushinoid. It was not clear what was happening to them as the drug was clearly entering the circulation. Do you have any experience of similar patients and do you have an explanation for these observations?

I.P. Hall:

There is a group of patients who are considered to have "glucocorticoid-resistant" asthma. I have never been convinced, because the distribution in terms of peak flow responses is not a bimodal distribution but unimodal. I think patients are labelled as glucocorticoid-resistant asthma if their response is less than a certain percentage. The difficulty obviously exists that is there may be some heterogeneity in the patients you are looking at, for example, some of these patients may not have asthma, they may have fixed air-flow obstruction. A group in

London sequenced the glucocorticoid receptor itself in half a dozen individuals who were said to be glucocorticoid resistant, and they did not find any polymorphic variance within it. However, there are a large number of downstream signalling molecules, which could potentially have some effect.

A. Breckenridge:
Most of your data was retrospective. Have you performed any prospective clinical trials with bronchodilators?

I.P. Hall:
We are performing a prospective study in standard clinical trial conditions. What we have not done is to examine whether knowledge of a patients genotype is going to affect a general practitioner's decision to treat the patients with salmeterol. Although these differences that I have described are probably real, they may not be clinically relevant, because they may not alter the way asthmatic patients are treated. Tasking a nihilistic view, this type of patient could be treated with salmeterol or fenoterol for a while and if there is no response, the dose of inhaled steroids could be increased. If genotype did determine response to long-acting β agonists, I would argue it is probably more cost-effective to genotype the patient first, but the size of the study required to reach this conclusion is a minimum of 100 individuals and we have not done such a study.

A. Breckenridge:
The other very interesting implication is the drug-regulatory one. If you designed your study with a smaller tighter group to show efficacy in this group for whom you might predict treatment would work, it would be a very interesting way ahead for drug regulation.

I.P. Hall:
One could argue that the pharmaceutical industry would not want to know about a group of individuals who are going to be non-responders. I think that that is probably wrong, because what you really want to know is how effective your drug is, and if you do small Phase-II or Phase-III studies and by chance include in them a number of non-responders, you will inevitably underestimate the efficacy of your drug. On the other hand, I am not aware that any of the licensing agencies to date have formally asked for genetic information, although I have heard rumours that the FDA has started to consider this. I have been asked by pharmaceutical companies to genotype individuals in β agonist studies. And I do not know what that information is being used for, but I suspect that the companies are preparing for possible requests from the regulatory authorities.

A.J.J. Wood:
Didn't Liggett's group find an association with nocturnal asthma, and also with the desensitisation phenomena *in vivo*?

I.P. Hall:
There is a retrospective study looking at individuals with nocturnal asthma (Turki J *et al.*, J Clin Invest, 1995) showing that they are more likely to have the down-regulating Gly 16 genotype. There is also a good biopsy study published (Turki J *et al.*, Am J Phys-Lung

Cellular & Molecular Physiology, 1995) showing reduced β adrenoceptor number in individuals with Gly 16 genotype after treatment.

P.B. Watkins:

I had an interesting experience recently as a consultant to industry. Clinical trials revealed that genetic polymorphism appeared to identify 50% of the individuals who responded to the drug, and this made sense on a physiological basis. In this situation, the head of clinical development suggested that with the follow-up compounds with same mechanism genotyping could be used to reduce the sample size of the clinical trials, improving speed and cutting costs substantially. A person responsible for regulatory affairs commented that if only studies on people who are genotyped are done, it is likely that the drug would only be approved in individuals who had genotyping. He pointed out that this would be reducing the market for the drug by 50%. He also pointed out the genotyping raised ethical issues that society has not completely dealt with. Interestingly, a decision was made in that discussion not to pursue the genotyping any further, but to save genomic DNA samples on every individual enroled in clinical trials in case this information became desirable or was required by the FDA at a later date.

A.J.J. Wood:

Would you approve a drug to be used in a group that had not been tested? If you had carried out your studies in a single genotype and showed that there was a beneficial safety-toxicity ratio in that group, would you approve it for use in a different genotype?

A. Breckenridge:

No, of course you would not. But the drug company needs to indicate whether it would only be submitting for approval in those patients who had been genotyped. It depends in part on the nature of the disease, but if we are going to take therapeutics any further forward, a group like this should be encouraging this kind of approach.

I.P. Hall:

The drug companies can develop the test and sell it. However, there may be a conceptual problem. We do not have any problems measuring theophylline levels in patients on theophylline, but we seem to have a major problem in taking a blood sample to obtain someone's genotype.

M.M. Reidenberg:

You said that, in your view, it would be cost-effective for the general practitioner to determine the β adrenergic genotype. Could you expand on the basis for that opinion, please?

I.P. Hall:

At the moment we do not know it specifically for β-receptor genotypes. I said that if you could say whether or not a patient was going to respond to salmeterol (for example) depended on genotype, then it would be more cost-effective to genotype an individual if you set up a service to do it, than to do a sort of informal trial in that patient. The reason for that is that the cost of genotyping, if it were widely available, could easily come down to a few pounds per sample.

E.M. Sellers:

One of the main reasons why most pharmaceutical companies do not analyse their data with respect to differences in gender response to drugs, is that they feel they will be restricted in their labelling, if they find any differences. Since studies are powered to detect a main group effect a subgroup analysis may give a type II error of non-efficacy. If that happens with gender, it is not surprising to see the same reasoning occurring for genotyping.

Variability in Human Drug Response
G.T. Tucker, Editor

Tolerance as a Modulator of Drug Response

Neal L. Benowitz

Division of Clinical Pharmacology and Experimental Therapeutics, University of California, San Francisco, CA (USA)

ABSTRACT

Development of tolerance to the effects of drugs is a common phenomenon in medicine. The development of tolerance has implications with respect to therapeutic outcomes and in planning medication regimens. This paper will focus on the development of tolerance to psychoactive and cardiovascular drugs, with an emphasis on methods for studying drug tolerance in humans.

Several pharmacokinetic-pharmacodynamic models have been proposed for studying drug tolerance. In various models tolerance is driven by time, drug concentration, or by the effect itself. The latter type of physiological model allows modelling of both tolerance and withdrawal effects.

Tolerance to different pharmacologic actions of a drug may develop at different rates and/or to different extents. Differences in the development of tolerance to different effects of a drug may provide insight into mechanisms of drug action and have implications for drug safety.

Key words: tolerance, pharmacodynamics, pharmacokinetics, modelling, nicotine, toxicity.

Correspondence: Prof. Neal L. Benowitz, Division of Clinical Pharmacology and Experimental Therapeutics, University of California, San Francisco, Box 1220, San Francisco, California 94143-1220, U.S.A., Tel. +1-415-206-8324, Fax: +1-415-206-4956, Email: nbeno@itsa.ucsf.edu

Funding acknowledgement: Research presented in and the preparation of this manuscript was supported by grants No. DA01696 and DA02277 from the National Institute on Drug Abuse, National Institutes of Health, and carried out in part at the General Clinical Research Center with the support of the Division of Research Resources, National Institutes of Health (RR-00083).

INTRODUCTION

The development of tolerance to effects of drugs is a common phenomenon in medicine. Tolerance develops to the actions of a variety of drugs, including psychoactive drugs, analgesics, and cardiovascular drugs. The development of tolerance has important implications with respect to therapeutic outcomes and for planning medication regimens. This paper will focus on the development of tolerance to psychoactive and cardiovascular drug effects, with an emphasis on methods for studying the development of tolerance in humans.

WHAT IS TOLERANCE?

A broad definition of tolerance is "a pharmacologically defined phenomenon that appears after one or several exposures to a drug, when the same dose or concentration of the same drug produces a smaller response than that which appears in appropriate controls" [1].

It is useful to consider examples of ways of measuring tolerance. 1) Decreased duration of a drug effect — for example, a progressive decrease in the duration of analgesia with repeated doses of narcotics. 2) Reduced intensity of response to a particular dose — for example, a reduced hypnotic effect of a sleeping pill taken on a regular basis. 3) Increased dose required to produce a given effect — for example, increased doses of nitroglycerin needed to vasodilate and control symptoms of angina pectoris. 4) Significant hysteresis in the plasma concentration time curve. The latter has been used in modeling short term tolerance to the acute effects of drugs [2].

WHY IS TOLERANCE IMPORTANT?

The development of tolerance may be important in a variety of ways. 1) The most obvious is that tolerance reduces the therapeutic effect of a drug given repeatedly over time. This is well illustrated by the development of tolerance to the anti-ischemic effects of transdermal nitroglycerin given to patients with angina pectoris, and to the effects of opiates given in chronic pain patients. 2) A second implication of toxicity is less toxicity after chronic exposure. An example of toxicity reducing tolerance is less sedation or respiratory depression with chronic opioid use. 3) The development of tolerance is also associated with the development of physical dependence, which is seen with a variety of substances of abuse. Physical dependence refers to the development of withdrawal symptoms when a drug is stopped after a period of drug administration. The same mechanism involved in the development of tolerance is often involved in producing withdrawal symptoms. Physical dependence is one element, although not a required element, in the development of addiction. Many psychoactive drugs are associated with the development of tolerance and physical dependence, including caffeine, nicotine, alcohol, heroin, and sedative hypnotics.

MECHANISMS OF DEVELOPMENT OF TOLERANCE

The general mechanisms of tolerance can be considered in several general categories including 1) dispositional or pharmacokinetic tolerance; 2) functional or pharmacodynamic tolerance; 3) behavioral tolerance, and 4) conditioned tolerance. Dispositional tolerance occurs when repeated doses of a drug results in accelerated metabolism. An example of this is with repeated administration of barbiturates or ethanol [3]. Dispositional tolerance is not a common mechanism of tolerance and can explain only moderate tolerance — that is, reducing the tolerant response to only two to three times compared to the initial response.

Functional or pharmacodynamic tolerance implies that there is a different response in the presence of the same concentration of drug at the receptor site or other site of action. There are several ways in which pharmacodynamic tolerance can develop, as discussed below. Behavioral tolerance is a particular type of tolerance seen with psychoactive drugs. In this case, when an organism is exposed to a drug in the context of some behavior, that behavior can be learned in the presence of the drug with improvement over time. Thus, the individual learns to compensate for a particular drug effect. An example of this is the effects of marijuana smoking while driving an automobile. Driving can be learned when repeatedly performed under the influence of marijuana, but this tolerance does not necessarily extend to the effects of marijuana in other behavioral situations. Conditioned tolerance refers to the development of tolerance to a drug effect in a particular environment, while exposure to the same drug in another environment may not be associated with tolerance. This is purported to occur with the abuse of drugs such as alcohol or heroin. After development of tolerance to these drugs in a particular environment, exposure to a placebo in the same environment will produce an effect apparently opposite to that of the drug action. That is, the cues of drug taking elicit a compensatory or adaptive counterregulatory response.

Functional tolerance implies that there is a change in response with a particular concentration of a drug present at the receptor site. A variety of types of functional tolerance have been described. 1) Depletion of an endogenous intermediary. An example is a drug that releases catecholamines from neuronal stores, such as amphetamine. In this case, the repeated dosing of amphetamine results in a diminished cardiovascular response related to a reduction of intraneuronal catecholamine stores. 2) Inactivation or reduction in numbers of receptors. Changes in receptor function and structure are associated with the development of tolerance to beta adrenergic agonists, as well as other drugs. Initial rapid tolerance development (also termed desensitization) is associated with phosphorylation of receptors and sequestration of receptors in a cellular compartment no longer accessible to the agonist. Subsequently, uncoupling of the receptor from the second messenger system and, finally, internalization of the receptor to intracellular sites occurs [4]. Thus, agonists no longer have access to the receptors and tolerance is apparent. Receptor binding studies show the presence of fewer receptors. An interesting exception to the phenomenon of the apparent downregulation of receptors with the development of tolerance is seen with nicotine [5]. Chronic exposure to nicotine is associated with increased numbers of nicotinic binding sites. In this case, nicotine, while initially activating receptors, subsequently desensitizes receptors, functionally acting as an antagonist. The response to receptor antagonism is upregulation of receptors. 3) A third category of functional tolerance is the development of homeostatic feedback responses, as described below.

Homeostatic feedback is a well described mechanism of the development of tolerance to cardiovascular drugs. For example, with continuous infusion of sodium nitroprusside (or a number of other vasodilator drugs), tolerance develops to vasodilatory and hypotensive effects owing to the retention of sodium with the expansion of plasma volume, as well as sympathetic neural activation resulting in increased heart rate, myocardial contractility, cardiac output, and vasoconstriction [6]. The resultant increase in cardiac output and vascular resistance counteracts the hypotensive effects of the vasodilator. Understanding this mechanism of tolerance is important because other drugs can be used to prevent the development of tolerance. For example, diuretics can prevent volume expansion and sympathetic blocking drugs can prevent the effects of endogenous sympathetic activation.

NICOTINE AS A MODEL DRUG TO STUDY TOLERANCE

The pharmacology of nicotine is of interest because nicotine mediates tobacco use, a major cause of premature death and disability. Nicotine is also being developed as a medication, both to aid smoking cessation and potentially for the treatment of other diseases, such as ulcerative colitis [7].

Tolerance is well known to develop to the noxious actions of nicotine that are experienced when a person smokes their first cigarette, but rapidly dissipates or disappears if smoking continues. The development of tolerance is associated with the development of physical dependence to nicotine and, as such, contributes to addiction. Rapid development of tolerance explains in part why delivery by routes such as smoking, that result in rapid absorption, are maximally reinforcing because the high resultant arterial concentrations can overcome tolerance [8]. Finally, tolerance is a key safety issue in considering the use of nicotine medications in aiding smoking cessation as well as in the development of nicotine for use in harm reduction, both situations in which smokers may continue to smoke cigarettes while receiving nicotine medications.

A brief review of the clinical pharmacology of nicotine is necessary to understand the studies of tolerance described later. Nicotine acts on nicotinic cholinergic receptors located in the brain, in autonomic ganglia, in the adrenal, and at the neuromuscular junction [7]. Nicotine acts, at least in part, presynaptically, such that nicotinic cholinergic activation augments the release of various neurotransmitters in the brain, including dopamine, norepinephrine, epinephrine, serotonin, and acetylcholine. Release of various neurotransmitters is thought to modulate the psychological effects of nicotine. Nicotine also produces generalized sympathetic neural activation, increasing circulating catecholamine levels, increasing heart rate and blood pressure, increasing metabolic rate, and stimulating lipolysis.

Animal and human studies have demonstrated substantial development of tolerance to various effects of nicotine. In animals, the development of tolerance has been associated with increased numbers of nicotinic cholinergic binding sites, as mentioned previously [5]. Two types of tolerance — acute and chronic tolerance — develop to the actions of nicotine. Within seconds of exposure to nicotine, acute tolerance develops related to conformational changes in the nicotine receptor [9]. Thus, the nicotine receptor appears to exist in both activatable and inactivatable states, with an equilibrium between the two, that is influenced acutely by exposure to nicotine. With prolonged nicotine exposure, the number of nicotine receptors increases, related primarily to a decreased rate of nicotine receptor catabolism [10]. While these receptors bind nicotine with normal affinity *in vitro*, *in vivo* these receptors are not as responsive to nicotine because of conformational changes, as discussed above.

PSEUDOTOLERANCE

A common method of examining tolerance is the use of plasma concentration-effect curves, also called hysteresis curves [2]. If a particular pharmacologic effect occurs at the same blood concentration as levels of the drug increase and decrease, then a concentration-effect curve will be superimposable on the ascending and descending limbs of the concentration effect curve (Figure 1). If the effects are greater as blood levels are rising, and lower as concentrations are falling, the concentration-effect curve shows a different profile in the rising and falling phases producing a loop, also called hysteresis. Clockwise hysteresis has been interpreted as indicating the development of tolerance. Clockwise hysteresis has been observed for the venous plasma nicotine-heart rate accelerating effect curve during and after intravenous nicotine infusion [11]. Counterclockwise hysteresis may be interpreted as a lag between the appearance of nicotine in the blood stream and the observed effect. Counterclockwise hysteresis has been reported for the relationship between plasma procainamide concentration and electrocardiographic effect [12].

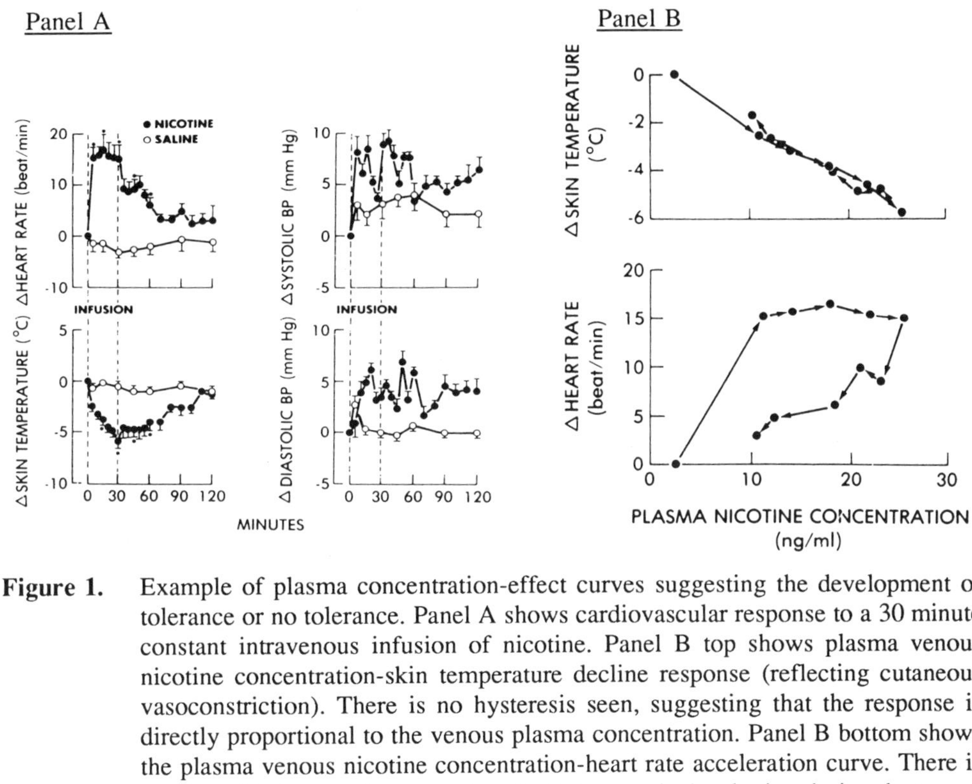

Figure 1. Example of plasma concentration-effect curves suggesting the development of tolerance or no tolerance. Panel A shows cardiovascular response to a 30 minute constant intravenous infusion of nicotine. Panel B top shows plasma venous nicotine concentration-skin temperature decline response (reflecting cutaneous vasoconstriction). There is no hysteresis seen, suggesting that the response is directly proportional to the venous plasma concentration. Panel B bottom shows the plasma venous nicotine concentration-heart rate acceleration curve. There is considerable hysteresis, suggesting that tolerance is developing during the course of drug exposure. Reprinted with permission from Benowitz *et al.* 1982 [11].

Clockwise hysteresis can also occur when the plasma concentration does not accurately reflect the concentration of drug at the receptor site, but rather the latter rises with a delay. This occurs when venous drug levels are used instead of arterial levels. With rapid dosing of a drug, arterial levels are higher and peak earlier than do venous levels. Nicotine, as well as many other drugs, exhibits significant arterial venous differences after rapid dosing, such as after smoking a cigarette, but even after a 30 minute intravenous infusion [13]. When arterial levels rather than venous levels are used in constructing a plasma concentration effect curve, no apparent tolerance was seen (Figure 2). The misinterpretation of the relationship between venous concentrations and effect as tolerance, has been termed dispositional tolerance [14].

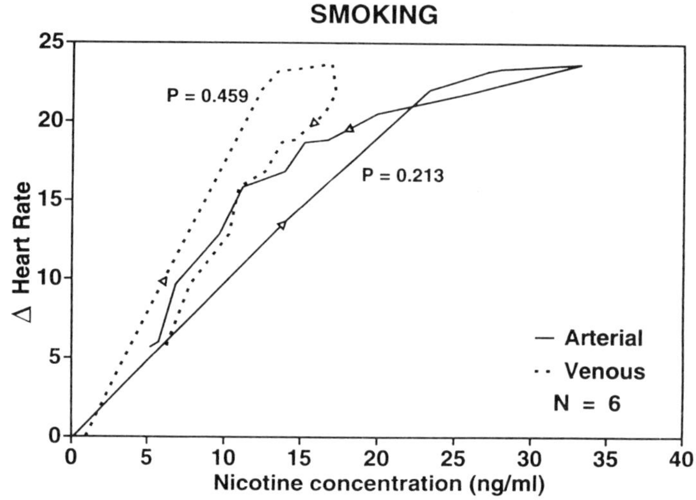

Figure 2. Illustration of dispositional tolerance. The figure shows mean arterial and venous heart rate response-concentration curves after smoking a cigarette. The dashed line representing venous plasma nicotine concentrations shows evidence of clockwise hysteresis, suggesting tolerance. However, the solid lines, indicating arterial plasma nicotine concentrations, show no evidence of hysteresis, indicating no evidence of tolerance. Reprinted with permission from Gourlay and Benowitz, 1997 [13].

EXPERIMENTAL PARADIGMS FOR STUDYING TOLERANCE

While it is difficult to define the extent of tolerance to the effects of a drug during the course of a single dose, owing to the problems of measuring arterial venous differences with rapid changes in drug levels, other dosing schemes can be used to assess tolerance. One approach is the use of repeated doses of a drug at varying intervals of time. When a second dose is administered in close temporal proximity to a previous dose, the extent of response will be lower due to the development of tolerance. If an adequate time is allowed between doses, tolerance will dissipate, resulting in a return of response of the challenge dose back to baseline. This approach has been used to examine the time course of development of tolerance to the effects of nicotine and caffeine (Figure 3) [15,16].

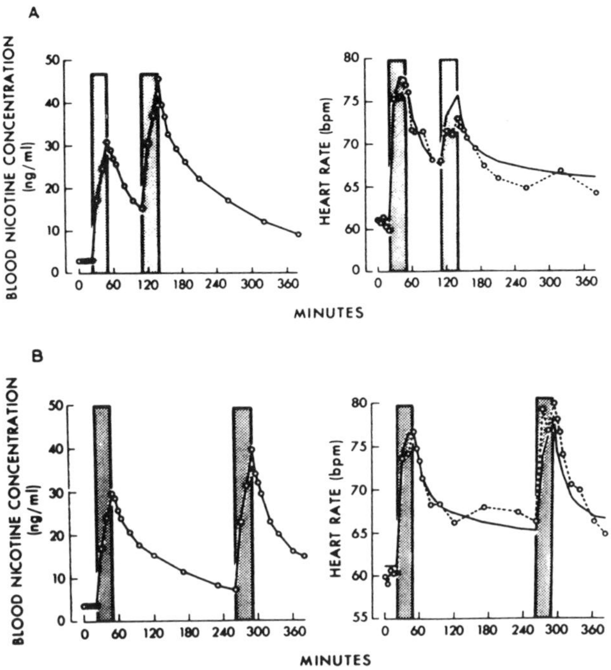

Figure 3. Mean blood concentrations of nicotine (Panel A) and the corresponding mean heart rate (Panel B) in eight subjects after two 30 minute intravenous infusions of nicotine separated by 60 minutes (A) or 210 minutes (B). The shadowed area indicates the period during which nicotine was infused. The solid line shows the fit of the model to the effect data. Reprinted with permission from Porchet *et al.*, 1988 [15].

Another approach is to infuse a drug to achieve and maintain a relatively constant plasma concentration over a prolonged period of time [17]. A decline of effects in a situation where blood concentrations are in steady state indicates the development of tolerance.

Both of these methods have been used to study the development of tolerance to the effects of nicotine, and have been used in constructing mathematical models for the pharmacodynamics of tolerance.

PHARMACOKINETIC-PHARMACODYNAMIC MODELS OF TOLERANCE

Several different types of pharmacokinetic-pharmacodynamic models have been proposed to characterize the pharmacodynamics of drug tolerance. All have the characteristics that the effects of the drug change over time. In the simplest model, the dependent variable is time (Figure 4). This model has been used to describe tolerance to heart rate acceleration following single doses of cocaine [18]. In this model, the drug effect declines over time, and this decline is determined by a mathematical construct called a "function generator". A limitation of this model is that there is no way for the model to adapt to different drug doses or different drug dosing schedules, or from prior exposure to the drug.

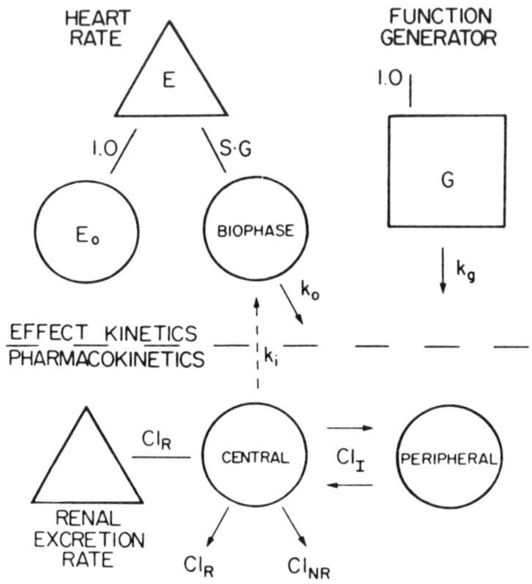

Figure 4. Pharmacokinetic-pharmacokinetic model used to model the development of tolerance to heart rate effects of cocaine. Tolerance is driven by time, via the function generator (G) that multiplicatively attenuates the function S that relates biophase cocaine concentration to effect. The function G has an initial value of 1.0 and an exponential decay rate, kg. E and E0 represent the observed and initial heart rate, respectively. The rate constants ki and k0 represent the relationship between cocaine concentration in the central compartment to that in the biophase compartment. Reprinted from Chow *et al.*, 1985 [18].

Another approach is where the drug concentration is the dependent variable that drives the development of tolerance. We have used such an approach in studying development of tolerance to the effects of nicotine and caffeine [15,16,17]. Others have used this type of model to study tolerance to morphine and furosemide [19,20]. In this case, the drug concentration drives tolerance either by postulating additive effect and tolerance functions, or by postulating the development of a response modifier equivalent to a competitive antagonist principle or metabolite (Figure 5). In the latter model, the hypothetical antagonistic metabolite is formed in proportion to the concentration of the drug in the central compartment, with elimination characterized by a particular rate constant that describes the rate of development and dissipation of tolerance. This type of model behaves such that the degree of tolerance increases as the concentration of the drug and the duration of the drug exposure increases. Such a model does not, however, predict withdrawal effects.

A third type of model is a more physiological model in which tolerance is driven by the effects of the drug. This type of model has been used to model tolerance to effects of alfentanil and nitroglycerin [21,22]. In this case, tolerance is modeled as occurring through the development of homeostatic responses or as a change in cellular mechanism of drug response (for example, a sequestration of receptors, change in second messenger systems, etc.) (Figure 6). These more physiological models have the potential to predict complete or partial tolerance, can incorporate differences in baseline physiological states (related, for example, to different levels of endogenous substances acting on the receptor system of interest) and can incorporate different mechanisms of tolerance development.

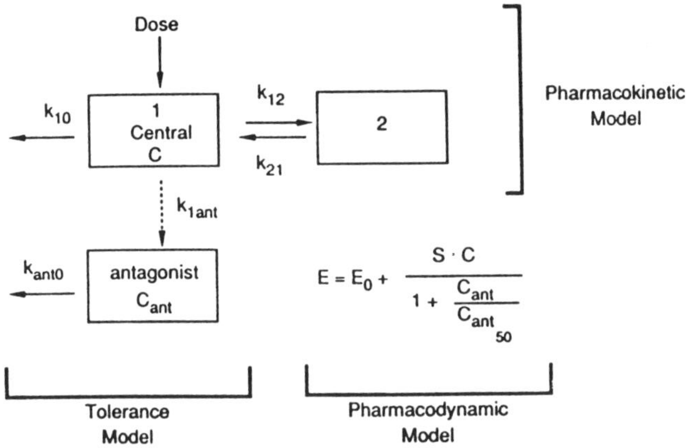

Figure 5. Inhibitory metabolite model of the pharmacokinetics and pharmacodynamics of nicotine tolerance. The k_{ij} are the intercompartmental and elimination rate constants, C is the concentration of the agonist, C_{ant} is the concentration of the hypothetical antagonist, S is the slope of the linear relationship between effect and concentration, E is the effect, and E0 is the baseline effect. Reprinted with permission from Porchet *et al.* [15].

STUDIES OF PHARMACODYNAMICS OF NICOTINE TOLERANCE

To illustrate the use of pharmacokinetic-pharmacodynamic models to study tolerance in humans, I will describe two studies from my laboratory on nicotine tolerance. The pharmacokinetic-pharmacodynamic model used is a drug concentration-driven "inhibitory metabolite" model, as previously described (Figure 4). In the first study, paired intravenous infusions of nicotine, separated by different intervals of time, were administered (Figure 3] [15]. Despite higher blood concentrations, heart rate acceleration and subjective effects were much less when a second infusion of nicotine was given at 60 or 120 minutes after the first infusion. With a 240 minute interval between infusions, however, the response was fully restored.

The pharmacodynamic parameters of most interest for characterizing tolerance are the half-life of development of tolerance and the concentration of drug at which 50% of the effect would have occurred compared to that which would have been seen without the development of tolerance (Cm50). Our study revealed a half-life of development and regression of tolerance to heart rate acceleration of 35 minutes. We found a Cm50 of 7.7 ng/ml, which implies that at a steady state concentration of 30 ng/ml, a typical concentration for a cigarette smoker, the response to another dose of nicotine would be attenuated to 20% of that which would have been seen without the development of tolerance. Tolerance is predicted not to be complete, which is what has been found in observational studies [23].

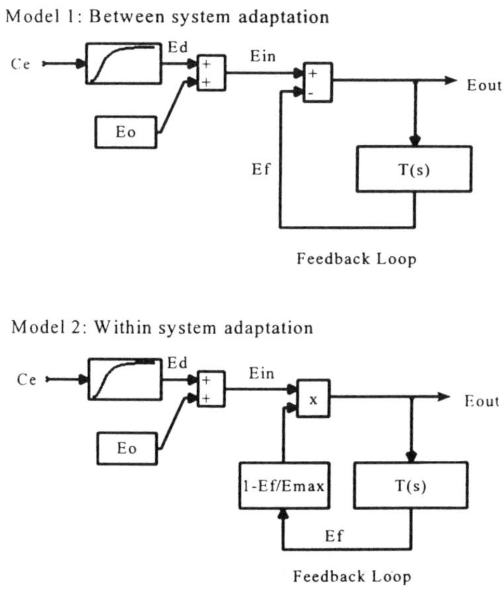

Figure 6. Tolerance models driven by pharmacologic effect. Model 1 illustrates between-system adaptation in which a pharmacologic effect elicits a compensatory or homeostatic effect that produces an action opposite to the initial drug effect, resulting in tolerance. Model 2 illustrates a within-system adaptation in which a pharmacologic effect triggers a regulatory response that changes one of the cellular components involved in producing the drug effect. Ce = effect site concentration; Ed = primary drug-induced effect; E0 = baseline effect caused by endogenous substances; Ein = sum of Ed and E0; Ef = opposing feedback response; T(s) = the transfer function that characterizes the regulatory mechanism; Emax = the maximum cellular regulatory response; Eout = net observed effect. Reprinted from Mandema and Wada, 1995 [21] .

A second study was performed using the same general pharmacokinetic-pharmacodynamic model. In this case, nicotine was infused rapidly to achieve a concentration of about 25 ng/ml, a level typical for smokers, followed by a computer controlled infusion to maintain this concentration for 180 minutes [17]. Tolerance to multiple nicotinic effects, including increases in heart rate, blood pressure, plasma epinephrine, and energy expenditure and free fatty acid concentrations were studied simultaneously. We found substantial differences in the rate and extent of development of tolerance to various responses. For heart rate acceleration, the half-life of tolerance development (22 minutes) and the Cm50 (8.9 ng/ml) were similar to that described in the first study. Rates of development of tolerance and Cm50 values for blood pressure and plasma epinephrine were reasonably similar to those seen for heart rate, consistent with the idea that these are all sympathetic neural responses. The concordance suggests that epinephrine may contribute to these other hemodynamic responses. In contrast to the heart rate and epinephrine responses, the effect of nicotine on energy expenditure showed extremely rapid and essentially complete tolerance within 30 minutes. The half-life of development of tolerance was estimated to be 3.5 minutes.

Table 1.
Pharmacodynamic model of tolerance: parameter estimates

$$E = E_0 + \frac{SC}{(1 + C_{ant}/C_{ant50})}$$

S = 1.31 bpm/ng per ml (12.8, C.V.%)

C_{ant50} = 7.72 ng/ml (18.8)

E_0 = 61.2 bpm (0.5)

$K_{ant0})$ = 0.0195 $\cdot$ min^{-1} (13.8)

$t1/2_{tolerance}$ = 35 min

E	=	effect
E_0	=	baseline effect
S	=	slope of linear relationship between effect and concentration
C	=	concentration of nicotine
C_{ant}	=	concentration of the hypothetical antagonist
C_{ant50}	=	concentration of the hypothetical antagonist that results in loss of 50% of the maximal effect due to tolerance
K_{ant0}	=	first order rate of appearance or disappearance of tolerance

* C.V.% = coefficient of variation

Of considerable mechanistic interest is that the free fatty acid response to nicotine did not demonstrate tolerance. Nicotine releases free fatty acids from triglycerides and adipose tissue, presumably via an adrenergic mechanism. Free fatty acids are rapidly cleared from the plasma, so in general free fatty acid levels reflect the release rate, and therefore would be a marker of nicotine-mediated lipolysis. The discordance between the pharmacodynamics of nicotine action on adipose tissue, that is, lipolysis, and that on epinephrine concentration suggests that epinephrine is not responsible for lipolysis. The discordance between nicotine effect on lipolysis and energy expenditure (metabolic rate) suggests that lipolysis with futile cycling of free fatty acids (proposed as a mechanism for adrenergically-mediated increases in energy expenditure) is not the mechanism for the nicotine action to increase metabolic rate.

The difference in rate and extent of development of tolerance to various nicotine responses may reflect nicotine acting on different nicotinic receptor subtypes, which have been reported to exhibit different rates of desensitization *in vitro*, and/or to different homeostatic responses [24].

IMPLICATIONS OF TOLERANCE

For drugs in general, findings of the development of tolerance have implications for the level or frequency of drug dosing. For example, narcotic analgesics need to be dosed at higher levels and either at greater frequency or using sustained release preparations in patients with chronic pain. For cardiac nitrates, continuous dosing with transdermal nitroglycerin is generally avoided [25]. Rather, intermittent doses of oral isosorbide dinitrate or isosorbide mononitrate, or the use of transdermal nicotine for only part of the day, leaving time to regain sensitivity, have become common practices. As mentioned previously, homeostatic tolerance to hypotensive effects of direct vasodilator drugs can be avoided by concomitantly administering diuretics and adrenergic blocking drugs.

Implications for the development of tolerance to nicotine provides other insights into the biological importance of tolerance. The development of tolerance to the noxious effects of nicotine exposure from smoking the first few cigarettes is essential for the continuation of smoking behavior. Without the development of tolerance to noxious effects, no one would smoke and there would be no smoking-related disease. As described previously, tolerance is linked to the development of physical dependence, which contributes to addiction. The temporal aspects of tolerance are likely to influence when a smoker smokes his or her next cigarette. Smoking cigarettes too closely together in time makes no sense when there is still a high degree of tolerance to the rewarding effects of the cigarette. Presumably, the smoker learns an optimal time to smoke the next cigarette when he or she can experience rewarding effects without a high level of residual tolerance, but also before he or she becomes uncomfortable due to withdrawal symptoms that occur when the intercigarette interval is too long. The use of the cigarette as a drug delivery system makes sense because rapid delivery of nicotine to the brain allows the effect to occur before there is time for the development of tolerance. In addition, smoking delivers transient high levels of nicotine to the brain which can overcome prior levels of central nervous system tolerance. Finally, the development of tolerance to cardiovascular responses to nicotine has implications for nicotine use as a medication. High levels of nicotine, such as those seen when one uses nicotine medication and smokes at the same time, is predicted not to produce greater cardiovascular toxicity [15]. This has been confirmed empirically in studies of cigarette smoking combined with intravenous nicotine or high doses of transdermal nicotine [26,27]. Tolerance to the toxic cardiovascular effects of nicotine makes it feasible to use nicotine as a potential harm reduction strategy, that is, using nicotine to decrease the level of cigarette smoking in people who are unable to quit.

CONCLUSION

Tolerance develops to the effects of many drugs, particularly psychoactive, analgesic, and cardiovascular drugs. The development of tolerance to drug action is an important consideration in optimizing medical therapy, both with respect to drug dosing and to toxicity. The development of tolerance can be quantitatively characterized in humans using pharmacokinetic-pharmacodynamic models, several of which have been discussed. Such quantitative studies may be useful in the design of medication regimens for patients who are likely to develop tolerance. Studies of tolerance may also provide mechanistic information on drug action and may provide clues to modifying the development of tolerance.

ACKNOWLEDGEMENTS: I wish to thank Ms. Kaye Welch for her editorial assistance in preparing the manuscript.

REFERENCES

1. Colpaert FC. Drug discrimination: No evidence for tolerance to opiates. Pharmacol Rev 1995;47:605-629.
2. Holford NHG, Sheiner LB. Understanding the dose-effect relationship: Clinical application of pharmacokinetic-pharmacodynamic models. Clin Pharmacokinetics 1981;6:429-453.
3. Kalant H, LeBlanc AE, Gibbins RJ. Tolerance to, and dependence on, some non-opiate psychotropic drugs. Pharmacol Rev 1971;23:135-191.
4. Insel PA. Adrenergic receptors - Evolving concepts and clinical implications. N Engl J Med 1996;334:580-585.
5. Marks MJ, Burch JB, Collins AC. Effects of chronic nicotine infusion on tolerance development and nicotinic receptors. J Pharmacol Exp Ther 1983;226:817-825.
6. Packer M, Meller J, Medina N, Yushak M, Gorlin R. Determinants of drug response in severe chronic heart failure. 1. Activation of vasoconstrictor forces during vasodilator therapy. Circulation 1981;64:506-514.
7. Benowitz NL. Pharmacology of nicotine: Addiction and therapeutics. Annu Rev Pharmacol Toxicol 1996;36:597-613.
8. Benowitz NL, Porchet H, Jacob P, III. Nicotine dependence and tolerance in man: pharmacokinetic and pharmacodynamic investigations. In: Nordberg A, Fuxe K, Holmstedt B, Sundwell A, (eds.) Progress in Brain Research, Vol. 79. Amsterdam: Elsevier Science Publishers, 1989;279-287.
9. Lena C, Changeux J-P. Allosteric modulations of the nicotinic acetylcholine receptor. Trends Neurosci 1993;16:181-186.
10. Madhok TC, Beyer HS, Sharp BM. Protein kinase A regulates nicotinic cholinergic receptors and subunit messenger ribonucleic acids in PC 12 cells. Endocrinology 1994;134:91-96.
11. Benowitz NL, Jacob P, III, Jones RT, Rosenberg J. Interindividual variability in the metabolism and cardiovascular effects of nicotine in man. J Pharmacol Exp Ther 1982;221:368-372.

12. Galeazzi RL, Benet LZ, Sheiner LB. Relationship between the pharmacokinetics and pharmacodynamics of procainamide. Clin Pharmacol Ther 1976;20:278-289.
13. Gourlay SG, Benowitz NL. Arteriovenous differences in plasma concentration of nicotine and catecholamines and related cardiovascular effects after smoking, nicotine nasal spray, and intravenous nicotine. Clin Pharmacol Ther 1997;62:453-463.
14. Porchet HC, Benowitz NL, Sheiner LB, Copeland JR. Apparent tolerance to the acute effect of nicotine results in part from distribution kinetics. J Clin Invest 1987;80:1466-1471.
15. Porchet HC, Benowitz NL, Sheiner LB. Pharmacodynamic model of tolerance: Application to nicotine. J Pharmacol Exp Ther 1988;244:231-236.
16. Shi J, Benowitz NL, Denaro CP, Sheiner LB. Pharmacokinetic-pharmacodynamic modeling of caffeine: Tolerance to pressor effects. Clin Pharmacol Ther 1993;53:6-14.
17. Fattinger K, Verotta D, Benowitz NL. Pharmacodynamics of acute tolerance to multiple nicotinic effects in humans. J Pharmacol Exp Ther 1997;281:1238-1246.
18. Chow MJ, Ambre JJ, Ruo TI, Atkinson AJ, Bowsher DJ, Fischman MW. Kinetics of cocaine distribution, elimination, and chronotropic effects. Clin Pharmacol Ther 1985;38:318-324.
19. Gardmark M, Ekblom M, Bouw R, Hammarlund-Udenaes M. Quantification of effect delay and acute tolerance development to morphine in the rat. J Pharmacol Exp Ther 1993;267:1061-1067.
20. Wakelkamp M, Alvan G, Gabrielsson J, Paintaud G. Pharmacodynamic modeling of furosemide tolerance after multiple intravenous administration. Clin Pharmacol Ther 1996;60:75-88.
21. Mandema JW, Wada RD. Pharmacodynamic model for acute tolerance development to the electroencephalographic effects of alfentanil in the rat. J Pharmacol Exp Ther 1995;275:1185-1194.
22. Bauer JA, Fung H-L. Pharmacodynamic models of nitroglycerin-induced hemodynamic tolerance in experimental heart failure. Pharmaceut Res 1994;11:816-823.
23. Benowitz NL, Kuyt F, Jacob P, III. Influence of nicotine on cardiovascular and hormonal effects of cigarette smoking. Clin Pharmacol Ther 1984;36:74-81.
24. Olale F, Gerzanich V, Kuryatov A, Wang F, Lindstrom J. Chronic nicotine exposure differentially affects the function of human α3, α4, and α7 neuronal nicotinic receptor subtypes. J Pharmacol Exp Ther 1997;283:675-683.
25. Parker JO, Amies MH, Hawkinson RW, Heilman JM, Hougham AJ, Vollmer MC, Wilson RR. Intermittent transdermal nitroglycerin therapy in angina pectoris. Circulation 1995;91:1368-1374.
26. Benowitz NL, Jacob P, III. Intravenous nicotine replacement suppresses nicotine intake from cigarette smoking. J Pharmacol Exp Ther 1990;254:1000-1005.
27. Zevin S, Jacob P, III, Benowitz NL. Dose-related cardiovascular and endocrine effects of transdermal nicotine. Clin Pharmacol Ther 1998;64:87-95.

Discussion: Tolerance as a modulator of drug response

M. Lader:
Some of the phenomena you have presented on nicotine studies could be very similar for benzodiazepines. For example, tolerance phenomena are observed quite quickly after an overdose of benzodiazepines. There is also evidence for the benzodiazepine receptors, that with continual use, different subunits are synthesised, and the sensitivity of the receptor changes. Do you think this has something to do with the type of the receptor, as a generic property of these trans-membranal receptors, or do you think it is specific for individual drugs?

N.L. Benowitz:
I do not know enough about the benzodiazepine receptor to answer that question.

U. Klotz:
Concerning the benzodiazepine receptors, many years ago there were several animal experiments, some of them in monkeys, where they could reset the receptors with the antagonist flumazenil. It was thought that the receptors could be reset to their original naive state by giving every second day an antagonist. Do you know if something similar has been tried later on with other drugs or receptors?

N.L. Benowitz:
It certainly has been done with opiates. There are people who have either been opiate addicts or have been chronically taking opiates in large amounts who have been brought into hospital, put under anaesthesia and given naloxone in high concentrations to resensitise them or to allow them to start on long-term opiate antagonists for therapy for opiate addiction. I do not know if flumazenil has been used in a similar manner for benzodiazepine dependence problems.

M. Lader:
There have been two studies. I did a pilot study which was successful in about 50% of cases. It was followed up in Sweden with a properly controlled study, which suggested that there was some benefit. Those patients who had persistent benzodiazepine withdrawal syndrome apparently continued after the acute withdrawal, and they seemed to benefit from this resetting. But the data are fragmentary and further studies are needed on this issue. The other thing you mentioned was rapid detoxification. This involves all sorts of commercial issues because people tried to patent it. There are also attempts now to do the same paradigm with the benzodiazepines as well, and I think that is much more dangerous. If you give an antagonist to an opioid user, you will get a reaction, but you will not get a potentially fatal one as could happen if flumazenil is given to someone who has been on high doses of benzodiazepines.

L. Aarons:
Although you describe them as mechanistic models, the antimetabolite model is essentially an empirical model. Could you comment on the use of empirical models for the management

or the interpretation of tolerance data, particularly if you move out of nicotine into some therapeutic area? Is it possible that you will take an incorrect decision if you do not know the full mechanistic basis of tolerance?

N.L. Benowitz:
Ours was equivalent to a receptor model. We were interested in using this model to study tolerance in individual subjects but this was not done because of the wide within subject variability in the response. One can model tolerance in an individual and can examine if the model can predict a perturbation in the system. A physiological model cannot be used for some of these responses. If you know there is a homeostatic response, for example, a compensatory vasoconstriction response to a vasodilator, one can develop a physiological (homeostatic) model. It is harder to test for some of the receptor models, because you do not know enough about the kinetics of drug-receptor interactions or the mechanism by which tolerance develops.

P. du Souich:
It should be taken into account that tolerance is not always bad, because sometimes we can induce tolerance to avoid an adverse effect. In the case of benzodiazepines, alprazolam for example, a slow release formulation can be used to decrease the sedative effect. On the other hand, we are all aware of the huge doses of morphine we need to administer to people with burns or in other painful situations. It was proposed that the presence of the 3-glucuronide metabolite could play a role in this tolerance. Do you know anything else about this morphine problem?

N.L. Benowitz:
I do not know about morphine with respect to tolerance. Certainly morphine-6-glucuronide has been thought to play a role in terms of persistence of opiate effects over time, effects such as unexpected respiratory depression occurring during long-term morphine exposure, even when morphine levels are constant. It has been suggested that morphine-glucuronide has a pharmacological role, but I am not aware of its contribution to tolerance.

P. du Souich:
The tolerance I mentioned must be a pharmacokinetic tolerance, because the 3-glucuronide metabolite of morphine is a much weaker agonist or even an antagonist.

Variability in human drug response. Age as a source of variability

Mark T. Kinirons

Clinical Age Research Unit, Guy's, King's & St Thomas' School of Medicine, Dentistry & Biomedical Science, London, United Kingdom.

ABSTRACT

Changes in liver size and volume, organ blood flow, enzyme activity and function, kidney function, receptor function, sensitivity, coupling mechanisms and second messenger responsiveness have all been elucidated and shown to influence responsiveness to ageing.

Phenotypic differences in drug handling were explained by genetic variations in drug metabolising enzymes such as the cytochrome P450 system (CYP). Using phenotypic probes for CYP2D6, CYP2C9 and CYP3A4 did not demonstrate any age related difference, yet CYP 2E1 has been shown to vary with age.

Recently, we have examined the impact of age and phenotype on CYP2D6 using propranolol as a model substrate. This showed a 55% decline in clearance of the propranolol in elderly PMs when compared to young EMs. This highlights the importance of the environment on differences in drug response.

More recently, frailty has been put forward to link the 'functional phenotype' with the 'physio-pharmacological phenotype'. Significant reduction in drug metabolism in frail elderly and not in well elderly has been noted. This separation based on function needs further research. Other areas include interaction studies to clarify the impact of genetics on drug response to such components as induction, inhibition and organ related age changes in CYP function.

Key words: age, pharmacokinetics, pharmacodynamics, variability, elderly.

Correspondence: Dr. M.T. Kinirons, Clinical Age Research Unit, GKT, Bessemer Road, London SE5 9RS, U.K., Tel: +44-171-346-3420, Fax: +44-171-346-3441

Funding acknowledgement: National Health Service

INTRODUCTION & HISTORY

This paper will summarise briefly the principle findings in relation to age as a co-variable in drug responsiveness. A detailed description is beyond the remit of this manuscript. The review will focus on both pharmacokinetic and pharmacodynamic aspects of human pharmacology.

PHARMACOKINETICS

There are no consistent clinically meaningful changes in relation to age in drug absorption. This is principally because of the enormous surface are for absorption overwhelms any changes (decline) in the ability of the small intestine to absorb drugs. Changes in gastric acid production for the large part do not impinge on drug absorption. Less is known of ageing and alternative routes of drug absorption such as skin and d nose.

DISTRIBUTION AND HALF LIFE

On of the earliest human studies on ageing was from the Dundee group. O'Malley and colleagues published a study of half-lives between young and elderly [1]. This showed a significant trend in half-life with age for antipyrine.

Half-life is directly related to volume of distribution and inversely related to clearance.

Volume of distribution increases with lipophilic drugs with advancing years. This understanding explained in part the pronounced effects of benzodiazepines with age due to increased half-life [2]. As half life was dependent on Vd, subsequent work shifted the emphasis from half-life to clearance of drug [3].

CLEARANCE

Clearance, (litre/min) is a measure of the efficiency of an organ (or organism) to irreversibly remove a drug from the perfusate [3]. Systemic clearance is independent of drug. The liver is the main metabolising organ in the body. Hepatic clearance is dependent the ability of the liver to extract the drug from the blood and the amount of blood delivering drug to the liver, (LBF). This can be expressed accordingly.

$$Cl_{hepatic} = \frac{Q\,[Ca - Cv]}{[Ca]} = QE$$

E	=	steady state extraction ratio
Q	=	liver blood flow
Ca	=	concentration of drug in portal vein and hepatic artery
Cv	=	concentration of drug in vein leaving liver in hepatic vein
$Cl_{hepatic}$	=	clearance by the liver

Clearance is therefore dependent on two physiological parameters: LBF and the extraction ratio (E). E is dependent on the hepatic metabolic enzyme capacity otherwise known as intrinsic clearance (Phase 1 and/or phase 2 enzymes). Standard pharmacokinetic studies can determine E for an individual drug. Drugs can be classified into three groups by their E into high 0.7, low 0.3 or intermediate 0.3 - 0.7.

LIVER SIZE AND BLOOD FLOW AND AGE

Liver volume declines by approximately 30 % [4,5] in the over 65 yr. LBF falls by 20% - 35% in healthy elderly compared to young [5,6,7]. As LBF is important in high E drugs such as propranolol, triazolam, and chlormethiazole predictable decline in hepatic clearance occurs.

INTRINSIC CLEARANCE AND AGE

Intrinsic clearance of a drug is a measure of the clearing organ to remove that particular drug. It is estimated by E. It is independent of blood flow [3]. Reduction in intrinsic clearance will produce significant changes in the clearance of low extraction drugs. This can be illustrated by equations below.

$$QE = \frac{Q \times Cl\ intrinsic}{Q + Cl\ intrinsic}$$

$$Cl_{intrinsic} = QE/1 - E$$

$Cl_{intrinsic}$ = intrinsic clearance of drug by the liver

Antipyrine is an example of a low extraction drug. Age related decline of 19% in the clearance of antipyrine has been reported [7]. This was due to reduction in intrinsic capacity. Therefore, low E drugs might be predicated to have reduced hepatic clearance. However, hepatic extraction does not translate into systemic clearance decline. Further the increasing complexity of the CYPs has raised the possibility of selective decline on one pathway can be compensated by metabolism down an alternate pathway. As such the role of alternate pathways needs to be considered.

CYPs AND AGE

In human metabolism there are six subfamilies responsible for most of human drug metabolism. These are CYP 1A, 2A, 2C, 2D, 2E and 3A. Of the range of subfamilies known, CYP1A1, CYP1A2, CYP2C9 & 19, CYP2D6, CYP2E1, CYP3A4 & 5 are the most important in terms of drug metabolism. The effect age has on the functional activity of the various CYPs has been an area of intense research since the 1970s [6,7]. Studies of *in vitro* enzyme levels (accepting the problems of sampling) have not documented a decline in CYP enzyme function and amount with age [8]. *In vivo* estimations are more problematic and surrogate markers such as plasma aspirin esterase activity has been used to suggest that there is no difference *in vivo* between the elderly compared to the young [9,10]. *In vivo* probes have documented a decline the dapsone recovery ratio in contrast to debrisoquine ratio for CYP2D6 and mephenytoin ratio for CYP2C9 [11]. Initially, dapsone was attributed to CYP3A4 but more latterly has been reassigned to CYP2E1 [12]. This data would therefore support a selective decline in CYP activity with age.

PHASE II REACTIONS AND AGE

There have been few studies examining age effects on conjugation because of the complex metabolism of many drugs. Nonetheless there are drugs exclusively metabolised by phase 2 reactions and these include lorazepam, oxazepam and paracetamol.

Studies with lorazepam did not find any significant reduction in the clearance of lorazepam with age following intravenous administration. [13]. Studies suggest that there is no age related decline in total clearance with oxazepam [2]. Yet a recent study of well elderly patients (80-94 yr.) noted a decline in unbound clearance compared to young. This was said to explain a pharmacodynamic difference in finger tapping between both groups [14].

Paracetamol conjugation is reduced in the elderly [15]. Similar data exists for the conjugation of metoclopramide in frail elderly but not healthy elderly. This difference persisted on correction for reduction in liver volume [16].

CYPs POLYMORPHISMS AND AGE

In a recent study, we examined the effect of age on both CYP2D6 and non-CYP2D6 pathways of propranolol's metabolism. Non-CYP2D6 pathways included conjugation of propranolol to its glucuronidated metabolite. We were unable to find any selective loss in capacity of either pathway when comparing young to elderly (65 - 81 yr.). However, the reduction in clearance of total propranolol in older patients who are deficient in CY2D6 pathway was greater than 50% compared to young subjects with functioning CYP2D6 (Kinirons *et al.* submitted). This indicates that elderly subjects who are deficient on CYP2D6 are at considerably greater risk of a drug related adverse effect because of increased demand on alternate pathways. This potential is further increased when the known changes in LBF and liver size further diminish the reserve in patients on chronic dosing of drugs metabolised by CYP2D6. All the elderly subjects studied in the above protocol where well healthy subjects.

There have been some interesting studies in frail elderly, a more clinically appropriate population to consider. Induction and inhibition in response to age is an area that needs to be re-examined in the light of our current understanding of the complexity of enzymes involved in drug metabolism.

ENZYME CHARACTERISTICS AND AGE

Based on only a small amount of data examining a few enzymes, no decline in Km and Vmax has been noted. In particular studies of the plasma esterase activity in the elderly has shown no difference compared to the young [10].

FRAILTY

Frailty has been defined as "persons over 65 yr., dependent on others for activities of daily living" [17]. Formal pharmacological studies on frail elderly have reported reductions in the metabolic activity of plasma aspirin esterase [9,10,18] and paracetamol conjugation [15] and in the metabolism of metoclopramide [16]. Studies with theophylline have documented increased variability in frail compared to healthy elderly [19]. These studies all emphasise the concept of frailty over age as a determinant of drug disposition and response.

Explanations for frailty might include greater reduction in liver volumes and /or blood flow compared to well elderly. This is supported by some studies. For example, Swift noted a decline in liver volume between well elderly and hospitalised elderly (990 ± 166 ml vs. 838 ± 242 ml) [4]. However, as mentioned above, correction for liver volume did not remove differences in phase 2 metabolism of metoclopramidde. There are no specific studies compared subjects with frail patients for liver blood flow.

ENZYME MODULATION AND AGE

Enzyme modulation is discussed in more detail by other speakers at the symposium and elsewhere [20]. Nonetheless, a few general points can be made.

The original studies on induction determined the inducibility of drug metabolising enzymes for antipyrine and propranolol's metabolism. This suggested that there was loss of inducibility with age [7,20,21]. By contrast, plasma esterase inducibility is not affected by age [22]. This would be consistent with differential selective inducibility with various enzymes based on our increased understanding of the complexity of CYPs.

Of note is the emerging data about the effects of diet on aspects of drug metabolism, induction and inhibition. An interesting report has reported significant inhibition of drug metabolism following changes in diet [23].

PHARMACODYNAMICS

Effects of ageing on the above are much less clearly defined. This is because of the problems in what to measure and what model to study. Frequently, altered drug pharmacodynamics are explained by some of the effects of ageing on pharmacokinetics. It is frequently difficult to disentangle one from the other. Further, one is not sure whether any reported changes are due to ageing or related to age-disease pathophysiology. Much of the data collected from animal models may not be applicable to humans. The main areas are in cardiovascular and in central nervous system pharmacology. I will therefore concentrate on this area for the remainder of this paper.

BETA RECEPTOR FUNCTION AND AGEING

The lymphocyte contains beta-receptors. This cell is accessible and therefore has been studied extensively. Initially, it was thought that numbers of receptors were lower in the elderly than the young and that this was the explanation for the [24]. However, more recent studies have not confirmed this [25]. The well-known decline in responsiveness with age is now felt to be due to decline in coupling with rather than a decline in maximal receptor activity. Because of the surplus capacity of the receptor-substrate coupling there is no discernible decline in maximal receptor activity with age. However, decreases in numbers may lead to a diminished response. This is may be termed redundancy in the signal amplification pathway. These findings demonstrate the difficulty in interpreting the pharmacodynamic data.

VASCULAR RESPONSIVENESS AND AGEING

More recently, studies have looked at ageing and the forearm vascular bed [26]. Various groups have either studied the hand vein or using phlethysmographic techniques in association with brachial artery infusions [27]. The data suggests that there is reduced responsiveness to beta agonists as estimated by changes in blood flow [28,29] consistent with the receptor data. More recent data from our unit has suggested in contrast, that there is impaired nitric oxide mediated vasodilatation with ageing. Further, ageing *per se*, was associated with reduced basal urinary nitrate excretion even when corrected for creatine clearance [30]. These finding mirror the findings of reduced acetylcholine-mediated vasodilation [31]. In regard to nitric oxide, changes in forearm responsiveness are reversible in disease states such as treated hypertension [27].

CONCLUSIONS

Ageing and understanding its effect on drug response is crucial to society. With the ageing of the population, the potential for future pharmacological problems will increase. This will most likely be seen in increased admissions to acute hospitals with drug related problems or in more serious and dramatic effects such as has been seen with terfenadine. Therefore, the need to pursue more aggressively the underlying aspects that distinguish the well young from the sick older person and to apply this understanding to improve selectivity and specificity of drugs is a challenge we must continue to pursue.

REFERENCES

1. O'Malley K, Crooks J, Duke *et al.* Effect of age and sex on human drug disposition. Br Med J 1971;3:607-609.
2. Greenblatt DJ, Harmatz JS, Shader RI. Clinical pharmacokinetics of anxiolytics and hypnotics in the elderly. Clin Pharmacokinet 1991;21:165-177.
3. Wilkinson GR, Shand D. A physiological approach to hepatic drug clearance. Clin Pharmacol Ther 1975;18:377-390.
4. Swift CG, Homeida M, Halliwell M, Roberts CJC. Antipyrine disposition and liver size in the elderly. Eur J Clin Pharmacol 1978;14:149-152.

5. Wynne H, Cope H, Mutch E, Rawlins M, Woodhouse K, James OF. The effect of age on liver volume and apparent liver blood flow in healthy man. Hepatology 1989;9:297-301.
6. Wood AJJ, Vestal RE, Wilkinson GR, Branch RA, Shand DG. Effect of ageing and cigarette smoking on antipyrine and iodocyanine green elimination. Clin Pharmacol Ther 1979;26:16-20.
7. Vestal RE, Wood AJJ, Branch RA, Shand DG, Wilkinson GR. Effects of age and cigarette smoking on propranolol disposition. Clin Pharmacol Ther 1979;26:8-15.
8. Schmucker DL, Woodhouse K, Wang R *et al.* Effects of age and gender on *in vitro* properties of human liver microsomal monooxygenases. Clin Pharmacol Ther 1991;48:365-374.
9. Yelland C, Summerbell J, Nicholson E, Herd B, Wynne H, Woodhouse KW. The association of age with aspirin esterase activity in human liver. Age and Ageing 1991;20:16-18.
10. William FM, Wynne H, Woodhouse KW, Rawlins MD. Plasma aspirin esterase: the influence of age and frailty. Age and Ageing 1989;18:39-42.
11. May G, Potter J, Wilkinson GR. Frequency distribution of dapsone n-hydroxylase: a putative probe for CYP3A4 activity in a Caucasian population. Clin Pharmacol Ther 1994;55:492-500.
12. Karesch J, Thummel K, *et al.* Cytochrome P450 2E1 is responsible for the metabolism of dapsone. Clin Pharmacol Ther 1996;59:231-237.
13. Krauss J, Desmond O, Marshall *et al.* effects of ageing and liver disease on disposition of lorazepam. Clin Pharmacol Ther 1978;24:411-419.
14. Sonne J, Sloft S, Dossing M, Boesgaard S, Andereasen F. Single dose pharmacokinetics in the very elderly institutionalised subjects. Br J Clin Phamacol 1991;31:719-722.
15. Wynne H, Cope LH, Herd MD, James OF, Woodhouse KW. The association of age and frailty with paracetamol conjugation in man. Age and Ageing 1990;19:419-424.
16. Wynne H, Yelland C, Cope LH, Boddy A, Woodhouse KW, Bateman DN. The association of age and frailty in the pharmacokinetics and pharmacodynamics of metoclopramide. Age and Ageing 1993;22:354-359.
17. Woodhouse KW, Wynne H, Baillie H *et al.* Who are the frail elderly? Q J Med 1988;68:505-506.18
18. Summerbell J, Yelland C, Woodhouse K. The kinetics of plasma aspirin esterase in relation to old age. Age & Ageing 1990;19:128-130.
19. Groen H, Horan MA, Roberts NA, Gulaki RS, Milijkovic B, Jansen EJ. The relationship between phenazone (antipyrine) metabolite formation and theophylline metabolism in healthy and frail elderly women. Clin Pharmacokinetics 1993;25;36-144.
20. Vestal RE, Norris AH, Tobin JD, Cohen BH, Shock NW, Andres R. Antipyrine metabolism in man: influence of age, alcohol, caffeine and smoking. Clin Pharmacol Ther 1975;18:425-432.
21. Twum-barina Y, Finnegan T, Habash AI, Cape RD, Carruthers SG. Impaired enzyme induction by rifampicin in the elderly. Br J Clin Pharmacol 1984;17:595-597.
22. George G, Wynne H, Woodhouse K. The association of age with the induction of drug metabolising enzymes in human monocytes. Age & Ageing 1990;19:364-367.
23. Walter-Sack I, Klotz U. Influence of diet and nutritional status on drug metabolism. Clin Pharmacokinet 1996;31:47-64.

24. Dillon N, Chung S, Kelly J, O'Malley K. Age and beta adrenoceptor-mediated function. Clin Pharmacol Ther 1980;27:769-772.
25. Kilfeather S, Collins D, McCormack P, Cotter T, O'Malley K. The effect of *in vitro* ageing on human receptor density, coupling and response. Mech Aging Dev 1992;63:247-256.
26. Martin SA, Alxiera S, Carruthers SG. The influence of age on dorsal hand vein responsiveness to norepinephrine. Clin Pharmacol Ther 1986;40:257-260.
27. Lyons D, Webster J, Benjamin N. The effect of antihypertensive therapy on local intra-arterial N-monomethyl-l-arginine in patients with essential hypertension. J Hypertens 1994;12:1047-1052.
28. Ford G, Dachmann WD, Blaschke TF, Hoffman BB. Effect of ageing on beta 2 mediated uptake of potassium phosphate, free fatty acids and glycerol in human forearms. Am J Physiol 1994;266:E659-665.
29. Ford G, James OFW. Autonomic blockade in healthy young, healthy and endurance trained elderly persons: haemodynamic responses and effect on cardiac beta receptor responsiveness Cli Sci 1994;87:297-302.
30. Lyons D, Roy S, Patel M, Benjamin N, Swift CG. Impaired nitric oxide mediated vasodilatation and total body nitric oxide production in healthy old. Cli Sci 1997;93:519-525.
31. Taddei S, Viridis A, Mattei P *et al.* Ageing and endothelial function in normotensive subjects and essential hypertensive patients. Circulation 1995;91:1981-1987.

<u>Discussion</u>: Variability in human drug response: age as a source of variability

P. Rolan:

In the Vanderbilt's University paper (May G *et al.*, Clin Pharmacol Ther, 1994) you have shown a reduced dapsone clearance, were people of both genders included in the results stratified by gender?

M . Kinirons:

Yes, both genders. I think there was an about 40-60% split in gender distribution. A relationship with age was present in both genders.

L Aarons:

You have shown that the trends of physiologic variables with age are not linear, because they remain constant up until a certain age and then they drop off. Nevertheless, all the relationships which you showed and which are ubiquitous in the literature, show linear relationships of clearance, volume of distribution, etc., with age. Firstly, I would just like to get your comment on that. And secondly, did you measure protein-binding in your propranolol study?

M. Kinirons:

It is very hard to explain that discrepancy. I only can mention the existence of an increasing loss in liver mass and decline in liver volume with age. Arbitrarily, people have chosen 65 years as older, but perhaps if there were more detailed longitudinal studies, you would find much greater variability. About your second question, we measured protein-binding and there was no difference.

M.M. Reidenberg:

Firstly, I think that your exploration of the idea of frailty versus chronologic age is important, and I hope you will expand on that a little bit. Secondly, I would point out that virtually all of the studies in this field are cross-sectional studies, looking once at each person and then stratifying by age. The only longitudinal studies I am aware of are from the Baltimore Longitudinal Study of Aging in renal function (Lindeman RD *et al.*, J Am Geriat Soc, 1985). Here it is very clear that some people have virtually no decline in renal function as they get older, where other people have a slow and still others, a more rapid decline. So, when you look at a cross-sectional study, it appears as if people have a decline in renal function as they age. But in fact, some do and some do not. Clinically we can see people of the same age, and some obviously are frail and these are the ones who have trouble therapeutically. Has your thinking gone farther in coming up with criteria for defining frailty, in terms of research studies?

M. Kinirons:

No, I am afraid not. We are currently trying to look at those people who get admitted to hospital with drug-related adverse reactions and trying to equate with frailty, just to see if this concept persist in a different selected population. It has not caught on, so people have not taken up the idea put forward by Ken Woodhouse to try and translate from socio-functional definition to a physiological definition. I have only tried to put forward some suggestions that there are links, because obviously changes in liver blood flow and liver mass cannot fully explain frailty.

G.T. Tucker:

You mentioned some work on debrisoquine suggesting that CYP2D6 activity does not change with age. This is based on constancy of the urinary metabolic ratio which, as I said, is also a function of renal drug clearance. What I believe happens with CYP2D6 with age is that enzyme activity and renal clearance tend to decline in parallel. Hence, the metabolic ratio does not change.

M. Kinirons:

It is very difficult sometimes to separate out those two aspects. Nonetheless, if you take debrisoquine as an estimate of CYP2D6 and you accept it for that, it is obviously important that we try to develop estimates or probe estimates for systemic clearance. What happens actually in the internal milieu is almost secondary because, even if it is important, the final line must be what comes out. So there could be a decline in hepatic metabolism, which is corrected by renal retention.

G.T. Tucker:

The fact is the enzyme may deteriorate with age, but you cannot see it with the index that you are using.

M. Kinirons:

From some of the data that I have shown, it is hard to imagine that if you get a 30% reduction in liver mass, the enzyme has upregulated with ageing, because you have now lost one third of all the cells that are metabolising CYP2D6. So in a sense one could speculate that this is what is happening, that there is some increased activity, but the individual data does not suggest that.

A. Breckenridge:

I would like to express the frustration of the drug regulator on this question of age and drug response. Nearly, every agency will have guidelines that a new drug should be studied in the elderly. But too often one gets results of investigations in what you might call geriatric "supermen". If a company came to you for advice on how to study a new drug, and they said they wanted to examine the effect of ageing, what advice would you give them?

M. Kinirons:

The pharmaceutical industry has failed to study the right population. The FDA's guidelines concerning studies in older people, have pushed up the age requirement as the realisation of the demographic trends have become apparent.There has got to be a need to study the real-world patients for your own practice. All the trials for donepezil in dementia were done in very clean patients, but the reality is that lots of these patients are on multiple drugs. Rivastigmine has moved forward in that because they have given the drug in their trials to a more varied population.

J. Urquhart:

The pharmacoepidemiology should inform regulators on what ought to be looked for in the studies with aged people. Because much of what you do as a regulator is to look at me-too drugs, so there are already drugs in the market-place that represent that class of therapy. It is possible to consult in data-bases those people who get that class of drug and to see what is the age distribution, and their current and past prescription drug histories profile. For example, basic community pharmacy records can give you a picture of what the dominant drug usage patterns are, how old the patients are, and what the gender distribution is. That is possible in the Netherlands where you have a reimbursement system, and where the basic system requires patients to designate a single pharmacy for their reimbursed prescriptions. If we are going to approve another drug in this class, we ought to have data in patients who have this and that sort of concomitant drug usage, age distribution, etc. And that will be representative of what is going to happen with the new product, because presumably it will go in unless the sponsor has compelling evidence for how they are going to label it differently and force the drug into a different usage pattern. But even in that situation you can look at it as soon as it goes in the market, to see where it goes, and then come back and hope for Phase IV studies to fill in the blanks. So I think that is a very realistic subject and it has not been done to my knowledge.

A. Breckenridge:

The role of the drug regulator is not to prevent a drug from coming to the market if it is going to benefit patients. The evidence of its safety must be gathered from wherever it can be obtained. However, one would submit that it is the role of the pharmaceutical company to produce that evidence, and a lot of them would be very happy to support it. If they produced evidence in what we were calling the geriatric supermen, the most severe comment would be that this drug had not been studied in an appropriate group of subjects, therefore it is not indicated in them. But most drug regulators would be unhappy about that, if it was seen not to be benefiting patients. But the plea that I was making is for more realistic studies to be carried out by the industry or better information to be obtained by them.

M.M. Reidenberg:

Let me ask for advice on issues I face as an editor. We will get a paper looking at either age or gender or some disease's effect on a drug. There will be 6 to 8 subjects in a group. The elderly people will range in age from about 60 to 69 with a median of perhaps 62 or 63. If the variability in a group is small, then sometimes a small difference can have a statistically significant $p<0.05$. If it is $p<0.1$, then they claim a trend has occurred. And the real issue I have as an editor is: Should these be rejected or am I simply contributing to publication bias? They are certainly not definitive, and if somebody does enough of these studies, some will have a $p=0.05$; and as you look at the data, it is because they were lucky and had small variability between one of the groups so that they could get statistical significance.

A.J.J. Wood:

The reason we study healthy elderly is to be sure we are studying only one variable, that is age and not frailty, ill health, nor other drugs. Similarly, if you were studying renal failure, presumably you would try and study patients who had renal impairment, but not other variables. Hence, we have to be careful that we do not get ourselves into a situation where we study patients who happen to be elderly, but have cardiac failure, ischaemic heart disease or whatever else.

M.M. Reidenberg:
I am unwilling to accept people between 60 and 65 as being an elderly group for the purpose of clinical decisions with respect to drug therapy.

J. Urquhart:
Why do not you set a policy for what age means ? I vote for 85 and up.

M.M. Reidenberg:
This is what I am inviting advice on. These are decisions that have to be made. For the journal, I would rather we do it publically than that I personally make an arbitrary decision.

M. Lader:
One group of drugs is often given to people in their 50s and then they are continued on a regular basis into old age. The hypnotic drugs are amongst the most widely used of all the medications. The elderly lose their tolerance to these medications and they then end up either with a broken hip or pseudo-demented. And this is another area where we need longitudinal rather than cross-sectional studies.

T. Salmonson:
What I meant by publication bias is that interesting data may not be published by industry, because of other reasons. If you do pick up an effect in a small number of 60-65 year old people, it would be very interesting to see how that would translate into an 85-year old one. But if we had all the time and resources that we wanted, I am sure we could do a lot of work on existing data. There is plenty of data in regulatory agencies, where you can look at the effect of age in a number of drugs, and perhaps get the magic age number or year you are after.

U. Klotz:
Recently, an article (Fliser *et al.*, Kidney Internat, 1997) about aging and creatinine clearance was published which comprised a sufficiently high number of subjects. Included were the so-called fit elderly, just to find out an age effect, and different patient groups (elderly with hypertension and elderly with congestive heart failure). I think this is the type of study you were looking for and you will be happy to accept it because it is the way to clearly distinguish age *per se* and the effects of diseases.

Variability in Human Drug Response
G.T. Tucker, Editor

Gender as a source of variability in human pharmacokinetics and pharmacodynamics.

Paul Rolan and Lynn McKeown

Medeval Ltd, Skelton House, Manchester, U.K.

ABSTRACT

The issue of gender as a clinically important source of variability has only received attention relatively recently. Most literature relates to possible pharmacokinetic differences. Where pharmacokinetic differences do occur, they are generally small and are unlikely to be clinically important. Gender-related dose-response differences are frequently reported for CNS-acting compounds but have also been reported for other classes such as corticosteroids. Whether such differences have a pharmacokinetic or pharmacodynamic basis is not clear but further investigation is warranted as the magnitude of some of the reported differences is clinically important. In women, the effects of phase of menstrual cycle, hormonal contraception, pregnancy and the interaction with age are additional potentially significant sources of variability and need to be considered in assessing gender differences in drug response.

Key words: gender, variability, pharmacodynamics, pharmacokinetics.

Correspondence: Paul Rolan, MD, Medeval Ltd, Skelton House, Lloyd Street North, Manchester M15 6SH, UK, Tel: +44-161-226-6525, Fax: +44-161-226-8936, Email: p.rolan@medeval.com

1. INTRODUCTION

The issue of gender differences between men and women has only been a significant component of clinical pharmacology literature in relatively recent years, approximately the last decade. Drugs were developed mainly using male subjects, because of the concern about potential effects of a new chemical entity on the embryo or foetus and fertility if given to women of child-bearing potential. This traditional view was challenged by women's rights groups because this approach had lead to women of child bearing potential being disadvantaged in not being offered early access to novel potential therapies. Partly in response to these concerns, the US FDA issued advice to pharmaceutical companies in 1993 [1], encouraging them to include women in early clinical studies but also encouraged the early exploration of gender-related and hormonal-treatment- related effects on drug handling and response. This advice led to a major increase in the literature on gender-drug interactions and related issues, such as interactions between drugs and hormonal treatment and contraception. In this article, we have reviewed and summarised such literature and assessed the likely contribution of such factors to variability in drug response.

2. GENDER DIFFERENCES IN PHARMACOKINETICS

2.1. Absorption/ bioavailability

Although there is evidence that gastric emptying and intestinal transport may be slower in women than men, evidence that this causes differences in drug absorption is lacking. Indeed, Aarons *et al.* [2] found that absorption of orally administered aspirin was faster in women than men, without a change in extent of absorption. Some studies have found an apparent slower absorption of "intramuscularly" administered drug to be slower in women, but the potential confounder of the administration actually being subcutaneous (due to the greater depth of adipose tissue) needs so be considered in interpreting such claims [2]. For drugs delivered by the inhaled pulmonary route, Knight *et al.* [3] found less respiratory tract deposition of aerosolised ribavirin in women compared to men. In contrast, Bennett [4] found a 30% greater deposition of 2 m particles of carnauba wax in women. The difference has been attributed to breathing patterns but the clinical significance is not clear.

In contrast to the inconsistent gender differences in drug absorption, significant differences in bioavailability with drug subject to first-pass extraction have been reported, mainly due to differences in hepatic enzyme activity (see section 2.3). Part of the gender difference in alcohol pharmacokinetics is attributed to lower gastric and/or hepatic alcohol dehydrogenase activity in women [5].

2.2. Distribution

Compared to men, women have a lower body weight and a higher percentage of body weight being adipose tissue. Higher body-weight adjusted distribution volumes have been reported in women for lipophilic drugs such as trazodone, diazepam and sufentanil [6] but a significantly lower volume of distribution for ethanol [5].

Although gender-related differences in plasma protein binding have been reported, the extent appears to be small and not of clinical relevance [7].

2.3. Metabolism

Most of the literature on gender-related differences in pharmacokinetics has reported differences in drug metabolism. This has recently been extensively reviewed by Harris *et al.* [7]. The available data have been summarised by individual metabolic pathways as there are no consistent trends for gender-related differences common to all pathways. The same lack of consistent trend can be said for drug classes: for examples, with benzodiazepines, some are cleared more quickly in men, some more quickly in women, and for some there is no gender difference.

When considering potential gender-related differences in drug metabolism, it is important to separate differences due to gender from those related to body weight, and so weight-adjusted clearances should be examined.

2.3.1. Hepatic cytochrome P450s

2.3.1.1. CYP 3A4

CYP 3A4 is the enzyme responsible for the metabolism of most therapeutic drugs. There is a consistent body of evidence that young women have a 20-40% higher clearance of CYP 3A4 substrates than young men. This has been shown for erythromycin, methylprednisolone, verapamil, diazepam, midazolam. Although there are some negative studies, small sample size and subject heterogeneity may have made the gender effect difficult to detect.

2.3.1.2. CYP 2D6

After CYP 3A4, CYP 2D6 is the next most important enzyme for metabolism of therapeutic drugs. Its activity shows a genetic polymorphism which is not influenced by gender. In contrast to CYP 3A4, the available data suggest that clearance by CYP 2D6-dependent pathways is higher in men than women. Higher rates have been found for clearance of desipramine, *(R)*-propranolol, and clomipramine hydroxylation.

2.3.1.3. CYP 2C19

CYP 2C19 is another important drug metabolising enzyme that displays genetic polymorphism, but which is independent of gender. Consistent effects of gender on clearance of CYP 2C19 substrates are lacking, but the trend is for faster clearance rates in men.

2.3.1.4. CYP 1A2

The available data on gender differences in clearance of CYP 1A2 substrates is lacking, with faster rates reported for men for caffeine and thiothixene but faster rates for women for theophylline. Smoking appears to induce CYP 1A2 to a greater extent in men than women.

2.3.2. Conjugation

Where gender-related differences in clearance by conjugation have been observed, the trend is for it to be faster in men than women by approximately 20-30%. Examples of drugs with faster clearance in men include temazepam, oxazepam, paracetamol and diflunisal. In contrast, no gender-related differences were detected for clofibric acid or ibuprofen, with conflicting data for salicylic acid conjugation with glycine.

2.3.3. Dihydrouracil dehydrogenase

The hepatic enzyme responsible for the metabolism of the anticancer drug fluorouracil is dihydrouracil dehydrogenase. Given its narrow therapeutic index and Michaelis-Menten kinetics at therapeutic concentrations, the markedly lower clearance in women is likely to be clinically important [7,8].

2.4. Elimination

Elimination of drugs by renal filtration is unlikely to be gender-dependent as GFR is comparable in men and women after adjustment for body weight. There are little data examining possible gender affects on tubular secretion or reabsorption, although differences have been found for the renal clearance of the diastereomeric cations quinine and quinidine which undergo significant tubular secretion [9].

3. GENDER DIFFERENCES IN PHARMACODYNAMICS

Many of the studies that report a possible gender-related difference in pharmacodynamics do not exclude pharmacokinetic differences or possible prescription and reporting bias as the explanation for the difference. However, as the differences may be clinically important, we attempt to summarise the available literature.

3.1. Psychotropic medication

The most compelling gender differences in pharmacodynamics appear to stem from psychiatric disease processes and their treatment [7,10,11]

3.1.1. Antipsychotics

When treated with the antipsychotic chlorpromazine, young women show a greater magnitude of response with more severe side effects [10,12]. In a study by Chouinard *et al.*, women are also prescribed approximately half the dose of the antipsychotic fluspirilene for men for the treatment of schizophrenia despite similarities in age and weight [13]. However, Simpson *et al.* [14] implied that the required therapeutic dose of fluphenazine was not significantly different between males and females. The differences in the dose-response relationship of antipsychotics may be a mirror of the pharmacokinetics as suggested by higher thiothixene clearance in males or higher plasma levels of chlorpromazine in women [13,15], but it is not known if other variables were taken into consideration e.g. menstrual cycle, smoking and oral contraception, during these trials.

A possible explanation for pharmacodynamic differences is the hypothesis that oestrogen can act as a dopamine antagonist, accentuating the effects of the antipsychotics [7,10] whilst the metabolites of progesterone may act on GABA receptors as agonists or antagonists, also inducing behavioural changes.

Tardive dyskinesia is an adverse effect of neuroleptics. Chouinard *et al.* [16] suggested that males had more severe forms and were more susceptible to the disorder. Conflicting data from Smith *et al.* stated that there was a higher prevalence in treated females [17]. In reviewing both sets of data, Smith concluded that age and gender should always be considered concurrently since the over 67s' age group appeared to have a significant gender difference and women over the age of 67 had much higher incidences of tardive dyskinesia [17]. This is thought to be due to dopaminergic denervation supersensitivity therefore if oestrogen were acting at dopamine receptors it would be consistent with a protective effect for premenopausal females not post menopausal. There are other factors that could complicate these effects and no studies have yet confirmed any hypothesis.

Oestrogen has not been studied for antipsychotic activity in humans only in animal models and the fluctuations of the menstrual cycle have not been examined for female intra-individuality. The extent to which schizophrenia and its treatment are affected by gender is still being studied.

3.1.2. Antidepressants

In the treatment of depression with panic attacks it has been suggested that men have a better response to the tricyclic antidepressants like imiprimine whilst young women have better responses to the monoamine oxidase inhibitors (MAOIs), e.g. phenelzine [7,10]. Raskin *et al.* [18] implied that older women (over 40) also responded well to imiprimine and therefore age must be considered together with gender.
Some studies that have shown women respond better than men to the selective serotonin reuptake inhibitors (SSRIs) e.g. fluoxetine [7,11].

In the prophylactic treatment of bipolar depression with lithium the incidence of hypothyroidism was higher in women but little research has been carried out in this area [10], this could be a reflection of the population as a whole where hypothyroidism is more prevalent in women.

3.2. Corticosteroids

In addition to the pharmacokinetic differences discussed in section 3.3.1.1, Lew *et al.* [19] found that premenopausal women were more sensitive to immunosuppressive action of methylprednisolone as evidenced by changes in circulating basophil and helper T cell counts. The women were all in the luteal phase of their cycle when hormone levels were relatively high and constant and none was taking oral contraceptives, which according to Gustavson *et al.* [20] can decrease clearance rates. It was postulated that either oestrogen or progesterone was responsible for the increased sensitivity or therefore the menstrual cycle will affect the pharmacodynamics of methylprednisolone, although because of the opposing pharmacokinetics (higher clearance) there is an overall similar net response in males and females.

3.3. NSAIDS

Walker *et al.* assessed gender variability in the response to NSAIDs and suggested that only men showed any analgesic response to ibuprofen when subjected to cutaneously applied stimulation as compared to premenopausal women. Baseline differences in pain threshold had been taken into consideration and plasma concentrations were similar in both genders[21].

3.4. Neuromuscular Blockers

Atracurium is a neuromuscular blocker used in anaesthesia. Parker *et al.* analysed its effects for gender related differences using electromyographic monitoring and measuring four different parameters [22]. The only statistically significant difference was that the rate constant for exit of the drug from the effect compartment (k_{eo}), was greater in women than in men. They speculated that this may be due to differences in muscle blood flow but there was no evidence to support this.

3.5. Antihypertensives

There is little medical literature on gender differences in the treatment of hypertension even though Kitler suggests that, on average hypertension is a more important risk factor for heart disease in women than in men [23]. Data from the Medical Research Council showed that stepped care hypertensive medication was not as effective in some women with moderate and severe diastolic hypertension [24] and that it could actually be harmful to white women [23]. However, Anastos *et al.* suggest that the evidence for all women is inconclusive and most of the findings on gender differences were incidental as the studies were not designed for this and did not include significant numbers of women [24].

4. INTERACTION BETWEEN GENDER EFFECTS AND AGE

Where gender-related differences in pharmacokinetics or pharmacodynamics have been observed, the most frequent causative factor offered as an explanation is the effect of the female hormones, particularly oestrogen. As oestrogen production declines substantially after the menopause, it could be anticipated that where gender differences are found between young men and young women, these differences should lessen in older subjects. Evidence consistent with this hypothesis is the disappearance of the gender-related differences in theophylline metabolism [25] and the antimigraine drug zolmitriptan [26], although the pathways responsible for the latter are not clear.

Unfortunately, this point does not appear to have been appreciated by some researchers, who after finding differences between young men and young women claim that this is a gender effect rather than a possible age/ gender interaction.

5. SPECIFIC ASPECTS OF FEMALE REPRODUCTIVE PHYSIOLOGY

Given that female hormones are often thought to be the causative factor in gender-related differences in drug handling and response, and that plasma levels of the hormones vary widely during the menstrual cycle, it is reasonable to anticipate that additional hormonal therapy (e.g. oral contraceptives or hormone replacement therapy), the timing of the menstrual cycle, pregnancy or menopause may affect drug kinetics or response.

5.1. Oral contraceptives (OCs)

Oral contraceptives can interfere with the metabolism or activity of numerous therapeutic agents.

5.1.1. Benzodiazepines

It has been shown in many studies that oral contraceptives can inhibit enzyme hydroxylation activity and reduce clearance of some benzodiazepines, e.g. diazepam and nitrazepam [27,28,29]. Ellinwood *et al.* [30] postulated that OCs decreased the rate of absorption of diazepam and during the week off hormones the plasma levels quickly rose and women became 'intoxicated' during the menses. This may lead to associated pharmacodynamic changes especially in motor and mental functions. However, some other benzodiazepams, bromazepam and clotiazepam do not have their metabolism impaired by OCs, but are not commonly used.

5.1.2. Methylxanthines

Abernethy and Todd [31] reported a reduction in the clearance of caffeine by up to 40% when taken with OCs, similarly Roberts *et al.* [32] suggested lower clearance rates and a longer half-life with theophylline. Although no clinically relevant effects dynamic changes were reported, a change in clearance of this magnitude is likely to be important for theophylline given its narrow therapeutic index.

5.1.3. Analgesics

Miners *et al.* [33] suggest that salicylic acid clearance was increased by 40% in OC users due to an increase in both the glycine and glucuronic acid conjugation pathways in pill users. They postulated that this could also be an explanation of why OCs may enhance morphine clearance.

5.1.4. Corticosteroids

There have been several studies of the possible inhibition of prednisolone metabolism by OCs. OCs can reduce clearance and prolong half life, but interpretation is confounded by the increase of the corticosteroid binding protein, transcortin, by oestrogen [28].

5.1.5. Antidepressants

OCs are reported to reduce clearance of imiprimine, amitryptyline and nortriptyline.

5.2. Menstrual cycle

The possible effects of the phase of the menstrual cycle of drugs have been reviewed recently by Kashuba [34]. Consistent effects of the menstrual cycle of drug absorption and distribution are lacking. Clearance of theophylline, caffeine and paracetamol is reduced in the luteal phase but the difference is not thought to be clinically significant. No consistent effect of the phase of the menstrual cycle has been detected for CYP 2C, 2D6, 2E and 3A4 substrates.

In addition to potential pharmacokinetic changes, there may be interactions between the target disease and menstrual cycle which could affect drug response. For example, it is well known that migraine is often more frequent in a female patient around the time of menstruation, and it has been suggested that such attacks are particularly resistant to treatment. However, the clinical response to zolmitriptan was unaffected by whether the attack was peri-menstrual [35].

5.3. Pregnancy

Pregnancy has been reported to increase the clearance of the antiepileptic drugs phenytoin, phenobarbital and carbamazepine [36] to a clinically important degree, which requires dose increase, presumable due to hepatic enzyme induction. In contrast, pregnancy reduces caffeine clearance. For some drugs used in pregnancy, e.g. zidovudine [37], no significant effect was observed

6. CLINICAL SIGNIFICANCE OF THE VARIABILITY DUE TO GENDER

With the recent interest in gender as a source of variability in drug response, the potential effect of gender on most important pharmacokinetic processes has been examined. Although there are consistent trends for differences between the genders, particularly for some drug metabolism pathways, the overall extent of a kinetic difference is small, and usually less than the general between-subject variability.

However, the same extent of data is lacking when examining potential pharmacodynamic differences. It is important to examine whether the concentration-response relationship differs, as a difference in dose-response can be due to pharmacokinetic factors.

For some categories, particularly psychotropic drugs, there may be clinically important gender differences. With such drugs, individual clinical response can be hard to judge and so it is important in the development of such drugs that potential gender differences are positively sought in a systematic manner, not only for the therapeutic effect but also adverse effects. Although the authors are unaware of any drugs for which the dosing recommendations differ for men and women (except for gender-specific conditions), it is possible that closer attention to potential differences in the dose-concentration-effect relationships between the genders may reveal the need for such labelling in the future.

REFERENCES

1. Dept. of Health and Human Services, Food and Drug Administration. Guideline for the study and evaluation of gender differences in the clinical evaluation of drugs. Federal Register. 1993;58:139.
2. Aarons L, Hopkins K, Rowland M. Route of administration and sex differences in the pharmacokinetics of aspirin, administered as its lysine salt. Pharm Res 1989;6:660-666.
3. Knight V, Yu CP, Gilbert BE, Divine GW. Estimating the dose of ribavirin aerosol according to age and other variables. J Infect Dis 1988;158:443-448.
4. Bennett WD, Zeman KL, Kim C. Variability of fine particle deposition in healthy adults: effect of age and gender. Am J Resp Crit Care Med 1995;153:1641-1647.
5. Thomasson HR. Gender differences in alcohol metabolism. Physiological responses to ethanol. Recent Dev Alcohol 1995;12:163-179.
6. Greenblatt DJ, Friedman H, Burnstein ES, *et al.* Trazodone kinetics: effects of age, gender and obesity. Clin Pharmacol Ther 1987;42:193-200.
7. Harris RZ, Benet LZ, Schwartz JB. Gender effects in pharmacokinetics and pharmacodynamics. Drugs 1995;50:222-239.
8. Ortiz de Montellano PR, Kunze KL. Self catalysed inactivation of cytochrome P-450 by ethynyl substrates. J Biol Chem 1980;255:5578-85.
9. Gaudry SE, Sitar DS, Smyth DD, *et al.* Gender and age as factors in the inhibition of the renal clearance of amantadine by quinine and quinidine. Clin Pharmacol Ther 1993;54:23-7.
10. Yonkers KA, Kando JC, Cole JO, Blementhal S. Gender differences in pharmacokinetics and pharmacodynamics of psychotropic medication. Am J Psychiatry 1992;149:587-595.

11. Dawkins K, Potter WZ. Gender differences in pharmacokinetics and pharmacodynamics of psychotropics: focus on women. Psychopharmacol Bull 1991;27:417-426.
12. Chouinard G, Annable L. Pimozide in the treatment of newly admitted schizophrenic patients. Psychopharmacology (Berlin) 1982;76:13-19.
13. Chouinard G, Annable L, Steinberg S. A controlled clinical trial of fluspirilene, a long acting injectable neuroleptic, in schizophrenic patients with acute exacerbation. J Clin Psychopharmacol 1986;6:21-26.
14. Simpson G M, Yakalam KG, Levinson DP *et al.* Single dose pharmacokinetics of fluphenazine after fluphenazine decanoate administration. J Clin Psychopharm 1990;10:417-421.
15. Ereshefsky L. Saklad SR, Watanabe MD, *et al.* Thiothixene pharmacokinetic interactions: a study of hepatic enzyme inducers, clearance inhibitors and demographic variabilities. J Clin Psychopharm 1991;11:296-301.
16. Chouinard G, Annable L, Ross-Chouinard A, Nestoros JN. Factors related to tardive dyskinesias. Am J Psychiatry 1979;136:79-83.
17. Smith JM, Dunn DD. Sex differences in the prevalence of severe tardive dyskinesia. Am J Psychiatry 1979;136:1080-1082.
18. Raskin A. Age-sex differences in response to antidepressant drugs. J Nerv Ment Dis 1974;159:120-130.
19. Lew KH, Ludwig EA, Milad MA, Donovan K, Middleton Jr. E, Ferry JJ, Jusko WJ. Gender-based effects on methylprednisolone pharmacokinetics and pharmacodynamics Clin Pharmacol Ther 1993;54:402-14.
20. Gustavson LE and Benet LZ. Menopause: Pharmacodynamics and Pharmacokinetics. Exp Gerontol 1994;29:437-444.
21. Walker JS, Carmody JJ. Experimental pain in healthy human subjects: gender differences in nociception and in response to ibuprofen. Anesth Analg 1998;86:1257-1262.
22. Parker CJR, Hunter JM and Snowdon SL. Effect of age, gender and anaesthetic technique on the pharmacodynamics of atracurium. Br J Anaesthesia 1993;70:38-41.
23. Kitler ME. Differences in men and women in coronary heart disease, systemic hypertension and their treatment. Am J Cardiol 1992;70:1077-1080.
24. Anastos K, Charney P, Charon RA, Cohen E, Jones CY, Marte C, Swiderski DM, Wheat M and Williams S. Hypertension in women: What is really known? Ann Intern Med 1991;115:287-293.
25. Cuzzolin L, Schinella M, Tellini U, *et al.* The effect of sex and cardiac failure on the pharmacokinetics of a slow-release theophylline formulation in the elderly. Pharmacol Res 1990;22:137-8.
26. Peck RW, Seaber E, Dixon R *et al.* The pharmacodynamics and pharmacokinetics of the 5-HT $_{1B/1D}$ agonist zolmitriptan in healthy young and elderly men and women. Clin Pharmacol Ther 1998;63:342-53.
27. Back DJ and Orme ML. Pharmacokinetic drug interactions with oral contraceptives. Clin Pharmacokin 1990;18:472-484.
28. Shenfield GM, Griffin JM. Clinical pharmacokinetics of contraceptive steroids: An update Clin Pharmacokin 1991;20:15-37.
29. Shenfield GM. Oral contraceptives. Are drug interactions of clinical significance? Drug Saf. 1993;9:21-37.

30. Ellinwood EH, Easier, Linnoila M, Molter DW, Heattherly DG, Bjornsson TD. Effects of oral contraceptives and diazepam induced psychomotor impairment. Clin Pharmacol Ther 1983;35:360-366.
31. Abernethy DR, Todd EL. Impairment of caffeine clearance by chronic use of low-dose oestrogen containing oral contraceptives. Eur J Clin Pharmacol 1985;28:425-428.
32. Roberts RK, Grice J, McGuffie C, Heilbronn L. Oral contraceptives impair the elimination of theophylline. J Lab Clin Med 1983;101:821-825.
33. Miners JO, Grgurinovich N, Whitehead AG, Robson RA, Birkett DJ. Influence of gender and OC steroids on the metabolism of salicylic acid and acetylsalicylic acid. Brit J Clin Pharmacol 1986;22:135-142.
34. Kashuba AD, Nafziger AN. Physiological changes during the menstrual cycle and their effects on the pharmacokinetics and pharmacodynamics of drugs. Clin Pharmacokin 1998;34:203-218
35. Rolan PE, Martin GR. Zolmitriptan: a new acute treatment for migraine. Exp Opin Invest Drugs 1998;7:633-652.
36. Lander CM, Eadie MJ,. Plasma antiepileptic drug concentrations during pregnancy. Epilepsia 1991;32:257-66.
37. O'Sullivan MJ, Boyer PJ, Scott GB *et al.* The pharmacokinetics and safety of zidovudine in the third trimester of pregnancy for women infected with the human immunodeficiency virus and their infants: phase I acquired immunodeficiency syndrome clinical trials support group study. Am J Obstet Gynecol 1993;168:1510-6.

Discussion: Gender as a source of variability in human pharmacokinetics and pharmacodynamics

A.J.J. Wood:

From the data that you have presented, the general idea was that there were not many gender-related differences. What would be your recommendation? Should we stop looking for gender-related differences or should we just include women randomly in trials?

P. Rolan:

If you exclude women, you are reducing your trial population unnecessarily. Additionally, at the moment, the regulatory climate is requiring to include women in the clinical trials, even though pharmacokinetic differences are unlikely to be important. I mentioned that pharmacodynamic differences are likely to be important, and if you do not include enough women in your trials, you will not see them. In conclusion, I believe it is quite important that you do include women as early as possible. From a practical point of view, it is not necessary to have young volunteer women in your first studies. I am still concerned that, despite all the care that you can bring about, people still get pregnant in studies. We know that perhaps 90% of molecules that go into Phase I do not get any further, and I would not suggest we have women in every early study. But not to include women in later studies is really shooting yourself in the foot from both the regulatory point of view, and because there are drugs with a gender-related difference in drug response.

A.J.J. Wood:

If we just include them as part of the regular population, should we stratify by gender?

P. Rolan:

Definitely. Because if you do not stratify, you cannot do the appropriate analysis.

J. Urquhart:

There are a couple of quite notable gender differences. One of them is that if you look at actuarial data or age-specific death rates, there is roughly a twofold difference in age-specific mortality, and this is at every stage of life from childbirth to very advanced age. The biology of that has got to be multifactorial because the biology is different at all those ages. If you look in the early 1920s there is an even bigger difference between the sexes attributable to accidental death in males because they drive crazier than women do. The other notable difference is on alcohol toxicity. The threshold for cirrhosis, estimated in daily alcohol intake, is about 50% lower in women.

P. Rolan:

I will only allude to the fact that the kinetic-gender differences in alcohol have been extensively studied. But they do not explain adequately this well-known difference in toxicity.

T. Salmonson:

I agree with you that we do not see gender differences very often and that differences tend to go away when they are studied in elderly women. However, I would not agree with the statement that differences do not exist. Possibly due to publication bias or to other reasons, there is a wish not to find these differences. We approved a stroke medicine which due to both pharmacokinetic and pharmacodynamic explanations was not effective in women. But there are also anti-migraine and other drugs that despite pharmacokinetic differences were recently approved. As Alasdair Breckenridge commented earlier, perhaps the regulators are not performing very well when it comes to these issues. From my subjective point of view the pharmaceutical companies do not want to see as important these gender differences, because they would restrict labelling. They are happy to change the dose for a twofold increase or decrease in clearance if it is a decreased kidney function, but not by gender differences. In migraine, for example, they have included women in Phase III studies and no difference in adverse effects has appeared. But obviously, these studies were not sized to pick up these types of differences. As long as you are not showing that this twofold difference in clearance lacks effect, you have to assume that there is an effect, just as you would do for a decreased kidney function.

P. Rolan:

There is an accepted culture to reduce the dose for decreased renal function but to avoid any gender label, However, pharmaceutical companies may be a bit more willing to accept the latter. When you get the dose wrong, what happens is that it incurs the company financial disadvantage. In this situation, the prescriber will halve the dose in those people and they will get as good a response. And the drug company only gets half the income from the female population. So the companies that try and use the wrong dose for a large slab of the population, it will actually be to their economic disadvantage.

T. Salmonson:

Time will tell if you are right. We have not been able to force them to have a different dosing. But I admit, when it comes to anti-migraine, it may be that we underdose men rather than overdose females.

Ethnic differences in drug response: A model for understanding interindividual variability

Alastair J.J. Wood

Division of Clinical Pharmacology, Vanderbilt University, Nashville, TN, USA

ABSTRACT

The mission of clinical pharmacologists is to understand interindividual variability in drug response in order to allow optimization of therapy for the individual patient. In the quest to improve such individualization it is important to identify patient groups whose characteristics put them at special risk from either excessive or reduced pharmacologic effects. It has long been recognized that such inappropriate response may be due to either pharmocokinetic or pharmacodynamic variability so that the individual may have an appropriate pharmacological response to an abnormal drug concentration at the effect site (pharmocokinetic variability), or may have an inappropriate response to a normal drug concentration at the effect site (pharmacodynamic variability). Recent advances in molecular biology have allowed us to understand many of the molecular mechanisms responsible for such interindividual variability in drug response and to explain the differences in drug response among different ethnic groups.

Key words: ethnicity, drug response, pharmacokinetics, pharmacodynamics, receptors.

Correspondence: Prof. Alastair J.J. Wood, Division of Clinical Pharmacology, Vanderbilt University, Nashville, TN 37232-6601, USA, Tel. +1-615-343-8701, Fax: +1-615-343-8701, Email: Alastair.Wood@mcmail.vanderbilt.edu

Funding acknowledgement: Supported by NIH Grants GM 31304 & HL56251

INTERETHNIC DIFFERENCES IN DRUG METABOLISM

Interethnic differences in drug metabolism may be due to one of the following:

- Interethnic differences in distribution of a polymorphic trait.
- Mutations which code for enzymes with abnormal activity which occur with altered frequency in different ethnic groups.
- Interethnic differences in metabolism within a phenotype.
- Interethnic differences in substrate specificity.

The effects of these differences will depend on whether the drug in question produces its effects directly or through a metabolite, examples of both situations have been found to result in interethnic differences in response.

Many of these differences are well illustrated by the effects of ethnicity on the analgesic codeine which is metabolized by CYP2D6 to morphine (Figure 1). Most of codeine's therapeutic effects are due to the production of this active metabolite, so that the therapeutic effect produced in an individual is dependant on the combination of that individual's CYP2D6 activity and their sensitivity to morphine. Individuals who lack active CYP2D6, poor metabolizers, produce minimal amounts of morphine (Figure 2) [1] and achieve little opiate effect [1] (Figure 3). Because of the interethnic differences in the distribution of the poor metabolizer phenotype (Table 1) the proportion of individuals who fail to produce morphine will also show marked interethnic difference.

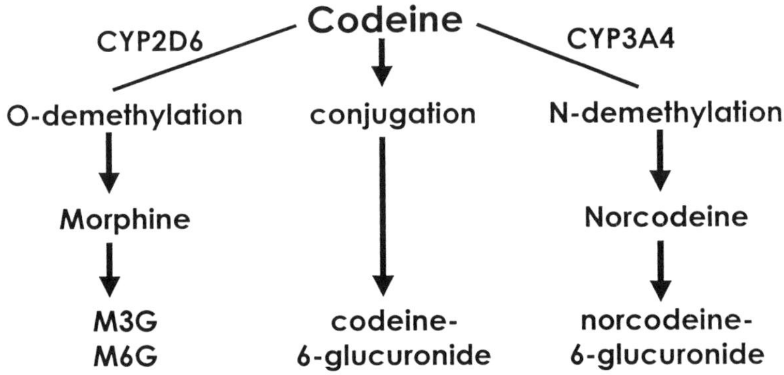

Figure 1. Routes of codeine metabolism

Table 1.
Frequency of CYP2D6 poor metabolizers in different ethnic groups [2]

Population	Poor metabolizer frequency
US Caucasian	7%
Nigerians	8%
Chinese	0,7%
Japanese	0,5%

Thus altered frequency of a polymorphic trait is an important determinant of interethnic differences in response. However even within a phenotype interethnic differences may occur. Again this can be illustrated with codeine. In Chinese extensive metabolizers the partial

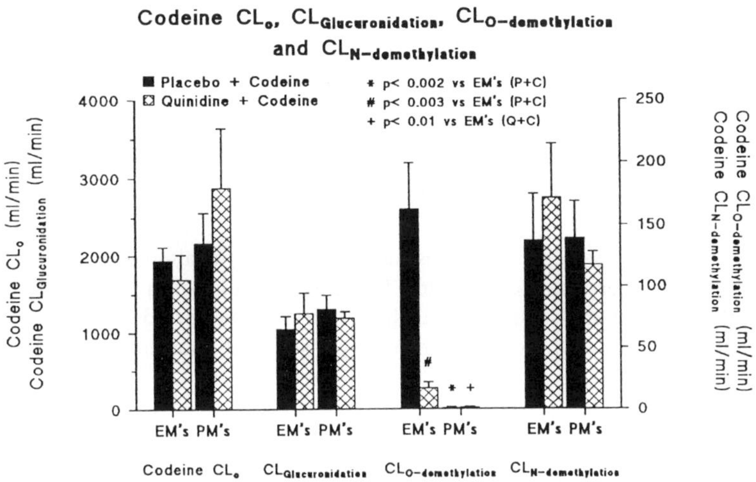

Figure 2. Partial metabolic clearance of codeine by various routes in extensive (EM) and poor metabolizers and following quinidine [1]

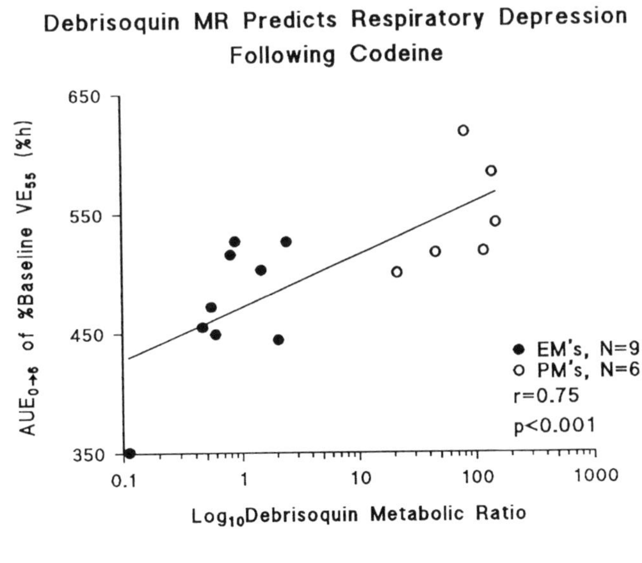

Figure 3.
Relationship between debrisoquin metabolic ratio and codeine induced respiratory depression[1]

metabolic clearance of codeine by the O-demetylation pathway (the pathway responsible for the production of morphine) was substantially lower in Chinese EMs than in Caucasians [3].

The explanation for this is also now clear and has a genetic basis. Chinese individuals have a high incidence of the allele CYP2*10 [4] which codes for an enzyme with reduced metabolic activity [5], so that even though they are phenotypically extensive metabolizers they have a lower enzyme activity.

ETHNIC DIFFERENCES IN DRUG SENSITIVITY

Ethnic differences in drug response also occur due to altered sensitivity at the receptor level even when corrections are made for drug concentration. Sensitivity to morphine is decreased in Chinese individuals [6] resulting in less respiratory depression in response to both direct morphine administration [6] and in response to the morphine produced by metabolism of codeine [3].

ETHNIC DIFFERENCES IN VASCULAR RESPONSE

It is well recognized that mortality and morbidity from hypertension and other vascular disease is higher in Blacks. This led us to investigate role of ethnicity in determining vascular response. Vascular tone is determined by both vasodilation and vasoconstriction and ethnic effects have been shown on both. The vasodilatory response to $beta_2$ stimulation by isoproterenol is impaired in African Americans [7] (Figure 4). Again exploration of the genetic

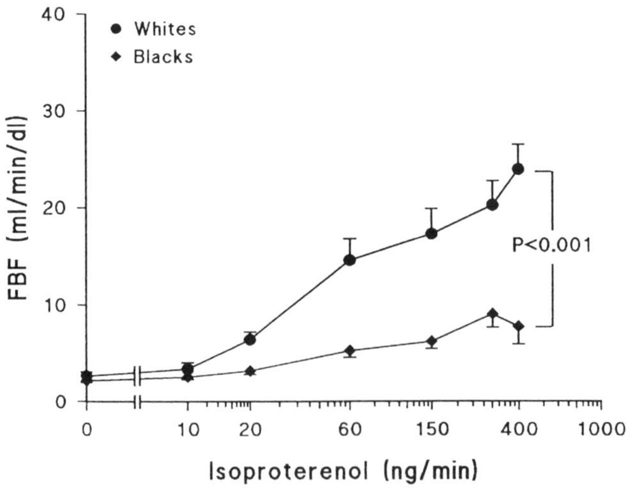

Figure 4. Impaired vascular response to $beta_2$ receptor mediated vasodiation [7]

basis for this difference has become possible, with recent data suggesting that this interethnic difference may be due to an altered frequency of a mutation for the $beta_2$ adrenergic receptor gene. Response to vasodilation induced by nitric oxide is impaired in Blacks whether the generation of NO is endogenous (produced following methacholine administration) or whether produced following sodium nitroprusside [8]. Vasoconstriction produced by intra-arterial administration of phenylephrine is markedly increased in Blacks so that the combination of impaired vasodilation accompanied by enhanced vasoconstriction will result in additive effects and increased vascular tone.

CONCLUSION

Thus in conclusion, understanding the basis for ethnic differences in drug response have significantly enhanced our ability to define the underlying basis for interindividual variability in responses to drugs.

REFERENCES

1. Caraco Y, Sheller J, Wood AJ. Pharmacogenetic determination of the effects of codeine and prediction of drug interactions. J. Pharmacol. & Exp. Ther. 1996; 278:1165-1174.
2. Wood AJ, Zhou HH. Ethnic differences in drug disposition and responsiveness. Clin. Pharmacokin. 1991; 20:350-373.
3. Caraco Y, Sheller J, Wood AJ. The impact of Ethnic origin and quinidine coadministration on Codeine's disposition and pharmacodynamic effects. "In Press JPET 1999.
4. Droll K, et al. Comparison of three CYP2D6 probe substrates and genotype in Ghanaians, Chinese and Caucasians. Pharmacogenetics 1998; 8:325-333.
5. Bertilsson L. Geographical/interracial differences in polymorphic drug oxidation. Current state of knowledge of cytochromes P450 (CYP) 2D6 and 2C19. Clinical Pharmacokinetics 1995; 29:192-209.
6. Zhou HH, Sheller JR, Nu H, Wood M, Wood AJ. Ethnic differences in response to morphine. Clinical Pharmacology & Therapeutics 1993; 54:507-513.
7. Lang CC, Stein CM, Brown RM, Deegan R, Nelson R, He HB, et al. Attenuation of isoproterenol-mediated vasodilatation in blacks. New England Journal of Medicine 1995; 333:155-160.
8. Stein CM, Lang CC, Singh I, He H, Wood AJ. Increased vascular adrenergic vasoconstriction and decreased vasodilation in Blacks: Additive mechanisms leading to enhanced vascular reactivity. Submitted 1998;

<u>Discussion</u>: Ethnic differences in drug disposition and response

P. du Souich:

Just to confirm some of the data presented, the Mexicans have shown that the need of nifedipine among them is almost half the dose of Caucasians. This fact has been associated to the widespread use of corn in their meals.

A.J.J. Wood:

We are currently looking at midazolam in Mexico and we are not seeing huge differences, though there have been data in the past that suggested that such differences might exist. When you are looking at ethnic differences it is difficult to know whether they are due to the environment or to the genotypic differences.

H.K. Kroemer:

Related to this morphine story in Chinese, it could be a pharmacokinetic phenomenon due to the production of glucuronides or to the P-GP transport through the blood-brain barrier. Do you have further details on how that works? My second question is: Do you know whether the development of tolerance to morphine effects in Chinese is different from in Caucasians?

A.J.J. Wood:

The point is that morphine is metabolised to an active glucuronide and that might explain these differences. We performed this study but the differences in morphine glucuronidation and in plasma glucuronide concentrations did not explain these differences. We also thought that morphine-3-glucuronide might be a P-GP substrate, but unfortunately through our studies *in vitro* we could not confirm that. The anaesthetic literature had said that Asians were much more sensitive to morphine than Caucasians, however this goes the wrong way with what we were led to expect. In fact, Asians appear to be much more sensitive to the nausea-producing effects of morphine than were Caucasians. But as the anaesthesiologists were not measuring CO_2 response curves, perhaps what they had was a different effect. We also do not know whether that is due to some different receptor responses.

M. Lader:

I am wondering whether we are not being a little over-facile with this issue. For example, one of the problems in the development of drugs for schizophrenia is the possible over-representation of Afro-Caribbean origin patients, who are treatment-refractory. They end up in locked wards and on high doses of anti-psychotic drugs. There may be an over-representation of Western African origin people but not for people of East African origin. We need to have much more precise ways of defining ethnic groups than talking about blacks and Caucasians. The same happens when you refer to about Indians, without taking into account that there is a great deal of ethnic difference here. I think we are in danger of missing important data if we just put all people together by geographical origin, instead of doing some more biological analyses to typify what these groupings are.

A.J.J. Wood:

I agree with that completely. On the other hand, I think part of our purpose as clinical pharmacologists is to try to identify factors that we, as physicians, can use to better individualise dose. That can range from genotyping people, some sort of intervention we make before we give someone a dose, to more superficial measures, which include gender, age, frailty or ethnic background. We ought not to ignore the opportunity to try to use these techniques. For example, knowing somebody is from China, Japan or Korea, tells you they are very unlikely to be a poor metaboliser of debrisoquine, and secondly, it tells you that they are likely to have a higher incidence of the alleles that metabolise CYP2D6 substrates more poorly. There are some data actually also from side-effects of different anti-psychotic agents that show quite marked differences in the frequency, which may reflect expectation in different ethnic groups. Therefore, we need to try to find clues.

I.P. Hall:

When you have a polymorphism which is fairly common in a given population, it is relatively likely to be distributed events across that racial group. That is true for the β-receptor polymorphisms, which have a similar prevalence in all black South Africans or Afro-Caribbean populations and also in Japanese population, which have been studied. I have also a question that refers to the work on vasodilator properties of isoproteronol. It always worries me that there is a circular argument in saying that there is a causality link when you have got a population with a reduced vasodilator response and with a different prevalence for polymorphism. You have got in your population the key individuals, which are those who have the Glu-27 polymorphism in the blacks. Would you predict that those people would have the same response as the white Caucasians?

A.J.J. Wood:

I do not know the answer, but that is precisely what we are studying. We are trying to evaluate the sensitivity to desensitisation in previously genotyped individuals of both populations. As you said, it is possible to predict that individuals of different ethnic backgrounds but of similar genotypes would respond to desensitisation similarly. And hence, would respond to vasodilation in desensitised or not desensitised states similarly. As you can imagine, it is not a trivial experiment to undertake, so we have to find the homozygotes, and we have to convince them to undertake a desensitisation experiment.

Variability in Human Drug Response
G.T. Tucker, Editor

Effect of disease on the pharmacokinetic and pharmacodynamic determinants of response to diuretics

D. Craig Brater

Division of Clinical Pharmacology, Department of Medicine, Indiana University School of Medicine, Indianapolis, IN (USA)

ABSTRACT

Loop diuretics are used in all edematous disorders, but each disease represents a different pathophysiology. As such, the mechanisms by which response to diuretics is altered in these disorders differ. In turn, these differences in mechanism translate to differences in therapeutic strategy. For example, the primary mechanism accounting for diuretic resistance in patients with renal insufficiency is pharmacokinetic wherein inadequate amounts of diuretic reach the site of action within the lumen of the nephron. The appropriate therapeutic strategy is to administer large doses of diuretics to attain effective amounts of diuretic at the site of action.

In contrast, in patients with cirrhosis or congestive heart failure, the mechanism of diuretic resistance is pharmacodynamic wherein the nephron has a submaximal response to the diuretic. Large doses of diuretic are not helpful in this circumstance; rather modest doses should be administered more frequently or combinations of diseases affect response to diuretics should be used. Understanding pharmacokinetic and pharmacodynamic mechanisms by which diseases affect response to diuretics allows more rational therapy.

Key words: diuretics, edema, renal insufficiency, cirrhosis, congestive heart failure.

Correspondence: D. Craig Brater, M.D., Indiana University School of Medicine, 545 Barnhill Drive, Emerson Hall 317, Indianapolis, IN 46202-5124, Tel: +317-274-8438, Fax: +317-274-1437, Email: dbrater@iupui.edu

INTRODUCTION

Diuretics are used in primary disorders of the heart (congestive heart failure), kidney (renal insufficiency and nephrotic syndrome), and liver (cirrhosis). The goal of therapy is the same in each of these disorders; namely, to cause negative salt and water balance. However, since each of these edematous disorders involves a different primary organ system, the pathophysiology differs among them. In all of the edematous disorders, resistance to diuretics occurs wherein natriuretic response is less than occurs in healthy persons. The mechanism for this altered response differs in all of the conditions enumerated above. Importantly, understanding these differences allows translation to therapeutic strategies to optimize use of diuretics.

DETERMINANTS OF DIURETIC RESPONSE

All diuretics except spironolactone exert their effects from the lumen of the nephron [1-3]. As such, they must reach the urine to cause a diuresis. Routes of entry into the urine vary among diuretics. Osmotic diuretics are filtered at the glomerulus whereas other agents are actively secreted from blood into urine at the proximal tubule. Acetazolamide, loop diuretics, and thiazide diuretics are secreted by the organic acid transporter [2,4] and amiloride and triamterene gain entry via the organic base transport pathway [5,6].

Determinants of access of a diuretic into the urine can be quantified by various pharmacokinetic parameters (Table 1). Urinary diuretic excretion rate is the product of the concentration of diuretic in serum and renal clearance of the diuretic. The determinants of each of these parameters are shown in Table 1. The influence of edematous disorders on these parameters will be discussed below.

Once diuretic reaches its tubular site of action, natriuresis is a function of response of the nephron to the diuretic, so-called pharmacodynamics of response. Such response is a function of the interaction between the diuretic and the solute reabsorptive transporter it inhibits. In addition, overall response is affected by activity at other nephron sites. For example, in a patient with heart failure a loop diuretic may "normally" inhibit the Na^{+}-K^{+}-$2Cl^{-}$ transporter, but overall natriuresis may be subnormal because of increased solute reabsorption at other nephron sites such as the proximal and/or distal tubule. Ways in which edematous disorders can influence the pharmacodynamics of diuretic response will also be discussed below.

Table 1.
Pharmacokinetic determinants of diuretic response

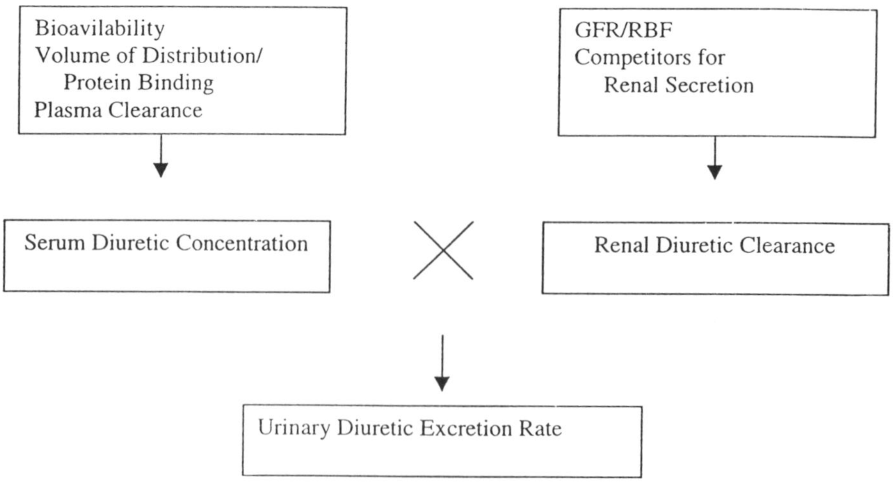

DISEASE EFFECTS ON PHARMACOKINETICS OF DIURETICS

Bioavailability

Presumably the edematous condition also includes edema of the intestinal wall, which might adversely affect drug absorption. However, several studies have shown that the bioavailability of loop diuretics is the same in patients with renal insufficiency, with both compensated and decompensated heart failure and in patients with cirrhosis [7-16]. Thus, the same quantity of diuretic is absorbed in edematous patients as compared to their healthy counterparts. The rate of absorption of loop diuretics is slowed in patients with edema, and this slowing appears to be greater in decompensated patients [13]. Whether this change in rate of absorption affects diuretic response is unknown. In general, it is unlikely that changes in absorption account for disease effects on diuretic response.

Volume of Distribution/Protein Binding

All loop diuretics are highly bound to albumin, which causes them to have small volumes of distribution, restricted in large part to the intravascular space [1-3,17,18]. In hypoalbuminemic conditions, such as nephrotic syndrome or cirrhosis, albumin binding diminishes, volume of distribution increases, and serum concentration is less [19,20]. However, it appears that the avidity of the proximal tubular secretory pathway is such that this small change in volume of distribution has negligible effect on delivery of diuretic to the active site in the lumen of the nephron. As such, patients with cirrhosis [20-23] and with nephrotic syndrome [19,24,25] deliver normal amounts of loop diuretic into the urine. Overall, then, changes in volume of distribution and protein binding are not causal of altered diuretic response in patients with edematous disorders.

Plasma Clearance

Edematous disorders affect the clearance of loop diuretics differently. Plasma clearance can be divided into that derived from the kidney and that from the liver. As will be discussed subsequently, renal dysfunction decreases access of diuretic to the site of action. Renal dysfunction, however, does not decrease overall clearance of bumetanide [26,27] and torasemide [14], because both of these loop diuretics have substantial hepatic clearance [14,26-29]. Hepatic elimination pathways compensate for declines in renal clearance. In contrast, for furosemide, renal pathways of elimination dominate so that decreases in renal clearance also result in declines in overall clearance and increases in half-life [1-3,17,18].

Conversely, in patients with cirrhosis or the congestive hepatopathy of heart failure, hepatic and total plasma clearance of bumetanide [27] and torasemide [16] decline while furosemide [20-23] is unchanged. The decreased overall clearance of bumetanide and torasemide with preserved renal clearance allows more of these two diuretics to be excreted into the urine [16,27].

Thus, diuretic resistance due to decreases in plasma clearance of a diuretic occurs when renal clearance declines.

Renal Diuretic Clearance

Renal diuretic clearance can be affected by overall declines in renal function and/or by blocking the active secretion of the diuretic into the urine. In patients with renal dysfunction, not only is GFR and RBF decreased, but the accumulated endogenous organic acids of azotemia compete with loop diuretics for active secretion [30,31]. Thus, by two mechanisms, decreased renal function results in diminished renal clearance of loop diuretics and concomitantly decreased access of loop diuretics to their site of action.

Overall, then, in terms of pharmacokinetic determinants of diuretic response, the edematous disorder in which pharmacokinetic factors are causal is renal insufficiency. In the other disorders, if renal function is satisfactory, adequate amounts of diuretic reach the site of action. The appropriate therapeutic strategy for patients with renal insufficiency is to administer sufficiently large doses to allow effective amounts of diuretic to reach the urinary site of action. In reference to Table 1, one is compensating for a decrease in renal clearance by increasing serum diuretic concentrations. This strategy is the rationale for the dosing algorithms that have been developed for patients relative to their level of renal function [32].

DISEASE EFFECTS ON PHARMACODYNAMICS OF DIURETICS

If one relates the amount of diuretic reaching the urinary site of action to natriuretic response, a sigmoidal concentration-response curve, as illustrated in Figure 1, is defined [1-3]. Changes in this relationship in edematous disorders reflect pharmacodynamic changes in response to a diuretic. Patients with nephrotic syndrome, cirrhosis, and congestive heart failure demonstrate downward shifts in this curve, as illustrated schematically in Figure 1 [1-3]. The maximal response or efficacy of the diuretic is diminished so that such patients will never have the same response as a healthy subject no matter how large a dose is administered. In

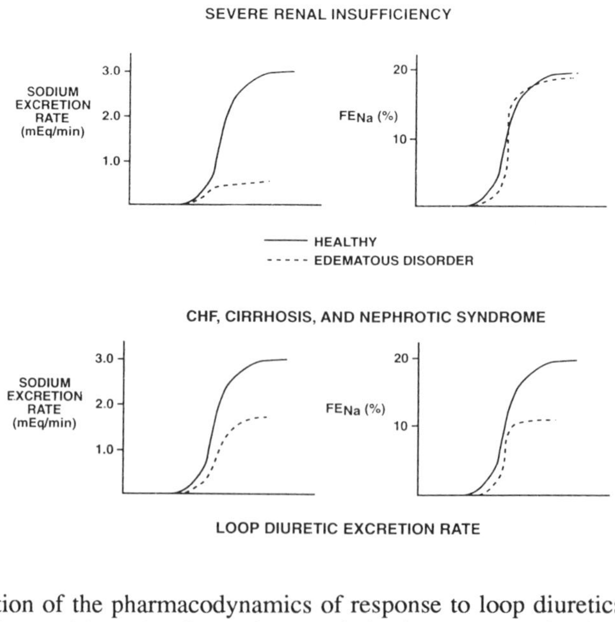

Figure 1. Illustration of the pharmacodynamics of response to loop diuretics and the change that occurs in patients with nephrotic syndrome, cirrhosis, or congestive heart failure.

fact, large doses should not be used in such patients. As discussed above, large doses are needed when there is decreased delivery of diuretic into the urine. Patients with nephrosis, cirrhosis, and heart failure do not have limitations of diuretic delivery if renal function is reasonably well preserved. Thus, large doses are superfluous. Rather frequent smaller doses should be given and/or combinations of diuretics should be used (vide infra).

The mechanism(s) by which changes in pharmacodynamics occur is unknown. Theoretically this could occur by a change in the interaction between the diuretic and the reabsorptive pathway it affects. Methods have not yet been developed that allow exploration of this possible mechanism. As noted previously, increased reabsorption of solute at either the proximal or distal tubule could also cause a diminished response to a loop diuretic. Though there has been no formal examination of these possible mechanisms, the fact that a synergistic response often ensues when a proximally or distally-acting diuretic is added to a loop diuretic implies that such mechanisms are indeed operative [33-38]. In turn, these observations suggest the utility of using combinations of diuretics in such patients. From a practical perspective, thiazide diuretics as distally-acting agents are the usual diuretics of choice since acetazolamide as the only currently available proximally-acting agent causes metabolic acidosis. In summary, then, in patients with pharmacodynamic causes of diuretic resistance, rather than using large doses of loop diuretics, combinations of loop and thiazide diuretics should be used.

SUMMARY

Changes in diuretic response can occur through pharmacokinetic or pharmacodynamic mechanisms. Renal insufficiency is the prototype of the former, which translates into a therapeutic strategy of administering large doses of loop diuretics. In patients with nephrotic syndrome, cirrhosis, and congestive heart failure, pharmacodynamic mechanisms dominate. The therapeutic strategy in these edematous disorders is to combine thiazide and loop diuretics. Thus, understanding the mechanisms by which disease affects response to diuretics extrapolates directly to therapeutics.

REFERENCES

1. Brater DC. Diuretic pharmacokinetics. IN: The *in vivo* study of drug action. Principles and applications of kinetic-dynamic modelling. Ed: CJ van Boxtel, NHG Holford, M Danhof. Elsevier Science Publishers, Amsterdam, 1992, 253-275.
2. Brater DC. Diuretics. IN: Principles of pharmacology. Basic concepts and clinical application. Ed: PL Munson, RA Mueller and GR Breese, Chapman and Hall, New York, 1995, 657-672.
3. Brater DC. Diuretic pharmacokinetics and pharmacodynamics. IN: Duretic agents: Clinical physiology and pharmacology. Ed: D. Seldin and Gieisch; Academic Press, San Diego, 1997, 189-208.
4. Odlind O. Relationship between tubular secretion of furosemide and its saluretic effect. J Pharmacol Exp Ther 1979;208:515-521.
5. Besseghir K and Rennick B. Renal tubule transport and electrolyte effects of amiloride in the chicken. J Pharmacol Exp Ther 1981;435-441.

6. Kau ST. Handling of triamterene by the isolated perfused rat kidney. J Pharmacol Exp Ther 1978;206:701-709.
7. Greither A, Goldman S, Edelen JS, Benet LZ, Cohn K. Pharmacokinetics of furosemide in patients with congestive heart failure. Pharmacol 1979;19:121-131.
8. Chaturvedi PR, O'Donnell JP, Nicholas JM, Shoenthal DR, Waters DH, Gwilt PR. Steady state absorption kinetics and pharmacodynamics of furosemide in congestive heart failure. Int J Clin Pharmacol Ther Toxicol 1987;25:123-128.
9. Bailie GR, Grennan A, Waldek S. Bioavailability of bumetanide in grossly oedematous patients. Clin Pharmacokinet 1987;12:440-443.
10. Van Meyel JJM, Gerlag PGG, Smits P, Russell FGM, Tan Y, Van Ginneken CAM, Gribnau FWJ. Absorption of high dose furosemide (frusemide) in congestive heart failure. Clin Pharmacokinet 1992;22:308-318.
11. Gottlieb SS, Khatta M, Wentworth D, Roffman D, Fisher ML, Kramer WG. The effects of diuresis on the pharmacokinetics of the loop diuretics furosemide and torsemide in patients with heart failure. Am J Med 1998;104:533-538.
12. Brater DC, Day B, Burdette A, Anderson S. Bumetanide and furosemide in heart failure. Kidney Int 1984;26:183-189.
13. Vasko MR, Cartwright DB, Knochel JP, Nixon JB, Brater DC. Furosemide absorption altered in decompensated congestive heart failure. Ann Intern Med 1985;102:314-318.
14. Gehr TWB, Rudy DW, Matzke GR, Kramer WG, Sica DA, Brater DC. The pharmacokinetics of intravenous and oral torsemide in patients with chronic renal insufficiency. Clin Pharmacol Ther 1994;56:31-38.
15. Vargo D, Kramer WG, Black PK, Smith WB, Serpas T, Brater DC. Bioavailability, pharmacokinetics, and pharmacodynamics of torsemide and furosemide in patients with congestive heart failure. Clin Pharmacol Ther 1995;57:601-609.
16. Schwartz S, Brater DC, Pound D, Greene PK, Kramer WG, Rudy D. Bioavailability, pharmacokinetics, and pharmacodynamics of torsemide in patients with cirrhosis. Clin Pharmacol Ther 1993;54:90-97.
17. Hammarlund-Udenaes M and Benet LZ. Furosemide pharmacokinetics and pharmacodynamics in health and disease — an update. J Pharmacokinet Biopharm 1989;17:1-46.
18. Beermann B and Groschinsky-Grind M. Clinical pharmacokinetics of diuretics. Clin Pharmacokinet 1980;5:221-245.
19. Rane A, Villeneuve JP, Stone WJ, Nies AS, Wilkinson GR, Branch RA. Plasma binding and disposition of furosemide in the nephrotic syndrome and in uremia. Clin Pharmacol Ther 1978;24:199-207.
20. Verbeeck RK, Patwardhan RV, Villeneuve JJP, Wilkinson GR, Branch RA. Furosemide disposition in cirrhosis. Clin Pharmacol Ther 1982;31:719-725.
21. Traeger A, Häntze R, Penzlin M, Krombholz B, Reinhardt M, Keil E, Jorke D. Pharmacokinetics and pharmacodynamic effects of furosemide in patients with liver cirrhosis. Int J Clin Pharmacol Ther Toxicol 1985;23:129-133.
22. Villeneuve JP, Verbeeck RK, Wilkinson GR, Branch RA. Furosemide kinetics and dynamics in patients with cirrhosis. Clin Pharmacol Ther 1986;40:14-20.
23. González, Arancibia A, Rivas MI, Caro P, Antezana C. Pharmacokinetics of furosemide in patients with hepatic cirrhosis. Eur J Clin Pharmacol 1982;22:315-320.
24. Keller E, Hoppe-Seyler G, Schollmeyer P. Disposition and diuretic effect of furosemide

in the nephrotic syndrome. Clin Pharmacol Ther 1982;32:442-449.
25. González-Martín G, Bravo I, Ibarra N, Arancibia A. Clinical pharmacokinetics of furosemide in children with nephrotic syndrome. Int J Clin Pharmacol Ther Toxicol 1983;21:598-601.
26. Howlett MR, Skellern GG, Auld WHR, Murdoch WR. Metabolism of the diuretic bumetanide in healthy subjects and patients with renal impairment. Eur J Clin Pharmacol 1990;38:583-586.
27. Marcantonio LA, Auld WHR, Murdoch WR, Purohit R, Skellern GG, Howes CA. The pharmacokinetics and pharmacodynamics of the diuretic bumetanide in hepatic and renal disease. Br J Clin Pharmacol 1983;15:245-252.
28. Brater DC, Leinfelder J, Anderson SA. Clinical pharmacology of torasemide, a new loop diuretic. Clin Pharmacol Ther 1987;42:187-192.
29. Schwartz MA. Metabolism of bumetanide. J Clin Pharmacol 1981;21:555-563.
30. Rose HJ, Pruitt AW, Dayton PG, McNay JL. Relationship of urinary furosemide excretion rate to natriuretic effect in experimental azotemia. J Pharmacol Exp Ther 1976;199:490-497.
31. Rose HJ, Pruitt AW, McNay JL. Effect of experimental azotemia on renal clearance of furosemide in the dog. J Pharmacol Exp Ther 1976;196:238-247.
32. Brater DC. Diuretic therapy. N Engl J Med 1998;339:387-395.
33. Sigurd B and Olesen KH. The supra-additive natriuretic effect addition of theophylline ethylenediamine and bumetanide in congestive heart failure. Am Heart J 1977;94:168-174.
34. Fliser D, Schröter M, Neubeck M, Ritz E. Coadministration of thiazides increases the efficacy of loop diuretics even in patients with advanced renal failure. Kidney Int 1994;46:482-488.
35. Knauf H and Mutschler E. Diuretic effectiveness of hydrochlorothiazide and furosemide alone and in combination in chronic renal failure. J Cardiovasc Pharmacol 1995;26:394-400.
36. Epstein M, Lepp BA, Hoffman DS, Levinson R. Potentiation of furosemide by metolazone in refractory edema. Curr Ther Res 1977;21:656-667.
37. Sica DA and Gehr TWB. Diuretic combinations in refractory oedema states: Clin Pharmacokinet 1996;30:229-249.
38. Dormans TPJ, Gerlag PGG, Russel FGM, Smits P. Combination diuretic therapy in severe congestive heart failure. Drugs 1998;55:165-172.

<u>Discussion</u>: Effect of disease on the pharmacokinetic and pharmacodynamic determinants of response to diuretics

J. Urquhart:

If you continue with the normal subject which you began with, and you do not replace the salt and you come back and do the same thing the next day, you get a minuscule response. How come?

D.C. Brater:

There are two forms of tolerance that have been described. One occurs very quickly. If you administer a continuous intravenous infusion of a loop diuretic, within hours the response relative to the amount of diuretic reaching the site of action becomes less. Studies have shown that development of acute tolerance can be prevented simply by restoring volume losses. Presumably, this is occurring by activation of homeostatic reflexes to protect us against volume depletion. These reflexes are multiple and include activation of the renin-angiotensin system, activating the sympathetic nervous system and perhaps other pathways. All these stimuli increase proximal tubular reabsorption of sodium. There is another form of tolerance that develops with chronic therapy. It has been shown to occur in rats, and probably occurs in humans. If you block the reabsorption of solute in the thick ascending limb, sodium floods downstream, bathing distal nephrons. Over time (in the rat this takes about a week), these distal nephrons hypertrophy, and their reabsorptive capacity for sodium increases four to fivefold. Importantly from a therapeutic perspective these nephrons are where the thiazide diuretics exert their effects. As such if this pathophysiology is occurring and a thiazide diuretic is added, then patients have a substantial diuresis; not only is response restored, but a truly synergistic effect can occur with a massive diuresis.

D.A. Smith:

It was just a query on the nephrotic syndrome experiments you performed in the rat. I guess the critical point is the concentration of the albumin you use, which I think was 3.8 M, which is about half the molar concentration of the drug. I was wondering how that was chosen. And secondly, when I looked at the response curve you showed at the end of your presentation, it appeared to be superimposable before going to a lower maximum, whereas my understanding of the albumin would be that you had actually shift it to the right.

D.C. Brater:

The chosen albumin concentration was based on creating a rat model of nephrotic syndrome by administering an aminonucleoside. In these animals nephrones can be micropunctured to measure the amount of albumin that is present. We used such values to determine how much albumin to use. We performed prior *in vitro* studies to determine albumin binding to furosemide. In other words, there was substantial background work that determined selection of these different concentrations we used. We wanted them to be concentrations that reflected what one would see in that clinical condition and with using standard doses of diuretics. In terms of the response curve in the nephrotic syndrome, indeed the binding ought to shift that curve to some degree. The data I shoed are published from another group and are not our studies, so I can not provide an explanation for that observations. In studies from the University of Michigan, a shift rightward in the relationship does occur.

L. Aarons:

I wonder whether you could comment on the use of creatinine clearance to mark active secretion, both for diuretics and, more generally, for other drugs?

D.C. Brater:

Creatinine clearance is a hybrid form of clearance, because there is a secretory component to creatinine's elimination in the urine. Its level of precision is quite low, and if you want to obtain a high-level of precision, one must use more gold standards such as inulin, GFR, or p-aminohippurate for renal blood flow. Usually GFR and RBF change in parallel. There are situations where this parallel relationship is disrupted. For example, probenecid blocks secretion of loop diuretics into the urine. In this circumstance the creatinine clearance has no relationship to the amount of drug reaching the site of action.

Effects of exercise on human drug response

Marleen A. van Baak

NUTRIM, Department of Human Biology, Maastricht University, Maastricht, The Netherlands

ABSTRACT

Increased physical activity is currently advised to many patients with a variety of diseases for therapeutic reasons, but also for reasons of general well being and health. Therefore, many patients on drug therapy are nowadays involved in regular exercise. In view of these large number it is surprising that relatively little is known about the interaction between exercise and the response to drug treatment in these active patients. On theoretical grounds both acute exercise and exercise training may be expected to influence the response to drugs by their effect on parameters involved in the pharmacokinetics of these drugs. The acute effects of exercise include changes in haemodynamics, enzyme activities, pH, plasma protein concentration, temperature and gastrointestinal function. Therefore, absorption, distribution and clearance may all be affected by acute exercise. In addition, exercise training may lead to more permanent adaptations that also pertain to the resting situation. The effects of exercise will vary among drugs, because of differences in physicochemical properties. Clinically relevant interactions between drugs and exercise are most likely in those drugs with a steep dose-response curve, a narrow therapeutic range, the need for continuous therapeutic efficacy and a short half-life.

Key words: pharmacokinetics, exercise, training, drug response, human, interaction.

Correspondence: Dr. Marleen A. van Baak, Department of Human Biology, Maastricht University, P.O.Box 616, 6200 MD MAASTRICHT, The Netherlands, Tel: +31-43-388-1630, Fax: +31-43-367-0976, Email: m.vanbaak@hb.unimaas.nl

INTRODUCTION

Interindividual variability in human drug response can result from pharmacokinetic as well as pharmacokinetic variability between individuals. For a long time it has been assumed that most of the variation in human drug response was due to interindividual pharmacokinetic differences. More recently it has become evident that pharmacodynamic variability, i.e. the variability in the relationship between pharmacological effect intensity and drug concentration,

may also be substantial and reproducible in humans, and often more pronounced than pharmacokinetic variability [1].
Exercise is one of the factors that may affect human drug response. On theoretical grounds both acute exercise and exercise training may be expected to influence the response to drugs by their effect on parameters involved in the pharmacokinetics of these drugs. Moreover, factors that may account for pharmacodynamic variability, such as receptor density and affinity, the concentration of endogenous ligands, postreceptor transduction processes, homeostatic responses and transport processes [1], may also be affected by exercise.

Increased physical activity and regular exercise are currently advised to many patients with a variety of diseases for therapeutic reasons, but also for reasons of general well-being and health. Therefore, many patients on drug therapy are nowadays involved in regular exercise. In view of these large numbers it is surprising that relatively little is known about the interaction between exercise and the response to drug treatment in these active patients.

ACUTE EXERCISE AND PHARMACOKINETICS

On theoretical grounds both acute exercise and exercise training may be expected to influence the response to drugs by their effect on parameters involved in the pharmacokinetics of these drugs. The acute effects of exercise include changes in haemodynamics, enzyme activities, pH, plasma protein concentration, temperature and gastrointestinal function. Therefore, absorption, distribution and clearance may all be affected by acute exercise. In addition, exercise training may lead to more permanent adaptations that also pertain to the resting situation. The effects of exercise will vary among drugs, because of differences in physicochemical properties.

In 1990 and 1991 the interaction between exercise and the pharmacokinetics of drugs has been extensively reviewed [2,3,4]. The reviews concluded that only few studies had really investigated the effects of exercise on pharmacokinetics and that more studies were needed to complete the picture. One review [2] stressed that although there are indications that acute exercise and exercise training may affect the pharmacokinetics of certain drugs, there is hardly any evidence for clinically relevant effects. Either because the drug showing an interaction would not be used in combination with exercise, or because the demonstrated effects were clinically insignificant. A notable exception is the effect of exercise on the absorption of insulin from subcutaneous or intramuscular injection sites, which is associated with increased plasma insulin concentration and reduced plasma glucose levels [5,6]. It was concluded that clinically relevant interactions between drugs and exercise are most likely in those drugs with a steep dose-response curve, a narrow therapeutic range, the need for continuous therapeutic efficacy and a short half-life. The literature on the interaction between exercise and pharmacokinetics since 1990 has been reviewed for this paper, in order to see whether any advances have been made and whether these conclusions are still valid.

Exercise and absorption

In 1990 it was concluded that exercise, if anything, was likely to reduce the gastrointestinal absorption of drugs, although there were no experimental data to support this [2,3]. In 1992 a study was published by Strömberg *et al* [7] investigating the effects of 50 minute aerobic treadmill exercise on the pharmacokinetics of orally administered midazolam and ephedrine. The absorption coefficient (K_a) of midazolam was significantly reduced by exercise (from 0.10±0.06 to 0.04±0.03 L/min), the K_a of ephedrine was also lowered (from 0.031±0.015 to 0.024±0.011 L/min), but this difference was not statistically significant. The T_{max}, time to reach peak plasma concentration, was increased by exercise in both drugs, although differences did not reach statistical significance. Both the decreased K_a and T_{max} are suggestive for a reduced rate of absorption with exercise.

In contrast to the effects on gastrointestinal absorption, the effect of exercise on subcutaneous and intramuscular absorption is relatively well studied, although the studies mainly concern the effect of exercise on insulin absorption. In the 70ties and 80ties it was shown that exercise increases the absorption of insulin from active tissues and this effect was due probably due to the massageing effect of muscle contractions rather than to changes in local blood flow [5,6,2]. An additional study showed that environmental temperature also affects insulin absorption. Although there was no synergism between exercise and environmental temperature, the most rapid absorption of insulin and the lowest plasma glucose concentrations were found during exercise at high environmental temperatures [8]. It was concluded that to avoid hypoglycemia after exercise at warm temperatures appropriate adjustments in diet and insulin dose should be made [8]. When comparing the effects of exercise on the absorption of insulin from subcutaneous and intramuscular injection sites in the thigh, it was shown that exercise affects absorption from intramuscular sites much stronger than from subcutaneous sites: the peak plasma free immunoreactive insulin (IRI) was 39 mU/L higher, the area under the IRI curve was 80% greater and the decrease in plasma glucose was 2mM greater after intramuscular than after subcutaneous injection [9]. It was concluded that the risk of accidental intramuscular injection of insulin should be minimised by injection into a skinfold or by use of shorter needles [9].

In most studies of transdermal drug administration, total drug absorption and plasma drug concentration have increased during heat exposure. This phenomenon appears to be mediated by acceleration of skin blood flow. Other contributing factors may be changes in the physicochemical properties of transdermal patches, sweating and increased humidity of the skin. At temperatures above 30°C 1.5 to 2.5-fold increases in plasma concentrations have been found [10]. Exercise also enhances skin blood flow, at least at relatively low exercise intensities, sweating and skin humidity and may therefore have similar effects on transdermal absorption as heat exposure [2]. Since the 80ties no further studies addressing the effect of exercise on transdermal absorption have been published.

Exercise and distribution

In the 1990/1991 reviews it was shown that the volume of distribution of drugs may increase or decrease during exercise, depending on the physicochemical properties of the drug (high or low plasma protein and tissue binding) and pH and blood flow changes during exercise [2,3]. Strömberg *et al* [7] demonstrated an increase in the apparent volume of distribution of midazolam after oral administration. It remains unclear whether this reduction is due to a reduced absorption/availability of midazolam or to an actual change in the volume of distribution. The apparent volume of distribution of ephedrine, on the other hand, did not change by exercise [7]. A study in horses showed that the steady-state volume of distribution of cortisol was significantly increased during a 56-km endurance exercise [11]. In contrast, the distribution volume of caffeine was found to be significantly reduced during exercise [12].

In rats acute exercise increased the rate of decarbamylation of physostigmine in red blood cells, brain and heart, but decreased it in diaphragm and skeletal muscle. Therefore, acute exercise reduced the central anticholinesterase efficacy of physostigmine treatment. The investigators suggest that the differences between the various tissues may be due to tissue-specific blood flow changes during exercise [13].

Exercise and clearance

Most studies reviewed in 1990/1991 [2,3,4] were unable to demonstrate an effect of exercise on the pharmacokinetics of drugs with a low hepatic extraction ratio. The only exception being a study on theophylline, where a 25% increase in clearance was found over an 8-hour period including 2 hours of exercise [14]. This finding had not been replicated or supported by additional studies. A study on the effect of exercise on the elimination of caffeine, a low extraction drug metabolised by liver enzymes, showed an unchanged clearance, assuming a 100% bioavailability after oral administration [12]. A recent review on the effects of environmental temperature on the elimination of low clearance drugs indicates that there is not much evidence for an acute effect of an increase in temperature on hepatic drug metabolism [10]. This suggests that it is also unlikely that the temperature elevation associated with exercise affects the clearance of low extraction drugs.

In contrast to low extraction drugs, the clearance of high extraction drugs by the liver is generally assumed to be reduced by exercise, due to the reduction of liver blood flow [2,3,4]. Nevertheless, significant reductions of clearance by exercise are often not found [2,3,15,16].

Renal elimination of drugs depends on filtration, secretion, reabsorption and urine flow, which may all be affected by exercise. In general the clearance of drugs by the kidneys is was found to be reduced during exercise [2]. Gillies *et al* [17] showed that the urinary content of pseudoephedrine measured over 6 hours, with or without a 40-km time trial on a cycle ergometer, did not differ, although the urinary pseudoephedrine concentration was increased on the exercise day. However, plasma pseudoephedrine concentration was increased during exercise, suggesting that renal clearance may actually have been reduced. On the other hand Strömberg *et al* [7] found that the apparent clearance of ephedrine, a drug largely excreted unchanged in the urine, was unchanged by exercise. Plasma ephedrine concentration and apparent volume of distribution were also unaffected. However, since the effect of exercise on the availability of ephedrine after oral administration is unknown, these results are difficult to interpret.

Clearance by extrarenal and extrahepatic mechanisms can also change during exercise, as shown by Lassourd *et al* [18] for the clearance of intravenously administered ^{3}H-cortisol in horses. The large increase of plasma cortisol clearance could not be explained by changes in clearance of classical organs such as liver, kidney and lungs. It was suggested that the muscles might have been responsible for the increased clearance of cortisol, in association with the increase in muscle blood flow during exercise.

In conclusion, since 1990 only a limited number of additional studies on the effects of acute exercise on pharmacokinetics of drugs has been published. These new data in general support the conclusions of previous reviews [2,3,4].

EXERCISE TRAINING AND PHARMACOKINETICS

In 1980 Frenkl and coworkers [19] introduced the concept of the 'trained liver'. They demonstrated that athletes had a higher antipyrine elimination rate than non-athletes. Antipyrine is metabolised extensively by the cytochrome P450 liver enzymes. It shows negligible protein binding and its elimination is not limited by liver blood flow. Other cross-sectional studies have confirmed these results [20,21]. The only longitudinal training study performed in humans showed that the hepatic clearance of aminopyrine and antipyrine increased by 13% and 12% respectively with training [22]. The increase in hepatic metabolism was correlated with the increase in VO_2max.

Furthermore, a small number of longitudinal training studies has been performed in rats. Frenkl *et al* [23] showed that liver P450 content and antipyrine elimination was increased after swimming training in Wistar rats. In contrast, running training for 8 weeks inhibited the microsomal metabolism of p-nitroanisole and aniline, whereas the metabolism of ethoxyresorufin was not significantly affected in Fisher-344 rats. This suggests that the various P450 isozymes have different sensitivities towards exercise training. The total P450 content was reduced 30% in exercised rats [24]. An additional finding in this study was that the hepatotoxic action of CCl_4 was completely prevented in rats after exercise training. CCl_4 is reduced to a trichloromethyl radical by the same P450 isozyme that is involved in aniline metabolism [24]. When exercise training by swimming and running were compared, running training was shown to reduce the hepatic microsomal P450 content and activity, whilst swimming training tended to increase P450 content and aniline metabolism [25]. It was suggested that it was the exposure to water rather than the exercise training that resulted in these changes in swimming rats [25]. A study which investigated the effects of running training on the clearance of ethanol at rest in Sprague-Dawley rats showed an increase in ethanol clearance. Since the in vitro alcohol dehydrogenase activity was not affected by training, other metabolic pathways, for instance stimulation of the hepatic cytochrome P450-dependent mixed-function oxidase system, may have been responsible for this increased ethanol clearance [26].

Only one study has looked at the effects of exercise training on renal drug metabolism. Piatowski *et al* [27] showed that running training increased the renal phase I drug metabolism without affecting phase II processes.

In conclusion, although in humans cross-sectional studies and a single longitudinal study all seem to indicate that exercise training increases the capacity of the liver for drug metabolism, the results from training studies in rats are equivocal. Clearly more studies are needed in this area to be able to fully understand the effect of exercise training on the pharmacokinetics of drugs.

EXERCISE AND PHARMACODYNAMICS

Pharmacodynamic variability can be defined as interindividual variability in the plasma concentration-effect relationship. Factors that may account for pharmacodynamic variability, such as receptor density and affinity, the concentration of endogenous ligands, postreceptor transduction processes, homeostatic responses and transport processes [1], may all be affected by exercise. However, no information on the effect of acute or chronic exercise on parameters of pharmacodynamic variability, such as the coefficient of variation of the EC_{50}, is available. Nevertheless, there are indications of pharmacodynamic interactions with exercise and some examples will be presented.

A 15 min treadmill running exercise at moderate intensity has been shown to increase the behavioral sensitivity to the carbamate cholinesterase inhibitor physostigmine in untrained and trained rats [28]. Exercise training reduced the behavioral sensitivity to carbamates due to an exercise bout, when the animals had been resting for at least 72 hours after the last exercise bout [28]. This suppressing effect of exercise training was also shown for other centrally acting drugs such as midazolam, scopolamine and benactyzine [29]. Whether this effect of acute exercise was due to the exercise *per se* or to the stress associated with exercise is not known. However, stress induced by forced swimming has been shown to disrupt the blood brain barrier for physostigmine and pyridostigmine in mice, resulting in CNS-mediated side effects [30]. Exercise training may decrease the stress of an acute exercise bout and thus partly prevent the central effects induced by acute exercise.

The response to β-adrenoceptor agonist stimulation before and after acute exercise has been compared in two studies. In one study the responsiveness of heart rate, diastolic blood pressure and lower extremity blood flow to the β-adrenoceptor agonist isoprenaline was found to be unchanged between 20 and 60 minutes after 1 hour exercise at low or high intensity [31]. In contrast, the systolic blood pressure response to isoprenaline was blunted after high intensity exercise which may be a manifestation of reduced cardioinotropic sensitivity. In the other study the dose of isoprenaline needed to increase heart rate by 25 beats/min was increased at 15 minutes after prolonged (95 min) exercise. The increase in dose was closely correlated with the reduction of the ejection fraction , suggesting reduced chronotropic sensitivity. Circulating lymphocyte β-adrenoceptor density and affinity and adenylate cyclase levels were unchanged after exercise [32]. Therefore, certain but not all β-adrenoceptor mediated responses may be blunted after acute exercise, but the mechanism remains to be elucidated.

Studies in rats suggest that exercise training may affect β-adrenoceptor densities, adenylate cyclase activity and G-protein content. However, the effects appear to vary among tissues and the data are far from consistent. For instance skeletal muscle β-adrenoceptor density has been found increased [33], unchanged [34], and reduced [35] after exercise training in the rat.

Cross-sectional and longitudinal studies indicate that endurance exercise training increases in vitro lipolytic responsiveness to catecholamines of adipocytes in humans. Since the density of receptors does not appear to change with training, the increased responsiveness appears to be a post-receptor adaptation, probably at the level of hormone-sensitive lipase [36]. β-Receptor density also does not change with training in human skeletal muscle [37]. In addition the heart rate and calf blood flow response to the b-adrenoceptor agonist isoprenaline did not change with training [31].

Exercise has been shown to improve the decreased response to a flicker fusion test after midazolam. The flicker fusion test is a sensitive test for measuring the sedative effects of psychotropic drugs. However, it could not be ascertained whether this effect was solely due to the pharmacokinetic changes or to the general alerting effect of exercise [7].

These examples show that it is likely that acute and chronic exercise influence drug response by pharmacodynamic mechanisms, although pharmacokinetic influences in some cases have not been fully excluded.

In summary, acute and chronic exercise may influence drug response by pharmacokinetic as well as pharmacodynamic mechanisms. Exercise and training status should therefore be considered in studies on human drug response. On the other hand, few clinically relevant effects of exercise or exercise training on drug response have been described up till now.

REFERENCES

1. Levy G. Predicting effective drug concentrations for individual patients. Clin Pharmacokin 1998;34:323-333.
2. van Baak MA. Influence of exercise on the pharmacokinetics of drugs. Clin Pharmacokin 1990;19:32-43.
3. Somani SM, Gupta SK, Frank S, Corder CC. Effect of exercise on drug disposition and pharmacokinetics of drugs. Drug Dev Res 1990;20:251-275.
4. Ylitalo P. Effect of exercise on pharmacokinetics. Ann Med 1991;23:289-294.
5. Koivisto VA, Felig P. Effects of leg exercise on insulin absorption in diabetic patients. New Engl J Med 1978;298:79-83.
6. Fernqvist E, Linde B, Östman J, Gunnarsson R. Effect of physical exercise on insulin absorption in insulin-dependent diabetics: a comparison between human and porcine insulin. Clin Physiol 1986;6:489-498.
7. Strömberg C, Vanakoski J, Olkkola KT, Lindqvist A, Seppällä T, Laitinen LA. Exercise alters the pharmacokinetics of midazolam. Clin Pharmacol Ther 1992;51:527-532.
8. Rönnemaa T, Koivisto VA. Combined effect of exercise and ambient temperature on insulin absorption and postprandial glycemia in type 1 patients. Diabetes Care 1988;11:769-773.
9. Frid A, Östman J, Linde B. Hypoglycemia risk during exercise after intramuscular injection of insulin in thigh in IDDM. Diabetes Care 1990;13:473-477.
10. Vanakoski J, Seppällä T. Heat exposure and drugs. A review of the effects of hyperthermia on pharmacokinetics. Clin Pharmacokin 1998;34:311-322.
11. Lassourd V, Gayrard V, Laroute V, Alvinerie M, Benard P, Courtot D, Toutain PL. Cortisol disposition and production rate in horses during rest and exercise. Am J Physiol 1996;271:R25-R33.
12. Collomp K, Anselme F, Audran M, Gay JP, Chanal JL, Prefaut C. Effects of moderate exercise on the pharmacokinetics of caffeine. Eur J Clin Pharmacol 1991;40:279-282.
13. Dube SN, Somani SM, Babu SR. Concurrent exercise alters central and peripheral responses to physostigmine. Pharmacol Biochem Behav 1993;46:827-834.
14. Schlaeffer F, Engelberg I, Kaplanski J, Danon A. Effects of exercise and environmental heat on theophylline kinetics. Respiration 1984;45:438-442.
15. Arends BG, Böhm ROB, van Kemenade JE, Rahn KH, van Baak MA. Influence of physical exercise on the pharmacokinetics of propranolol. Eur J Clin Pharmacol 1986;31:375-377.
16. Mooy J, Arends B, van Kemenade J, Böhm R, Rahn KH, van Baak M. Influence of prolonged submaximal exercise on the pharmacokinetics of verapamil in humans. J Cardiovasc Pharmacol 1986;8:940-942.

17. Gillies H, Derman WE, Noakes TD, Smith P, Evans A, Gabriels G. Pseudoephedrine is without ergogenic effects during prolonged exercise. J Appl Physiol 1996;81:2611-2617.
18. Lassourd V, Gayrard V, Laroute V, Alvinerie M, Benard P, Courtot D, Toutain PL. Cortisol disposition and production rate in horses during rest and exercise. Am J Physiol 1996;271:R25-R33.
19. Frenkl R, Györe Á, Mészáros J, Szeberényi Sz. A study of the enzyme inducing effect of physical training in man. The "trained liver". J Sports Med 1980;20:371-376.
20. Orioli S, Bandinelli I, Birardi A, Chieca R, Buzzelli G, Chiarantini E. Hepatic antipyrine metabolism in athletes. J Sports Med Phys Fitness 1990;30:261-263.
21. Villa JG, Cuadrado G, Bayón JE, González-Gallego J. The effect of physical conditioning on antipyrine clearance. Eur J Appl Physiol 1998;77:106-111.
22. Boel J, Andersen LB, Rasmussen B, Hansen SH, Døssing M. Hepatic drug metabolism and physical fitness. Clin Pharmacol Ther 1984;36:121-126.
23. Frenkl R, Györe Á, Szeberényi Sz. The effect of muscular exercise on the microsomal enzyme system of the rate liver. Eur J Appl Physiol 1980;44:135-140.
24. Day WW, Weiner M. Inhibition of hepatic drug metabolism and carbon tetrachloride toxicity in Fischer-344 rats by exercise. Biochem Pharmacol 1991;42:181-184.
25. Day WW, Chesky JA, Weiner M. Differential effects of swimming and running on microsomal metabolism in middle-aged and aged Fischer 344 rats. Mech Ageing Dev 1992;63:275-286.
26. Ardies CM, Morris GS, Erickson CK, Farrar RP. Both acute and chronic exercise enhance in vivo ethanol clearance in rats. J Appl Physiol 1989;66:555-560.
27. Piatowski TS, Day WW, Weiner M. Increased renal drug metabolism in treadmill-exercised Fischer-344 male rats. Drug Metabol Dispos 1993;21:474-479.
28. McMaster SB, Finger AV. Effects of exercise on behavioral sensitivity to carbamate cholinesterase inhibitors. Pharmacol Biochem Behav 1989;33:811-813.
29. McMaster SB, Carney JM. Chronic exercise produces tolerance to muscarinic antagonists in rats. Pharmacol Biochem Behav 1986;24:865-868.
30. Friedman A, Kaufer D, Shemer J, Hendler I, Soreq H, Tur-Kaspa I. Pyridostigmine brain penetration under stress enhances neuronal excitability and induces early immediate transcriptional response. Nature Med 1996;2:1382-1385.
31. Martin III WH, Spina RJ, Korte E, Ogawa T. Effects of chronic and acute exercise on cardiovascular β-adrenergic responses. J Appl Physiol 1991;71:1523-1528.
32. Eysmann SB, Gervino E, Vatner DE, Katz SE, Decker L, Douglas P. Prolonged exercise alters β-adrenergic responsiveness in healthy sedentary humans. J Appl Physiol 1996;80:616-622.
33. Buckenmeyer PJ, Goldfarb AH, Partilla JS, Pineyro MA, Dax EM. Endurance training, not acute exercise, differentially alters b-receptors and cyclase in skeletal fiber types. Am J Physiol 1990;258:E71-E77.
34. Fell RD, Lizzo FH, Cervoni P, Crandall DL. Effect of contractile activity on rat skeletal muscle beta-adrenoceptor properties. Proc Soc Exp Biol Med 1985;180:527-532.
35. Nieto JL, Diaz-Laviada I, Malpartida JM, Galve-Roperh I, Haro A. Adaptations to the beta-adrenoceptor-adenylyl cyclase system in rat skeletal muscle to endurance physical training. Pflügers Arch 1997;434:809-814.

36. Nicklas BJ. Effects of endurance exercise on adipose tissue metabolism. Exerc Sport Sci Rev 1997;25:77-103.

Discussion: Effects of exercise on human drug response

M. Lader:

There are some natural disease states which are essentially mimicking some of the effects of exercise, such as generalised anxiety disorder. Forearm blood flow in these patients, even at rest, is something like five to tenfold over the normal resting levels, so it is quite a dynamic circulation. You will need a higher dose of a sedative drug, a barbiturate or a benzodiazepine, in order to reach a sort of sedation end-point.

M. van Baak:

I do not think that you can characterise the human dynamic state that you reach by exercise training as a hyperkinetic state at rest, because usually the system is depressed a little bit in well-trained people. This activated system only appears during the exercise, although this period is so short compared with the half-life of drugs. It is hard to study the effect of drugs during exercise itself, because exercise has such a profound effect on its own that it is very difficult to find out what is the effect of exercise and what is the drug response.

M.M. Reidenberg:

Is it your judgement that few clinically relevant effects have been identified because there are few or because we are missing them?

M. van Baak:

I think there must be big pharmacodynamic effects because the exercise-trained individual really is very different, metabolically and hemodynamically, from an untrained individual. But, on the other hand, there are not many patients on drug therapy that will be that well trained. I think the reason that this area has not attracted much attention may be because people are just not triggered to it, but also that the effects that have been shown until now are really not clinically important.

N. Benowitz:

Acute effects of exercise on transdermal drug absorption have been shown, at least for nicotine. When temperature of the skin goes up and blood flow goes up, you can anticipate a faster absorption. In some situations, maybe clonidine or other drugs, that could matter.

M. van Baak:

It has been shown that plasma concentrations of nitroglycerin after transdermal administration are very much increased during and after the exercise. If you compare for instance to sauna, the increases are even higher. There have been no clinical effects measured in these studies, so it is hard to extrapolate any data on resulting drug effects.

A.J.J. Wood:

We have previously seen frailty as an index of extreme aging and now some data in which the elderly are trained. There are studies looking at the effects of training in the elderly on cardiovascular and osteoporosis indices. Perhaps it may be a relevant link to the training, because presumably we could make some of the elderly less frail if we trained them better.

There have been attempts to do that in some studies. Does Mark Kinirons want to comment on that?

M. Kinirons:

Mary Tinetti in Connecticut has published consistent data showing that multidisciplinary exercise programmes can improve cardiovascular responsiveness in those kind of frail elderly who fall (Tinetti M *et al.*, N Engl J Med, 1994), and that training can reduce the risk of falling. It is possible to predict that would also change their sensitivity to drugs that impair balance.

Variability in Human Drug Response
G.T. Tucker, Editor

Benefit risk evaluation of medicinal products - an epidemiological approach

Carlos Martinez

Hoechst Marion Roussel, Inc, Bridgewater, NJ, USA.

ABSTRACT

A fair comparison of the benefit/risk of drugs requires a separate estimation of both benefit and risk of each drug. Prerequisites before evaluation are: definition of the perspective of evaluation, definition of indication for drug use and definition of alternative treatment strategies. The benefit measure corresponds to the efficacy which strictly depends on the indication for drug use. Comparative estimates can only be obtained from randomized clinical trials. The evaluation of drug-attributed risks includes the following steps: define profile of ADRs of drug and comparator(s), obtain background incidence of each ADR, define common outcome measure and ADR-specific values, estimate excess incidence rate of each ADR by treatment strategy, select a common outcome unit and determine weights to permit comparison across ADRs, estimate adjusted excess incidence of each reaction with the weighting factor, sum weighed excess incidence rates for each treatment strategy, calculate net risk difference of drug-attributed risks, discuss validity of results and update evaluation when new eligible studies become published. Drug specific benefit/risk estimates could be expressed as the difference between benefits and risks, if the unit of measurement of benefits and risks is identical for all treatments only or by the benefit/risk ratio otherwise.

Key words: risk, benefit, adverse drug reaction (ADR).

Correspondence: Carlos Martínez, MD, MSc, Hoechst Marion Roussel Inc, Route 202-206, P.O.Box 6800, Bridgewater, NJ 08807-0800, USA, Tel: +1-908-231-5667, Fax: +1-908-231-4827, Email: carlos.martinez@hmrag.com

INTRODUCTION

A fair comparison of benefits risks of drugs requires a separate estimation of both the benefit and the risk of each drug. A fair comparison also implies that the medicines are comparable. The indications for drug use, the patient population including age and gender distribution, and the duration of treatment need to be alike for drugs aimed at such conditions as postoperative pain, community-acquired pneumonia or type I diabetes.

The following methodological framework elaborates the means to weigh the benefits and risks of new medicines against standard treatment. This framework intends to standardize the procedure of benefit and risk assessment from the point of view of health authorities or pharmaceutical firms, and to serve as a guidance for health authorities whose intention is to maximize health. Furthermore, the benefit-risk assessment is of primary importance to manufacturers, whose responsibility is to assess continually the benefit-risk balance of new medicines, particularly after marketing when the indication of new medicines is broadened or after new drug-attributed adverse events are identified.

This approach will result in a benefit-risk assessment that in most cases will be comparative. Since benefit-risk evaluations are only valid for drugs given for a single defined illness, this approach will not supply a benefit-risk score that will be valid for medicines used for different indications. The methodological approach will provide a score that could be used for competing drugs given for a defined indication or illness.

Although the risk of medicines can be measured, the safety of drugs is considered to be a judgment. The safety of drugs is a composite measure of benefits and risks. Our approach does not intend to change the current practice in clinical trials. It intends to use the knowledge that is already available.

BENEFIT ESTIMATION

Clinical efficacy of new compounds is usually not demonstrated by the proportion of prevented or postponed deaths, life-years gained or quality-adjusted life-years gained, i.e. direct measures of benefit. Primary endpoints in randomized clinical trials are intermediate parameters (surrogate endpoints) believed to be correlated with measures of direct benefit.

In this section the different measures of benefit as used in randomized clinical trials are reviewed and the potential benefits discussed.

1. Benefit measured as an intermediate parameter

Randomized clinical trials are the gold standard to test the efficacy of new medicines compared to placebo or commonly used effective medication. Randomization reduces bias and variability between randomized groups. Randomization generates comparable heterogeneous cohorts, i.e. the likelihood that patients in each cohort possess a given characteristic is similar. Thus, any difference in the frequency of outcomes in each group is attributable to the effect of the clinical intervention, i.e. the allocated treatment strategy.

Randomized clinical trials can have three results: (1) the new medicine is less efficacious than the comparator, (2) the new medicine is equivalent - the most common situation in real life and (3) the new medicine is more efficacious than the comparator.

Traditional measures of efficacy are intermediate parameters or surrogate endpoints that depend on the indication for drug use. Surrogate endpoints include diagnostic procedures, e.g. laboratory tests for such things as blood glucose level, cholesterol level or antibiograms; functional status such as blood pressure or ECG changes after exercise tolerance tests and forced expiratory volume at one second (FEV_1) in asthmatics; imaging procedures such as X-ray, CAT scan, ECG or ultrasound; symptom relief (particularly for pain, fever, inflammation), quality of life and other important disease-specific measures of efficacy. Advantages of cohorts can include information regarding time dependent variables such as changes in daily dose of any medication or smoking habits and total cumulative dose and the defined dose for which a clinical benefit is claimed.

For intermediate clinical endpoints an association with quality of life, morbidity or mortality is assumed; however, it is not routinely demonstrated as in morbidity or mortality studies, e.g. decreased mortality of cardiovascular events after secondary prevention of myocardial infarction with cholesterol-lowering medicines. As a consequence, long treatment duration and observation, differential loss to follow-up, patients' compliance and large sample sizes necessary to detect a significant difference would require expensive and time-consuming studies that could withhold efficacious medicines from patients.

2. Benefit measured as cumulative mortality or mortality rate

In mortality studies clinical benefit is measured by the number of prevented or postponed deaths. Mortality rates obtained in cohort studies are comparative and can either be compared with a do-nothing strategy such as aspirin in primary prevention of myocardial infarction (Physicians Health Study) [1], or with standard treatment or another medicine of interest. The measure of clinical outcome such as death is attributed to the treatment strategy as allocated by randomization. In any case, mortality studies provide strategy-specific cumulative mortalities or mortality rates, i.e. number of deaths in each treatment strategy divided either by the respective population at risk or by the accumulated person-time exposure in an intention-to-treat analysis. Total person-time exposure corresponds to the sum of person-time accumulated by individuals according to the primary assignment to a treatment strategy with the assumption that all subjects were compliant with the study protocol.

The differences and ratios of cumulative mortalities or mortality rates provide an estimate of the comparative benefit of the medicines studied. Differences provide a more informative estimate than ratios since differences inform us of the amount of prevented or postponed deaths in a defined population, i.e. provide an estimate for the number of prevented or postponed deaths attributable to a particular medicine in a defined population.

3. Benefits measured as life-years gained

Life-years gained is usually not a primary endpoint in studies submitted to registration authorities. Non-registration clinical studies have increasingly been used as a vehicle for pharmacoeconomic studies in which the clinical efficacy of a new medicine is translated into more useful natural units such as life-years gained, which are inherently built into mortality studies. Life-years gained could be calculated either from mortality data by modeling or directly from raw data (area between two Kaplan-Meier curves corresponds to the time, e.g. life-years, gained by the treatment strategy corresponding to the upper curve). The number of life-years gained attributable to a medicine could be considered as the benefit of a medicine from a societal viewpoint. The difference in life-years gained attributable to a medicine, however, does not consider the quality of life of patients whose death was prevented or postponed.

Example: In cancer therapy a new drug may postpone death, but may result in a lower quality of life because of the adverse events and repeated regimens of radiotherapy or chemotherapy.

4. Benefit measured as quality-adjusted life-years

Quality-adjusted life-years (QALYs) is a composite index that reflects the number of life-years gained, weighted by the quality of life of each of these years. Quality of life is the individual's subjective perception of his or her physical, emotional and social well-being, after taking the effects of a disease and its treatment into account. The components of quality of life differ by the scale used but in general include physical, social, emotional and functional well-being. The evaluation of new therapies to measure health outcomes have three principle components: (1) detection of changes of health status by defining the key domains of interest (description), (2) comparative quantification of quality of life changes by determining the means of weighting elements within the descriptive system (valuation), and (3) the determination of aggregate (dis)benefit.

Quality of life measures yield a profile or an ordinal or cardinal index. Indices can be used to quantify quality of life changes, a very important measure in benefit-risk evaluation. Health utility scores rank from 0 to 100. Complete health is anchored as 100 and death as 0. The advantage of health utility scores is that drug-related mortality and drug-related morbidity are integrated into one risk score. The patient's change of quality of life is integrated as well.

Benefits can be measured in QALYs. Different methods can be used, e.g. the time-trade-off method, standard gamble, or any quality of life scale that allows the generation of an index in a cardinal scale. The underlying principle is that different health outcomes can be valued in terms of the individual's preferences under conditions of uncertainty. Individual's preferences (choice) for a hypothetical health state yields a mathematical value. The individual's preference corresponds to a ranking of health utility scores. Although standard gamble and time-trade-off methods generate ordinal utilities, there is the tendency to use them as cardinal measures. There are no alternatives or other theories.

QALY measurements inherently contain the profile, the frequency and the value of respective adverse effects of a drug. In this case one unique measure provides the benefit-risk difference of a new compound without having to estimate the benefit and risk separately. The number obtained then needs to be compared with the standard of another alternative treatment. The compound with the higher number, i.e. larger QALY gained, has the better benefit.

5. Benefit measured as a morbidity rate

In addition to primary or secondary prevention studies, morbidity can be a primary endpoint in the study of treatments for chronic diseases, e.g. non-fatal cardiovascular events (myocardial infarction or stroke) in the treatment of hypertension or retinal hemorrhage in the treatment of type I diabetes.

RISK ESTIMATION

Until the start of drug marketing, clinical trials are the exclusive source of human efficacy data, and also provide high-quality data on the risk of medicines. The primary goal of clinical trials is to collect data on drug efficacy. The frequency of drug-attributed adverse events, however, depends on their nature. Adverse events which are a result of the pharmacological action are dose-dependent and likely to occur frequently, e.g. symptomatic hypotension in antihypertensive treatment or hypoglycemia in insulin-treated diabetes. In some treatment strategies each patient may have adverse events, e.g. neutropenia in anticancer treatment.

Other adverse events such as allergic reactions are believed not to be dose dependent and therefore not to result from the intended pharmacological action of a new medicine, e.g. dry cough in ACE-inhibitor treatment (less than 10% of patients) or allergic reactions. Potentially fatal adverse events attributable to drugs, e.g. anaphylactic shock, agranulocytosis, upper gastrointestinal bleeding or acute renal failure, are rare and occur far less than 1:1000. Since premarketing clinical trials involve about 3000 patients, potentially fatal adverse events are unlikely to occur, and if they do occur, further drug development would be questioned. Whether an adverse event can be statistically attributed to a medicine depends on the background incidence and the observed frequency of each adverse event. Potentially fatal adverse events observed in the postmarketing phase require hypothesis testing in epidemiological studies. Most data are generated by clinical studies, spontaneous reporting or epidemiological studies. Table 1 provides an overview of the origins of these data.

Table 1. Overview of the origins of data for risk estimation

	Clinical studies	Spontaneous reports	Epidemiological studies
Profile of adverse events	X	X	
Excess cumulative incidence	X ($<10^{-3}$)		X ($<10^{-3}$)
Duration of adverse event	X	X	X

Epidemiological studies are not routinely performed. They are often restricted to the investigation of certain serious adverse events. A case-control study can investigate one adverse event at a time. Therefore, epidemiological data on the frequency of other potentially serious adverse events may not exist. Published studies may therefore be biased in the sense that potential drug risks may not have been investigated.

The proposed measure of risk is drug-attributed loss of quality-adjusted life-years (DALQALY). DALQALYs can be either transient or permanent. Transient DALQALYs take into consideration (1) the drug-specific profile of adverse events, (2) the excess frequency of each adverse event, (3) the duration of each adverse event and (4) a health utility score based on each adverse event. As a consequence, the overall drug risk attributable to transient adverse events corresponds to a composite risk score synthesized from the following parameters:

$$DALQALY_i^{trans} = \sum_{j=1}^{nj} U_{ij} \times d_{ij} \times CI_{ij},$$

where

n is the number of all drug-attributed adverse events of the medicines to be compared,
U is the health-state utilities for each adverse event that has a potential impact on health status,
d is the duration of each considered adverse event,

CI is the excess cumulative incidence of each adverse event,
i corresponds to each medicine to be compared, and
j corresponds to each adverse event.

In the case of permanently disabling adverse events (e.g. stroke) or death, DALQALYs result from (1) the drug-specific profile of adverse events, (2) the excess frequency of each permanently disabling adverse event, (3) the mean life expectancy of the target population and (4) a health utility score based on each adverse event. The overall drug risk attributable to permanent adverse events corresponds to a composite risk score synthesized from the following parameters:

$$DALQALY_i^{permanent} = \sum_{j=1}^{nj} U_{ij} \times LE_{ij} \times CI_{ij} \,,$$

where LE corresponds to life expectancy.

The mean life expectancy of the target population receiving standard therapy can depend on the underlying disease, age, gender or other factors, e.g. life expectancy in patients with heart failure NYHA IV depends on age and gender. Data on life expectancy can be retrieved from published epidemiological studies if the life expectancy is disease specific and from national statistics when an otherwise healthy population is of interest, e.g. analgesic treatment for acute and transient pain.

The total DALQALY is the sum of transient and permanent adverse events:

$$DALQALY_i = DALQALY_i^{trans} + DALQALY_i^{permanent} = \sum_{j=1}^{nj} U_{ij} \times d_{ij} \times CI_{ij} + \sum_{j=1}^{nj} U_{ij} \times LE_{ij} \times CI_{ij}$$

Data on the qualitative profile of all drug-attributed adverse events of a medicine can be obtained from clinical trial data, observational studies and spontaneous reporting. Another prerequisite is the generation of health utility values for each adverse event. Utility values represent preferences for the health state and can be generated by the general population. There are established methods for utility assessment such as visual analog scales, standard gamble or time trade-off [2-4].

Alternatively, utility values could be generated by the costs of treatment of adverse events, where costs represent the patient's need of treatment. Treatment costs due to adverse event could be translated into a utility scale from 0 to 10, where the highest treatment costs correspond to 10 and no treatment costs to 0. The highest cost corresponds to death. The costs of death could be generated by the loss of life-years, as estimated from the expected life expectancy of the target population, and the annual costs of treatment of a chronic and severe disease, e.g. renal dialysis. Both the costs of transient and permanent adverse events would be translated into the utility scale. This would circumvent the problem of who is most suited to estimate utility values: patients, a random sample of the general population or experts. In many cases common sense dictates that the general population is best suited.

HOW BENEFITS AND RISKS CAN BE CONSIDERED IN A BENEFIT-RISK EVALUATION

There are several scenarios which need to be considered: the new medicine is more efficacious, equivalent or less efficacious than the comparator. In each case the new medicine may have a lower risk, the same risk or an increased overall risk. This is shown graphically in Figure 1. It is obvious that drugs that fall into category II, i.e. less benefit and higher risk, are of no interest from a public health perspective. Drugs that fall into category IV are ideal drugs, i.e. breakthrough drugs with lower risk than standard therapy. For drugs that fall into categories I or III a benefit-risk comparison is necessary, since an increased benefit is associated with an increased risk or a decreased benefit associated with a decreased risk. Figure 1 also conveys information of three other scenarios. First, if the benefit difference is zero, the medicine with the lower risk is favorable. Second, if the risk difference is zero, then the medicine with the higher benefit is favorable. Third, if both the benefit and risk difference are zero, then the medicines have the same benefit-risk balance and the new medicine is of no particular public health value. The problem is, however, that the benefit-risk category cannot be assessed in advance, and a benefit-risk assessment is essential.

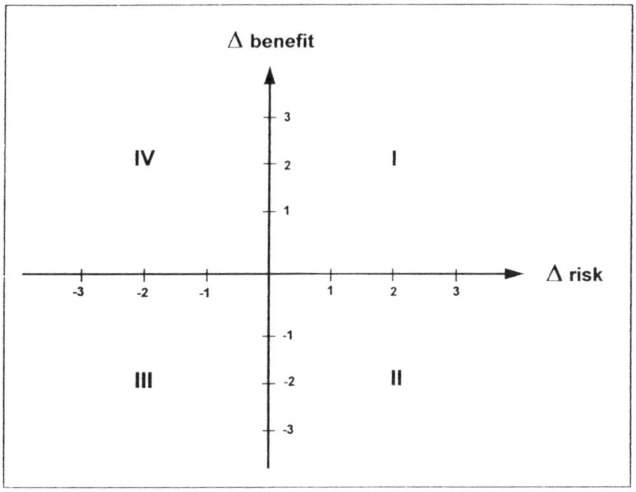

Figure 1. Benefit-risk evaluation scenarios

For the benefit-risk evaluation the following procedure is suggested:

1. Evaluate the benefit by quantifying the efficacy from randomized clinical trials.
    - Identify the comparators of the new medicine.
    - Identify the primary endpoint of registration studies.
    - Quantify the efficacy of the new compound comparatively.
2. Evaluate the overall risk from randomized clinical trials.
    - Identify all drug-attributed side effects for each drug.

- Estimate the cumulative incidence of each adverse event.
- Derive a utility value for each health state according to each adverse event.
- Estimate the duration of each adverse event.
- Estimate the life expectancy of the target population.
- Calculate the DALQALYs of each drug.

HOW BENEFITS AND RISKS OF DRUGS CAN BE BALANCED

To elaborate the benefit-risk balance evaluation, different benefit measurements are considered separately: (1) intermediate endpoints, (2) morbidity studies, (3) mortality studies, (4) life-years gained and (5) QALYs.

1. Benefits measured as an intermediate endpoint

When intermediate endpoints are measured to demonstrate clinical efficacy, then clinical efficacy and risk are not measured in the same units. To avoid the calculation of ratios such as the difference between benefit divided by the difference in risks, it is suggested that clinical efficacy be translated into a utility value, i.e. drug-attributed gain of QALYs (DAGQALYs). The medicine's benefit-risk balance could then be expressed as the difference between DAGQALYs and DALQALYs, each measured in the same units. As with risk estimation the translation of clinical efficacy into QALYs could be derived from a patient or general population.

If the new medicine and standard treatment are equivalent in clinical efficacy, then the risk difference measured in DALQALYs becomes important. The medicine with the smaller DALQALY is the more favorable.

If the new medicine and standard treatment have a different clinical efficacy but have an equivalent risk, then the medicine with the better clinical efficacy is more favorable, without translating intermediate endpoints into DAGQALYs.

2. Benefits and risks measured by morbidity frequencies

When the frequency of morbidity is the measure of clinical efficacy, then the clinical efficacy needs to be translated into a utility value, i.e. DAGQALYs. The medicine's benefit-risk balance could be expressed by the difference between DAGQALYs and DALQALYs. As with risk estimation the translation of morbidity into QALYs can be derived from a random sample of the general population.

3. Benefits and risks measured in deaths

In mortality studies new medicines are compared with standard treatment. An incremental benefit-risk analysis provides the difference in the overall cumulative death incidence. The net difference in overall mortality is already an expression of the benefit-risk balance. Non-fatal adverse events should also incorporated in the benefit risk balance by using morbidity data.

4. Benefits and risks measured in life-years gained

Information of life-years gained is inherent in mortality studies. When the overall mortality is considered, then the net difference in life-years gained is already an expression of the benefit-risk balance.

5. Benefits and risks measured in QALYs

If benefits and risks have the same unit, then the benefit-risk assessment is the difference between benefits and risks for each drug, e.g. DAGQALYs minus DALQALYs. The difference between DAGQALYs and DALQALYs corresponds to the net drug-attributed quality-adjusted life-years (DAQALYs). Any positive DAQALY is beneficial. The medicine with the higher DAQALY is more beneficial.

CONCLUSIONS AND DISCUSSION

The creation of a common measure of drug-attributed benefits and risks is proposed, i.e. drug-attributed gain of quality-adjusted life-years (DAGQALY) and drug-attributed loss of quality-adjusted life-years (DALQALY). The difference between these values can provide a comparative measure of the benefit-risk balance of medicines. The drugs to be compared, however, need to be comparable. Therefore, among other characteristics age and gender distribution, dose and duration of treatment and underlying disease have to be similar. The proposed measure of DALQALYs encompasses both transient and permanent adverse events. Transient DALQALYs take into consideration (1) the drug-specific profile of adverse events, (2) the excess frequency of each adverse event, (3) the duration of each adverse event and (4) a health-utility score based on each adverse event. For permanent adverse events information on the mean life expectancy of the target population is also necessary. For this purpose a registry of side-effect-attributed utility scores needs to be created. For each newly discovered adverse event, such a "utility register" would provide the respective utility value and allow the calculation of the updated value of the overall benefit-risk score by adding the side-effect-specific $DALQALY_{ij}$ to the previous equation. For this purpose use of an arbitrary population of 100,000 individuals as a standard is advised, i.e. $DALQALY_{ij}$ per 10^5.

The overall risk score must be compared with competing treatment strategies for which the same approach is necessary. Clinical efficacy data and adverse event data on competing treatment strategies are usually collected in randomized clinical trials.

A simplified risk analysis of non-narcotic analgesics, for example, might consider only drug-related mortality, assuming that all analgesics are equivalently efficacious and that there is only concern about potentially fatal adverse events. In this case, the drug-related mortality of each analgesic needs to be considered, thereby taking the different profiles of adverse events into account.

REFERENCES

1. Belanger C, Buring JE, Cook N, Eberlein K, Goldhaber SZ, Gordon D, Hennekens CH, Mayrent SL, Peto R, Rosner B, Stampfer MJ, Stubblefield F and Willett WC: Final report on the aspirin component of the ongoing physicians' health study. New Engl J Med 1989;321:129-135.
2. Froberg D, Kane R: Methodology for measuring health-state preferences - I: measurement strategies. Journal of Clinical Epidemiology 1989;42:345-354.
3. Froberg D, Kane R: Methodology for measuring health-state preferences - II: measurement strategies. Journal of Clinical Epidemiology 1989;42:459-471.

4. Torrance G, Feeny D: Utilities and quality-adjusted life years. International Journal of Technology Assessment in Health Care 1989;5:559-575.

Discussion: Benefit and risk evaluation of medicinal products - An epidemiological approach

J. Urquhart:

How did you ascertain drug exposure? You used the word 'on', which is a two-letter preposition that usually carries a lot of baggage in pharmacoepidemiologic studies.

C. Martínez:

These studies come from 1970s. Nowadays, the information that we are getting from the studies is more precise and complete. Overall, in all the studies, patients were asked by a questionnaire which drugs did they take last week, which dose and how often.

J. Urquhart:

I would suggest that the thing to do with studies done with meagre methods of ascertainment of exposure, is just to junk them, because they are not worth talking about. You get misled so badly by imbalanced exposure. Another point is the existence of two relevant issues when you try to do risk assessment: One is, what is the probability that the bad thing is going to occur?, and the other one, what is the bad thing? And probability runs on a common metric, but the nature of the bad things are all over the map, as you pointed out. You can find stunning differences in individual patient's preferences, about their fears, phobias, etc. Some people have a morbid fear of dying of cancer and will accept a sky-high risk of death from coronary heart disease rather than a very low risk of death from cancer for their own peculiar reasons. I think the attempt to try to homogenise the qualitative nature of adverse reactions is doomed to fail, once you confront the patient, because you find too much diversity.

C. Martínez:

I said at the beginning that a prospective is necessary, because the prospective for such an evaluation is crucial. I have done this study from a population base, from the healthcare or from a regulatory standpoint: If we had no paracetamol today, none at all, but we had to replace this drug with any other, that is what I would expect in this population. So that is crucial, because otherwise you are doing such an evaluation, and someone would say that is nonsense because my patient would also decide differently. Referring to your first point, I think that most of the reactions, besides gastrointestinal (GI) bleed, are not dose-dependent. They are idiosyncratic reactions or more of an allergic origin. And there is no difference if someone is taking probably 500 or 1000 mg of paracetamol in the last days. It would matter in GI bleed because is a type-A reaction, where there is a dose-dependence relationship. But if you see the order of magnitude at the end for this example, it is almost 80 times more. That means that even if we had patients complying fully with the drugs that were given to them, we will not really expect a higher difference. Therefore, I do not think this would invalidate this risk assessment. The order of magnitude would still be there, no matter if they had taken half of them, one-fourth or maybe double of it.

T. Salmonson:

Your approach is very interesting, and certainly a step forward to just comparing frequencies. But, did I understand you correctly when you said that you only include significant adverse events? Is there not then a risk that you would penalise well-established drugs with one or two major adverse events, compared to a less studied drug with more severe adverse events? If that is the case, why not use for instance the upper 95% confidence interval level instead? In this way, it is possible to take into consideration the uncertainty in something that is not very well-established instead of using just the things that we know exist.

C. Martínez:

If we use the upper limit of the confidence interval, then you can imagine that for drugs that maybe have a relative risk of one, but mentioned in studies that had almost no power, the point estimate could be going from 0.1 to maybe 95, and this 95 would go incompletely and overwhelm all the other reactions. I had to make this decision when we extensively discussed this problem, and the final decision was to say I will only take those adverse reactions where we had studies with the power to detect a difference.

T. Salmonson:

That is precisely what worries me, because you are saying that with your approach there is not a risk. You are neglecting this, when you know that there is a potential, at least from the statistical point of view, that it could be 95. But now you are saying that if it does not exist, you do not take that into consideration. The more conservative approach, which I suggest, would in fact give credit to the more established drugs, where we better know the problems.

C. Martínez:

It is a quite interesting point, and if I were to recalculate all these data, it would distort the whole evaluation, going probably in a different way. And this would also harm the drugs that have been very well studied. Where we have much more power, we have thousands of cases often, and the drug which is established and known to cause for example GI bleed like diclofenac, would have a small confidence interval, where another one could not be studied because it is not that often used, just because of the power problem, it would go completely up in value and give a value to other. If you remember the incidence rates of those reactions that were very rare, they would have more value than the ones that are occurring quite frequently.

E.A. Kalso:

You referred to assessing also the benefit and, for a clinician who is looking after pain patients, assessing the risk/benefit ratio is of utmost importance. The drug doses you have analysed are not equi-analgesic. Therefore we should assess the risk for the benefit, and if the patient does not get any benefit from paracetamol, it is no use even if it has no risks, whereas ibuprofen, which is safer than diclofenac, is significantly more potent.

C. Martínez:

The reason I had to choose these doses was, as I said at the beginning, driven by what is published. If we had studies that would clearly differentiate, let's say, less than 500 mg or more than 2 g of paracetamol, it would be much easier. But I think in the publications we were happy to find anything dose-dependent, age-dependent, sometimes gender, but I could not go more in that, because the numbers were too small and the confidence intervals would go very far apart. You decide which drugs you think the patient would benefit and then among those you look at the risk, if you have a choice. If you have no choice then there is no reason of comparing.

M. Pirmohamed:

I think you do a disservice to drugs such as aspirin, because clearly some of the reactions are dose-dependent. On the other hand, the risks that you estimated are dependent, to a great extent, on the quality of data that is available to you from the published studies. And clearly there are a lot of data out there which have not been published. For example, with aspirin you said there is a small additional excess risk of death from agranulocytosis, but aspirin is not usually associated with agranulocytosis. I was surprised to see there was no increased risk of Stevens-Johnson syndrome or toxic epidermal necrolysis with non-steroidal anti-inflammatory drugs such as diclofenac. If you look at some of the studies which have been done with non-steroidal anti-inflammatory drugs, (Roujeau JC *et al.*, N Engl J Med, 1995), you will see that NSAIDs are high up on the list of drugs causing these side effects.

C. Martínez:

If you take the Jean-Claude Roujeau's paper, you will not see an increased risk there for diclofenac or aspirin. Steroids do have, and the paracetamol-increased risk is taken from this paper. This is the only major epidemiologic study that we have so far for severe skin reactions for the drugs that we have looked at. I have not looked at all the drugs that they studied, so I have looked at those I wanted a priori to compare with each other. But the numbers are taken from there.

M.M. Reidenberg:

Is there a statistical way to correct for your risk estimate from the doses that are in the literature to what most of us would accept as equi-effective doses?

C. Martínez:

A short answer would be no. And the second answer would be, what would it mean? Even if the doses were not correct, what would you expect to change from the risk profile?

M.M. Reidenberg:

Using a different example, where the increase of risk was dose-dependent, then one could readily see that it would change.

C. Martínez:

That would be true for the drugs that have anti-inflammatory action through a COX inhibition. If the choice is between an anti-inflammatory drug and a non anti-inflammatory drug for the risk, then no matter which doses are used; if the drugs are both effective, then the drug without anti-inflammatory would be preferential. But if you are generalising your concept outside of this class of drugs, I had to go by what was published. Most studies, because of power problems, needed to make some cut point, although they are not equipotent from the activity, unfortunately. And I cannot imagine any measure to say we can adjust for, as we have no dose-dependency to certain defined adverse reactions.

Pain - How to standardize a subjective measure

Eija Anneli Kalso

Pain Relief Unit, Department of Anaesthesia, Helsinki University Central Hospital, Helsinki, Finland.

ABSTRACT

Pain is defined as "an unpleasant sensory and emotional experience associated with actual or potential tissue damage or described in terms of such damage". Consequently, pain as experienced by the patient itself is always a subjective measure and its quantification is not as straightforward as measuring blood pressure. However, good tools have been developed for clinical and research purposes. The sensitivities of various visual analogue and categorical verbal rating scales to measure both pain intensity and pain relief have been validated. In order to standardize these measurements the pain intensity and pain relief are examined at a certain state i.e. either at rest or during that activity that is most likely to produce the worst pain. Pain questionnaires have been developed to provide more information about the different qualities of pain: sensory-discriminative, affective-motivational and cognitive-evaluative.

The sensory qualities of pain can also be analyzed using standardized stimuli to evaluate mechanical allodynia (von Frey hairs), thermal hyperalgesia (thermotest) or pressure pain thresholds. These methods have shown to be useful diagnostic tools. They are also used to assess treatment effects in both acute and chronic pains. More sophisticated neurophysiological and neuroimaging techniques are available but not for routine use.

Key words: visual analogue scale, verbal rating scale, McGill Pain Questionnaire.

Correspondence: Dr. Eija Kalso, Pain Relief Unit, Department of Anaesthesia, Helsinki University Central Hospital, Haartmaninkatu 4, P.O. Box 260, FIN-00029 HYKS, Finland, Tel: +358-9-471-5640, Fax: +358-9-471-5641, Email: Eija.Kalso@huch.fi

INTRODUCTION

Pain is by definition "an unpleasant sensory and emotional experience associated with actual or potential tissue damage or described in terms of such damage" and therefore always a subjective measure. Several tools have been developed to measure pain. In order to use these tools adequately we have to understand of what components the total pain experience is made of. The quantity and also the quality of tissue injury is an important factor: more extensive trauma causes more pain which also takes longer to heal. The final report of pain is further modified by the patient's previous pain experiences and by the current emotional state.

TOOLS TO MEASURE PAIN

The sensory qualities of pain can be analyzed using standardized stimuli to evaluate mechanical allodynia (von Frey hairs), thermal hyperalgesia (thermotest) or pressure thresholds. These methods have been shown to be useful diagnostic tools. Sophisticated neurophysiological and neuroimaging techniques can quantify the neurophysiological responses of painful stimuli and localize the respective brain areas that are activated. However, the total experience of pain, as a subjective experience, can only be evaluated by the subject of pain, the patient.

The sensitivities of various visual analogue and verbal rating scales to measure both pain intensity and pain relief have been validated [1].

Verbal rating scales

The oldest of the standard measures is the four-point pain intensity category scale (Table 1). However, it may not have enough levels to allow the patients to accurately describe their pain level. In addition, the numerical scores for the categories are arbitrarily set to equal step integers without evidence that the levels of pain to which they correspond are spaced apart an equal number of discernible difference units. It has been suggested that there is a greater difference for patients between severe and moderate pain than between moderate and slight. More extensive lists of pain descriptors have therefore been developed (Table 1) [2,3].

Table 1.
Categorical scales for pain intensity

4-point scale	8-point scale
none	no pain
mild	just noticeable
moderate	weak
severe	mild
	moderate
	strong
	severe
	excruciating

Pain relief category scales have been reported to be more sensitive to small reductions in pain compared with the pain intensity category scales [4]. Categorical pain relief scales rely on the patient's memory of pain at the baseline period. This does not seem to be a problem in short studies (a few hours) but may reduce reliability of relief data in longer studies for reasons that will be discussed later.

Visual analogue scales

A visual analogue scale is a line with "least possible pain" labelled at one end and "worst possible pain" at the other. The patient is asked to mark the line at a point corresponding to his present pain level [5]. Visual analogue scales are continuous and thus relatively free from some of the biases that may complicate category scales such as patients using as much of the range of words as possible. Uninformed and especially older patients may, however, have difficulties in understanding the meaning of a visual analogue scale. Horizontal VAS scales [6] between 10 and 15 cm in [7] have been suggested to be the most reliable. Visual analogue scales can be used to measure both pain intensity and pain relief.

Wallenstein *et al.* [8] compared the ratings of 257 patients using the four category pain scale to the VAS pain scale and showed that the four categories were not far from equal spacing. Also the pain relief category scales were shown to be rather evenly spaced, relative to their equivalent VAS ratings [8].

Littman *et al.* [4] compared the pain intensity category, relief category and pain intensity VAS scales in 20 clinical trials with about 1500 patients receiving analgesics or placebo. The sensitivities of the scales to detect a treatment difference decreased in the following order: the relief category, the VAS pain scale and the pain intensity category scale. The three scales gave the same overall conclusion in 17 of the 20 studies.

In the same study Wallenstein *et al.* [8] showed that a very simple measure "pain is at least 50% relieved" is highly correlated with both the categorical and VAS ratings. The use of this simple measure as part of the analysis of pain relief would enable the combination and comparison across different studies using meta-analytical methods.

The McGill Pain Questionnaire

The McGill Pain Questionnaire (MPQ) was designed to assess the multidimensional nature of pain experience, not just pain intensity, of chronic pain problems. The Pain Rating Index (PRI) of the MPQ includes 20 groups of pain descriptors [9]. Each group assesses a different quality of pain experience. These subclasses are further grouped into three subscales designed to assess the sensory-discriminative, affective-motivational and cognitive-evaluative dimensions of pain [10, 11]. Because the PRI provides quantitative measures of multiple pain dimensions it can be used to evaluate the effectiveness of pain treatments.

Escape medication

Consumption of escape medication is often used as a primary measure in analgesic studies. In many clinical studies the protocols for taking escape medication have serious flaws. The escape medication should be clearly defined as to which drug should be given and when. If the decision is left to the nurse as "when needed" significant delays may take place. An important improvement in this respect is the use of patient controlled analgesia (PCA) which allows the patient to self administer opioids when needed intravenously. This method has been used to test the effectiveness of local anaesthetic blocks or non-steroidal anti-inflammatory drugs in postoperative analgesia [12-14]. A few words of warning are necessary, however. If the consumption of morphine is regarded as a measure of pain experienced by the patient then all patients should aim at a similar state of pain relief. If the VAS-values are different between the two study groups, the value of the consumed dose of morphine is less reliable. The patients may prefer pain to nausea caused by morphine. It should also be taken into account that analgesics may potentate each others' effects.

MEASURES TO STANDARDIZE THE ANALYSIS OF PAIN

As acute and chronic pain states represent pathophysiologically very different entities these conditions are discussed separately.

The noxious stimulus

The interindividual variation in response to noxious stimuli is great. Individual pain thresholds (when a potential injury is noticed as painful) and pain tolerance (how much pain the person can stand before taking a pain killer) are controlled by the individual's physiological, behavioural and cultural factors. Even if most of the demographic variables are controlled e.g. age, gender and ethnicity the variation still remains significant. Thus it is essential to standardize the noxious stimulus. Nerve compression pain is very intense as is ischaemic pain. Wound pain is less severe and can be almost absent when the patient is at rest. Thoracotomies are very painful postoperatively whereas operations for inguinal hernias rarely cause severe pain. Postoperative pain is the most commonly used set up to study acute pain. Molar extraction is perhaps the most commonly used model. As the operation is often performed to both sides the patient can serve as his own control. In the next examples, however, pain following thoracic surgery is used to show how pain measurement can be standardized.

Some of the factors that need standardizing in studies on postoperative pain are given in Table 2.

Table 2.
Factors affecting postoperative pain measures

type of surgery
surgical technique
premedication
type of anaesthesia
escape medication
timing of pain measurement
measurement of pain at rest/during movement
who performs the measurements

The significance of the type of surgery is shown in Figure 1. Thoracic surgery can be performed either by opening the chest wall (thoracotomy) or as videoaoassisted thoracoscopic surgery which causes significantly less trauma than thoracotomy. Figure 1 shows the evolvement of pain after these two types of thoracic operations. In both groups the patients were able to self administer as much intravenous morphine as they needed using a PCA device. In spite of this and the fact that the thoracotomy patients were given intercostal nerve blocks before closure of the thoracotomy, the mean VAS-pain intensity ratings were significantly lower in the thoracoscopy group.

Even today many studies on postoperative pain do not mention whether pain was measured at rest or during movement. Figure 2 shows the striking difference in pain intensity after thoracotomies when the pain is asked either at rest, when the patient moves or coughs. It is not only that the patient's report on pain intensity varies between these three measurements but these situations also analyze two different pathophysiological states of pain. The pain at rest usually represents the dull constant C-fibre-mediated pain whereas the pain which is evoked by movement or coughing is connected to hyperalgesia. As modern analgesics have more selective targets for actions these aspects of pain analysis become increasingly important

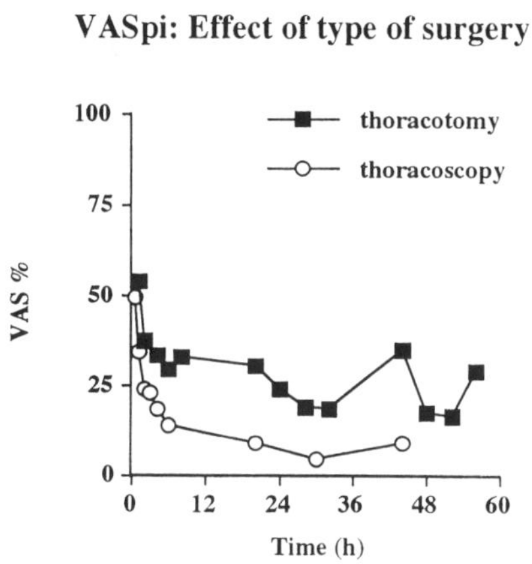

Figure 1. Pain intensity (% of the maximum on a VAS scale of 0-100) after thoracotomies and video-assisted thoracoscopies. Intercostal nerve blocks were performed at the end of surgery following thoracotomies. The patients were able to self administer morphine intravenously using a PCA (patient controlled analgesia)-device. Data has been combined from Perttunen *et al.* [12,14].

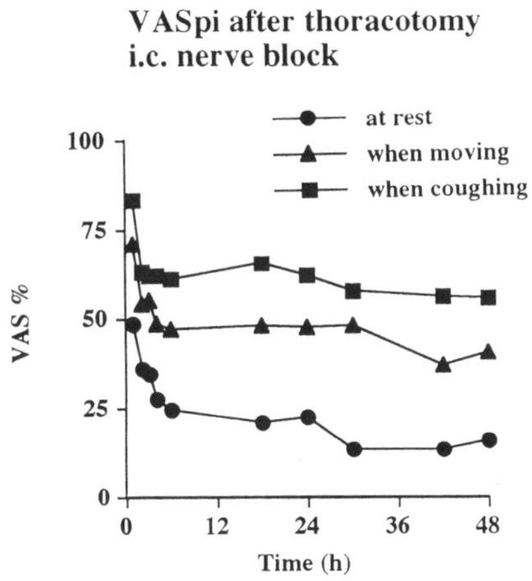

Figure 2. Pain intensity (% of the maximum on a VAS scale of 0-100) after thoracotomies. Intercostal nerve blocks were performed at the end of surgery. The patients were able to self administer morphine intravenously using a PCA (patient controlled analgesia)-device. Pain was asked when the patient was at rest, during movement and when coughing. Data is from Perttunen *et al.* [13].

Standardizing the painful state is equally if not even more important in chronic pain. The pathophysiological mechanisms behind different chronic pain states may be quite different [15]. A good example is neuropathic pain. Contrary to nociceptive pain neuropathic pain usually does not respond well to non-steroidal anti-inflammatory drugs or opioids. Instead, pain relief is achieved with antidepressants and anticonvulsants. Drugs that reduce hyperalgesia may have no analgesic effects in nociceptive pain.

In acute pain the time from tissue injury is important as pain decreases with time. In chronic pain the constant pain usually stays and is aggravated by different factors. The patients should therefore keep a pain diary and mark the intensity of pain 2-4 times a day. Again, in order to appreciate how much variation the individual patient may have in the pain experience the pain intensity is assessed as present pain, average pain, least and most intense pain. The time of the day when the pain analysis is made can also be important. Patients with rheumatoid arthritis suffer from stiffness and pain particularly in the morning. Many other chronic pain patients, however, report that their pain gets worse in the early evening hours.

Both the patient and the person who assess pain and pain relief should be trained to use the tools of measurement.

Standardizing initial pain intensity

Assay sensitivity and test power can be increased by selecting patients with sufficiently high initial pain intensity. A good example is a study by Bjune *et al.* [16] who studied pain relief after Caesarean section in a randomized, double blind, single oral dose parallel group comparison of paracetamol+codeine, paracetamol only or placebo. Of the total of 108 patients who completed the study 49 patients had moderate initial pain (visual analogue scale 40-60/100) and 59 severe pain (VAS >60/100). The latter group showed both good upside sensitivity i.e. two active drugs were differentiated, and downside sensitivity i.e. the active drugs showed better pain relief than placebo. On the other hand, no differences were revealed between the three groups in any of the efficacy variables in the group of patients who had moderate baseline pain. Similar results have been published recently [17,18].

PRESENT VS PAST PAIN

The present pain should always be included in the analysis as the situation can be standardized and as the intensity of present pain may affect the patient's estimation of previous pain. Present pain is usually asked in studies on acute pain and during the patient's visits in studies on chronic pain. The reason for not relying on the patient's memory for previous pain are discussed below.

Memory for pain

Memory for pain is often implied in assessment instruments used in research.
Current pain states seem to influence estimates of past pain intensity in a systematic manner. In a study on breast cancer patients [19] the women were allocated into two groups according to whether they had or did not have chronic treatment related pain at 12 months from surgery. Those patients who did not have chronic pain ($n = 69$) remembered their past postoperative pain at 12 months as significantly ($p<0.001$) less severe compared with how they remembered it at 1 month. The patients who had developed chronic treatment related pain ($n = 15$), however, remembered the past postoperative pain as significantly more severe when asked at 12 months from surgery compared when asked at 1 month after surgery. Similar results have previously been reported by Eich and colleagues [20] who studied patients with chronic headaches of myofascial origin. When the present pain was high, patients rated their maximum, usual and minimum levels of pain as being more severe than what the hourly pain diaries indicated. When their present pain intensity was low, the same patients remembered all 3 levels of prior pain as less severe than they actually had been. Linton *et al.* [21] have suggested that chronic pain patients may significantly overestimate recalled baseline pain ratings.

Modulation of memory by emotions

Emotions exert strong assimilative effects on memory [22] and could therefore be important in the processing of pain memory. Hunter *et al.* [23] have indicated that high affect may lead to a distortion and overestimation of pain in memory. Kent [24] examined the role of affect in memory for pain in dental patients. He found that anxious and non-anxious patients reported similar pain intensities when asked immediately after surgery. However, both the expected pain intensity levels before surgery and the recalled pain intensities at 3 month follow-up as reported by the anxious patients were significantly higher than the actual pain or the respective values reported by the non-anxious patients

Redelman and Kahneman have shown that individuals vary substantially in the total amount of pain they remember from painful medical treatments. Patients' judgment of total pain seems to be strongly correlated with the peak intensity of pain ($p<0.005$) and with the intensity of pain recorded during the last 3 minutes of the procedure ($p<0.005$). The duration of the painful procedure, however, does not correlate with the future memory of the past pain.

CONCLUSIONS

Only some of the factors that are important when attempting to standardize pain measurement have been discussed above. An excellent summary with a comprehensive list of references on this topic has been provided by the International Association for the Study of Pain [25].

REFERENCES

1. Max MB, Laska EM. Single-dose analgesic comparisons. In: Max MB, Portenoy R, Laska E (Eds), Advances in Pain Research and Therapy, The Design of Analgesic Clinical Trials, Raven Press, New York, 1991;18:55-96.
2. Gracely RH, McGrath P, Dubner R. Validity and sensitivity of ratio scales of sensory and affective verbal pain descriptors: manipulation of affect by diazepam. Pain 1978;5:19-29.
3. Tursky B. The development of a pain description profile: a psychophysical approach. In: Weisenberg M, Tursky B, eds. pain: new perspectives in therapy and research. New York: Plenum Press, 1976;171-194.
4. Littman GS, Walker BR, Schneider BE. Reassessment of verbal and visual analog ratings in analgesic studies. Clin Pharmacol Ther 1985;38:16-23.
5. Scott J, Huskisson EC. Graphic representation of pain. Pain 1976;2:175-184.
6. Sriwatanakul K, Kelvie W, Lasagna L *et al.* Studies with different types of visual analog scales for measurement of pain. Clin Pharmacol Ther 1983;34:234-239.
7. Price DD. Psychological and neural mechanisms of pain. New York: Raven Press, 1988, 28-38.
8. Wallenstein SL, Heidrich G, Kaiko R, Houde RW. Clinical evaluation of mild analgesics: the measurement of clinical pain. Br J Clin Pharmacol 1980;10:319S-327S.
9. Melzack R. The McGill Pain Questionnaire. In: R. Melzack (Ed.), Pain Measurement and assessment, Raven Press, New York, 1980, 41-48.

10. Melzack R and Casey KL. Sensory, motivational central control determinants of pain: a new conceptual model. In: D. Kenshalo (Ed.), The Skin Senses, Thomas Springfield, IL, 1986.
11. Melzack R. Measurement of the dimensions of pain experience. In: B. Bromm (Ed.), Pain Measurement in Man, Neurophysiological Correlates of Pain, Elsevier, 1984, 327-348.
12. Perttunen K, Kalso E, Heinonen J, Salo J. I.v. diclofenac in post-thoracotomy pain. Br J Anaesth 1992;68:474-480.
13. Perttunen K, Nilsson E, Heinonen J, Hirvisalo E-L, Salo JA, Kalso E. Extradural, paravertebral and intercostal nerve blocks for post-thoracotomy pain. Br J Anaesth 1995;75:541-547.
14. Perttunen K, Nilsson E, Kalso E. I.v. diclofenac and ketorolac for pain after videoassisted thoracoscopic surgery. Br J Anaesth (in press).
15. Arnér S, Arnér B. Differential effects of epidural morphine in the treatment of cancer-related pain. Acta Anaesthesiol Scand 1985;29:32-36.
16. Bjune K, Stubhaug A, Dodgson M S, Breivik H. Additive analgesic effect of codeine and paracetamol can be detected in strong but not moderate. pain after Caesarean section. Acta Anaesthesiol Scand 1996;40:399-407.
17. Stubhaug A, Grimstad J, Breivik H. Lack of analgesic effect of oral tramadol 50 mg and 100 mg after orthopaedic surgery. Pain 1995;62:111-118.
18. Houmes R-J M, Voets MA, Verkaaik A *et al.* Efficacy and safety of tramadol versus morphine for moderate and severe postoperative pain with special regard to respiratory depression. Anesth Analg 1992;74:510-514.
19. Tasmuth T, Estlander A-M, Kalso E. Effect of present pain and mood on the memory of past postoperative pain in women treated surgically for breast cancer. Pain 1996;68:343-347.
20. Eich E, Reeves JL, B Jaeger B, Graff-Radford B. Memory of pain: relation between past and present pain intensity. Pain 1985;23:375-379.
21. Linton S, Melin L. The accuracy of remembering chronic pain. Pain 1982;13:281-285.
22. Bower GH. Mood and memory. Amer Psychol 1981;36:129-148.
23. Hunter M, Philips C, Rachman S. Memory for pain. Pain 1979;6:35-46.
24. Kent G. Memory of dental pain. Pain 1985;21:187-194.
25. Fields HL (ed.). Pain Measurement in Humans. Core Curriculum for Professional Education in Pain. IASP Press, Seattle, 1995.

Discussion: Pain - How to standardize a subjective measure

L. Aarons:
Is it true that the pain relief scale and the pain intensity scale measure different things?

E.A. Kalso:
In a way these scales measure different things, because one is for intensity and one is for relief. But if you mean that they do not correlate with each other, there is evidence to show that intensity and relief go in opposite directions. To validate the pain relief scales against pain intensity scales it is possible to calculate the pain intensity difference, which you can use in more chronic trials if you want to assess the present pain before treatment and then at different time points during the treatment.

M.M. Reidenberg:
These methods that have been presented have enabled the scientific work on pain to advance very well. Our experience when trying to translate these into useful day-to-day patient care in a medical service is that they don't work because of staff attitudes of doctors and nurses towards pain. For most other areas of medicine and clinical pharmacology, procedures that were developed for research purposes can move over into clinical care with reasonably effective utilisation in daily care. Pain is different and the challenge that we have in addition is to come up with ways to assess pain in ordinary routine medical care that will be accepted and used by doctors and by nurses.

E.A. Kalso:
That is a very important point. In Sweden these scales have been introduced in daily practice. Following the quality programme at the Karolinska Hospital in Stockholm, for any patient who shows more than three times per day a pain intensity of 4 out 10 on the visual analogue scale, a pain specialist should be consulted.

M.M. Reidenberg:
After the requirement was instituted, did the frequency at which the pain levels were recorded at this height change?

E.A. Kalso:
I do not have this information.

J. Urquhart:
One of the great teachings to come out of the hospice movement, confirming observations of good doctors from long before that, was that the continuity of pain analgesia is a very important aspect and one has to consider that pain recurs in cycles. I wonder if you could comment on that.

E.A. Kalso:
This is a very complicated situation. If the pain is constant, then slow-release drugs or drugs that are given on a regular basis are fine. But most of the patients also have pain which is

aggravated by certain movements, or what we call insidious pain. And therefore the patients also need medication which they can take when they feel the pain. On the other hand, the patients want to balance between adverse effects and pain relief. The most important thing is that the patient is in control over the pain relief, and the drug is available when he needs it. And that is why, for example, it has been shown that the consumption of morphine can be decreased using patient controlled analgesia.

P. Rolan:

In our headache clinic, we routinely ask our patients to fill in a diary before their first appointment. We started that because we found it very difficult to reconcile some of the patients' histories. They are completed very well, but it is almost always that the diary shows less pain than the patients report to me. This is the opposite direction to the findings you presented. My interpretation is that patients have often waited a long time to see the doctor, and they want to really impress him how much they are suffering, so that the doctor will take them seriously and give them good treatment. And that is why I found the diary is absolutely essential. It is obviously looking at different populations and these are not really chronic pains, but recurrent acute pains.

E.A. Kalso:

This is true in most of the patients, but it really goes in both directions. We did a study for patients who had been operated for breast cancer and some of them developed chronic pain and others did not. We followed these women from the time before surgery and for a year after surgery. Those women who had chronic pain at one year remembered that their previous acute post-operative pain had been actually much more severe than it had been, whereas those women who had no chronic pain remembered their previous acute post-operative pain had been much less than what it had actually been.

G.T. Tucker:

Where are we now in terms of using biochemical indices of measurement of pain, like endorphins or encephalins? One expects an inverse relationship between their levels and the degree of drug requirement.

E.A. Kalso:

I do not think we have advanced much since the original studies done in Sweden in the early 80s, where it was shown that there is an inverse correlation between the levels of endorphins in the cerebro-spinal fluid and the amount of analgesics the patients needed. Nevertheless, biochemical markers are very insensitive, because they may not only correlate with the pain, but they also are released by stress factors and other factors not connected to pain.

A. Breckenridge:

Could you please add some data on this intriguing statement about the different cultural and ethnic backgrounds to the perception of pain?

E.A. Kalso:

The study which is most often quoted compared a Northern European population, a Southern European population, and a Jewish population. The expression of pain varied significantly. It was less in the Northern European population, the highest in the Southern European population, and in the Jewish population it changed, first it was high, but when the population realised what the question was about, their pain expression went down.

Variability in Human Drug Response
G.T. Tucker, Editor

Variable patient compliance as a source of variability in drug response

John Urquhart

Pharmaco-epidemiology Group, Maastricht University, Maastricht, The Netherlands

ABSTRACT

Patient compliance varies widely, but with what effect on drugs' actions?... beyond the obvious fact that drugs can't work when patients don't take them. Electronic monitoring shows that one-, several-, or many-day lapses in dosing are, in that order, the most common forms of noncompliance. How rapidly drug action fades during a multi-day lapse in dosing is usually not studied, but a slow off-response can allow drug action to persist during shorter lapses. On-responses, usually studied, often do not predict off-responses: some drugs with fast onset of action have slow off-responses, and vice-versa. Thus experimental data on off-responses are needed. Other factors that lessen the impact of shorter dosing lapses are: (a) zero-slope portions of hyperbolic concentration-effect (C-E) relations; (b) intermittent flattening of the entire C-E relation with some types of long-acting drugs. Either way, C can vary within a flat segment of the C-E relation without effect on E. Within limits, these nonlinear mechanisms contribute to the reliability of some drugs' responses, despite variability in dosage form functionality, compliance, and/or PK.

Key words: patient compliance, variability in drug response, pharmacodynamics, concentration-effect relations, rebound effects, first-dose effects.

Correspondence: John Urquhart, M.D., 975 Hamilton Avenue, Palo Alto, California 94301, USA, Tel: +1-650-321-3961, Fax: +1-650-324-9739, Email: urquhart@ix.netcom.com

INTRODUCTION

Variable patient compliance is a leading source of variability in drug response. This fact is reflected in the Harter-Peck (H-P) model of the sources of variability in drug response [1], which is a landmark in the analysis of variability in drug response and its sources. H-P used °theophylline to illustrate the main sources of variability and the mathematics that describe how each source contributes to overall variability in drug response when all components have linear kinetics or dynamics. The model is an informative starting point for analyzing drugs with more typically nonlinear pharmacodynamics (PD), which create a rather different situation than the all-linear case of the H-P model. The need to understand the clinical implications of the common patterns of noncompliant dosing, particularly the multiday lapse in dosing (the "drug holiday"), has put new light on some of the nonlinearities in PD, especially those that determine the persistence of drug actions during lapses in dosing.

The H-P model presents pharmacokinetics (PK) and patient noncompliance with prescribed drug regimens as the two greatest sources of quantitative variability in drug response. Since the H-P model was formulated, much has been learned about both PK and patient compliance. The latter is the focus of this paper. Electronic medication event monitoring (EM) and reliable chemical marker methods have revealed the spectrum of variable drug exposure due to poor and partial compliance, and EM has shown the variety of temporal patterns of drug exposure that occur and recur in ambulatory patients [2-4].

DEFINING THE CLINICAL CONSEQUENCES OF COMMON LAPSES IN DOSING

The need to know the clinical impact of lapses in dosing has exposed a frequently missing element in clinical drug development: few drugs come to market with data on how long drug action persists when dosing is interrupted. The time course of a drug's actions after dosing halts is conveniently referred to as the drug's "off-response". In contrast, most drugs have a well- characterized time-course of action as dosing begins, conveniently referred to as the drug's "on-response". Many drugs have a well-described response to a single dose, which is an amalgam of on- and off-responses, but the duration of response to a single dose rarely allows time for the body to develop full counter-regulatory responses to the drug's actions. Counter-regulatory responses can play a dominant role in off-responses, but are not a prominent topic in pharmacology, which often ignores the fact that drugs act within a rich meshwork of homeostatic, physiological feedback mechanisms.

A further consequence of the need to understand the clinical impact of lapses in dosing is a relatively new clinical study design: the controlled substitution of placebos for active drug. First used with oral contraceptives, as reviewed in [5], this design has recently been applied to anti-hypertensive agents [6-9], and to selective serotonin reuptake inhibitor (SSRI) antidepressants [10]. Of course, in many conditions the controlled placebo-substitution is too hazardous to impose on trial volunteers. Then one must make do with observational data on the clinical correlates of dosing lapses as they occur on the patient's own initiative.

Why have off-responses been neglected in clinical development? One reason is that it has only been in the past decade that EM has shown that dosing lapses are too common and too big to ignore. Previously, off-responses had been seen as one-time events that occurred when the prescriber ordered the drug's discontinuation. Another factor has been perseveration in linear thinking carried over from PK to PD, bringing the linear assumption that on- and off-responses are symmetrical, mirror images of each other. Examples of major asymmetries make it imprudent to assume dynamic symmetry in on- and off-responses. PK/PD models could be seriously unreliable when unconstrained by actual data from off-responses.

Three key points arise out of the foregoing considerations:

(a) Off-responses, which are basic to understanding the impact of the most common patterns of noncompliant dosing, must be determined experimentally; they are not reliably predicted from on-responses.

(b) Certain pharmacodynamic nonlinearities create *qualitative* as well as quantitative variability in the response to variations in drug exposure, especially to the holiday pattern, which recurs sufficiently frequently (see below) to complicate trials analyses.
(c) Certain other PD nonlinearities may beneficially attenuate the propagation of variability that arises from drug formulations, compliance, or PK.

These three points and their implications are the main topics of this paper. Their practical relevance follows from the fact that variability in drug response is the inverse of reliability in use, which is a key value-parameter for any product.

Before we consider these three points, it is useful to review the main points of the H-P model and its assumption that variable compliance is a leading source of variability in drug response.

BRIEF REVIEW OF THE HARTER-PECK MODEL

The H-P model has four components, serially arrayed, each with its own variability, represented with a coefficient of variation (CV, standard deviation as a percentage of the mean), the magnitudes of which Harter and Peck estimated from available data and educated guesses. The serially-arrayed components, through which drug passes from packaged dosage form to receptor-initiated drug action, are: drug formulation, compliance, PK, and lastly, PD.

COMPONENT	ESTIMATED CV(%)	SQUARED CV	TRANSFORMATION
drug formulation	20	400	drug quantity into release rate
compliance	50	2500	prescribed intake into actual intake
PK	50	2500	release rate into concentration(s)
PD	30	900	concentration(s) into effect(s)
	SUM OF SQUARES	6300	
	OVERALL CV	79%	

In the linear H-P model, the CV for the overall response is the square root of the sum of the squares of the CVs of the individual components, as tabulated above. The column entitled "transformation" denotes the changes in physical dimensions effected by each component. "Concentration(s)" are those of drug and/or active metabolites in plasma or other apt fluid.

SOME IMPLICATIONS OF THE H-P MODEL

H-P constrained their model by the estimate that patients' responses to a dose of theophylline intended to give a half-maximal response have a CV of 80%. Such variability is akin to an elevator in a 20-story building that is likely to go to any floor when "10" is pressed, which would promptly terminate its use, until repaired. Theophylline continues in clinical use, but its unreliability is one of the factors that has limited its use.

PD is the final process in the serial structure of the H-P model. Thus, PD can, depending upon the shape of the concentration-effect relation, amplify or attenuate quantitative variability arising from the first three processes, as Levy has noted [11]. One means of attenuation arises from the familiar hyperbolic dose-response relation, which can be approximated by three segments:

i. a zero-slope segment at concentrations too low to elicit any drug action
ii. a finite-slope segment in a mid-range of concentrations
iii. an essentially zero-slope segment at concentrations greater than needed for maximal action.

In reality the slope in segment iii may not be literally zero, but close thereto; the approximation as zero is convenient for this discussion. As a result, drug concentrations can vary within segments i or iii and make little or no change in the magnitude of drug action characteristic of the respective segment, i.e., zero within segment i, or essentially maximal action within segment iii. This functional characteristic is important in limiting the propagation of variability arising from drug formulation, compliance, or PK. In contrast, the slope of segment ii not only passes variability but may even amplify it: with a very steep slope in segment ii, a small percentage fluctuation in drug concentration can swing response between zero and maximum.

A limiting case is provided by drugs that have so-called "hit and run" actions, e.g., omeprazole and reserpine, which can totally inactivate, by irreversible binding, a key component of the mechanism upon which the drug acts. Omeprazole, e.g., irreversibly binds to the H+/K+ ATPase that is responsible for gastric acid secretion; once bound to drug, this enzyme ceases to function, and 3-5 days are required for new enzyme to be synthesized [12]. Thus, while omeprazole's on-response is fully developed within about an hour, its action continues for 3-5 days, signifying that the slope of segment ii is reduced essentially to zero. As a result, variations arising from drug formulation, compliance, and PK have little or no effect during the long off-response [13]. These long periods of attenuated propagation of variability contribute to omeprazole's high degree of reliability in use, which is reflected in the strength of its therapeutic claims [12]. Of course, some drugs achieve long action from their PK, not their PD, and can be represented by familiar linear mechanisms that create frequency-dependent attenuation of variability [14].

The H-P assumption that variable patient compliance plays a leading role in the variability of drug response makes compliance a topic to reconsider now, especially as the model was published shortly after EM methods for measuring compliance were introduced. In the intervening decade, many studies based on EM methods have been published, showing various patterns of variable drug exposure, some of which can trigger qualitative as well as quantitative variability in drug response.

THE COMMONLY OCCURRING PATTERNS OF NONCOMPLIANT DOSING BY UNSELECTED AMBULATORY PATIENTS

The methods used to gather these data are reviewed elsewhere [3]; key points are summarized here. EM and slow-turnover marker methods make it very difficult for patients to censor evidence for delayed or omitted doses, in contrast to older methods, which allow easy censoring: returned tablet counts, interviews, histories, diaries, and spot checks of drug concentration in plasma, all of which overestimate compliance [3], often grossly so [15].

Marker and EM methods are complementary: markers prove ingestion of drug, and give a measure of aggregate intake of drug, but cannot show when doses were taken; EM shows when doses were taken and thus the temporal patterns of drug exposure, but cannot prove ingestion, which has turned out not to be a substantive limitation. Thus, the simpler and lower-cost EM methods have become the standard for reliable assessments of drug exposure in clinical research. A recent cost-reduction makes EM practical for distinguishing pharmacological non-responders from noncompliers in various practice settings. For pharmacometric studies, the time-history of drug intake, which only EM can provide, is crucial for defining the effects of variable compliance on drug response.

DEFINING COMPLIANCE

EM data support a precise definition of compliance: the extent to which the patient's actual drug dosing history corresponds to the prescribed drug regimen [3].

What compliance is not: the three phases of ambulatory pharmaco-therapy

Ambulatory pharmaco-therapy has three distinct phases, of which compliance, as defined, applies to the second phase.

The first phase is the patient's acceptance of the concept of treatment and agreement to execute the prescribed regimen. Patients naturally have the right to reject the proffered treatment, but some do it covertly by not having the prescription filled, or by not collecting or not starting to take dispensed medicine. Prescribers who fail to recognize non-acceptance are likely to interpret the ensuing non-response as drug-refractory disease, which can be a costly error.

The second phase, applicable to those who start treatment, is execution of the prescribed regimen. It is an ongoing process, with opportunities for errors of both omission and commission, whence the definition of compliance given above. It is in this phase that various temporal patterns of drug intake contribute to dose-dependent fluctuating magnitudes of drug responses, and, in some circumstances, pattern-dependent, qualitatively different drug responses.

The third phase is discontinuation of treatment, which may occur on medical advice or on the patient's own initiative. Either way, early discontinuation of treatment is a common occurrence. It is much in need of study, as recommended durations of treatment are often not met. Early discontinuation may bring avoidable hazard to the patient, and has several kinds of economic impact.

One could, of course, lump both non-starting and early discontinuation as "noncompliance", but it mixes up two usually one-time events with the ongoing process of regimen execution. It seems preferable to use "adherence" as the blanket term covering all three phases, of which the first and third - adoption and continuation - are dichotomous, usually one-time occurrences; the second - drug regimen compliance - encompasses a spectrum of often recurrent deviations from the prescribed dosing regimen.

DOSING PATTERNS DEFINED BY ELECTRONIC MONITORING

EM data define subgroups of patients according to dosing patterns, including some subgroups likely to enrich the understanding of the drug's exposure-dependent actions, e.g., --

- About a third of unselected patients have full, unrelenting exposure to drug, and thus can be expected to show full effects of the drug, both beneficial and adverse.
- Another third of unselected patients have recurring drug holidays and thus reveal potentially hazardous effects of sudden stopping or restarting of dosing; holidays recur ca. monthly in half these patients, and ca. quarterly in the other half, as reviewed in [3].
- The remaining third of unselected patients take appreciably less drug than called-for by the recommended regimen, though without lapses in dosing long enough to be classed as holidays; their responses constitute a "reality check" on whether the recommended dosing regimen calls for needlessly frequent or high doses.

"Unselected" means that the patients' prior medical history has not been such as to selected for unusually good or poor compliance, a topic discussed in [3].

The drug holiday -- key source of mischief

EM reveals drug holidays, defined as three or more days of interrupted dosing [16], during which drug actions fade and eventually disappear, if dosing is halted long enough, but then resume after dosing resumes. This is the quantitative aspect of variability in drug response created by drug holidays.

Qualitative variability arises because drug holidays also serve as the trigger for rebound or acute withdrawal effects, which differ qualitatively from the drug's usual actions. Rebound effects appear in the days following a sudden halt in dosing, following a period of more or less well-maintained dosing. Some rebound effects are hazardous, as discussed below. Resumption of dosing may also trigger recurrent first-dose effects, which also differ qualitatively from primary effects [3].

KEY PHARMACODYNAMIC POINTS

A. Off-responses not predictable from on-responses

Several currently best-selling pharmaceuticals illustrate this point. Already described are the asymmetrical on- and off-responses of omeprazole, the drug with largest-ever sales. One might caricature its on- and off-responses as "fast-on, slow-off". In contrast, the opposite pattern - "slow-on, fast-off" - prevails for the SSRI antidepressant, paroxetine, also a leading product. Like other anti-depressants, paroxetine takes 10 days or more of dosing before any anti-depressant action is evident, and a further week or so before anti-depressant action is fully developed; in contrast, when paroxetine dosing suddenly halts, mood deteriorates within 2-3 days [10]. Thus, on- and off-responses can be markedly asymmetrical in either direction, making it essential that both on- and off-responses be studied experimentally. Without such data, assumptions about off-responses are too unreliable to project the clinical impact of the common lapses in dosing. Simulation of clinical trials and computer-assisted trials design may be similarly unreliable when based on PD models unconstrained by experimental data on off-responses.

Off-responses determine the parameter called "forgiveness", defined as the drug's post-dose duration of therapeutically useful action (D_a) minus the recommended dosing interval [3]. Long-acting drugs can forgive occasional lapses in dosing that do not exceed the drug's D_a. In practical terms, a drug that can forgive the occasional occurrence of two sequentially omitted doses will make variable compliance a non-issue in 70-80% of patients. In contrast, a drug with only a few hours of forgiveness can be expected to have recurring lapses of action in a majority of patients, with likely negative impact on treatment outcome [13,17].

B. Qualitative variations in drug responses due to variable dosing

A well-recognized form of qualitative variability in drug response arises from the familiar concept that the most desirable drugs have dose-dependent beneficial effects occurring at relatively low doses, with side-effects occurring at considerably higher levels of dosing. By keeping the dose in the proper range, only the desired, therapeutic effects of the drug are elicited; in the face of variability in PK, it may be necessary to adjust the dosing level to stay within a desired range of drug concentrations in plasma to achieve selective action. In some instances, however, the trigger for undesirable side-effects is not the amount of drug taken, or the concentration of drug in plasma, but sudden stops or starts in dosing.

Examples of rebound effects

The two best-known rebound effects are the withdrawal syndrome that occurs when long-maintained dosing with a narcotic analgesic is suddenly discontinued, and the coronary spasm, hypertension, tachycardia, and increased risk of incident coronary disease that occur when a sudden halt occurs in long-maintained dosing of beta receptor antagonists of the non-ISA category. Rangno and Langlois [18] showed how the response to exogenous isoproterenol changes in the days following cessation of beta blocker dosing: the initially small response, characteristic of receptor blockade, is reversed within several days to a level of response far higher than that which prevailed prior to the start of beta blocker treatment. Then gradually, over a 10-14 day period, response returns to the pre-treatment baseline. These changes signify changes in receptor sensitivity, a counter-regulatory response to receptor blockade that is revealed during the off-response because the beta blocker disappears and beta blockade fades much sooner than hyper-responsiveness to catecholamines. The drug's off-response is an amalgam of the two processes. During periods of catecholamine hyper-responsiveness, the patient runs a gauntlet of elevated risk of incident coronary disease and/or coronary spasm [19,20].

Recurrent first-dose effects - likely examples

Many drugs have prominent first-dose effects [3], but their recurrence when dosing resumes after drug holidays has not yet been studied.

Overview

The holiday pattern of drug dosing can trigger rebound effects and probably also recurrent first dose effects that differ qualitatively from the drug's usual effects. Some of these pattern-dependent effects are hazardous, but the safety problems are obscured by intention-to-treat analysis, which ignores drug exposure, and simply averages qualitatively diverse data from all randomized patients. The result is an underestimate of risk in those patients who are actually at risk, and a misattribution of diluted risk to the majority who are not at risk.

C. CERTAIN NONLINEARITIES IN PD CAN ATTENUATE THE PROPAGATION OF VARIABILITY

The means by which the PD of omeprazole can attenuate variability have already been discussed. Another example is reserpine, which, along with hydralazine, was used in the VA Cooperative Trial that first demonstrated the value of treating hypertension [21,22]. Reserpine has about a two-week D_a, so, with its once-daily dose, it is extremely forgiving, which arises, as with omeprazole, from its nonlinear PD; there are many-day intervals in which the drug's concentration-effect relation is completely flat, and thus unable to propagate variability originating from drug formulation, compliance, or PK. It is also noteworthy that the compliance of patients in the VA trial had been screened, pre-randomization, by a marker method that probably served to exclude from the study non-acceptors and the worst of the poor compliers. In summary, several extra-ordinary aspects of this trial had the effect of markedly attenuating variability that usually prevails in trials of other types of drugs, at the cost of statistical power.

The results of the VA Cooperative Trial have been a landmark in the hypertension field, which has been subsequently beset by many ambiguous trial results with agents whose forgiveness is measured in hours, not days. There are doubtless multiple reasons for the singular clarity of the VA Cooperative Trial results, but clarity can only have been enhanced by use of an extremely forgiving agent and exclusion of non-acceptors and patients whose compliance was too poor to be offset even by the extreme forgiveness of reserpine. These qualitative considerations of course need to be translated into quantitative terms, which could be done by retrospective simulation of this and other trials, focused on the sources of variability in drug response. Indeed, it would seem that meta-analysis of complicated fields like hypertension can be enriched by retrospective computer simulations of key trials. A principal objective of this kind of "dynamic meta-analysis" would be an examination of the role of differential degrees of forgiveness and how their associated attenuation of variability may have influenced trial outcomes.

CONCLUSION

Variability in drug response is the inverse of reliability in use, which is a key value-parameter for any product, pharmaceuticals included: reliability is a powerful competitive advantage. Accurately differentiating noncompliance from nonresponse as the basis for poor outcomes of treatment is a basic step, and has been done in the oral contraceptive field since its beginnings. Best is to understand the sources of variability in drug response and to design drug formulations, regimens, and individualized dosing schemes that maximize forgiveness, minimize variability, and minimize the propagation of variability. As Sir David Cox recently noted [23], variable patient compliance, as we now understand it, has major implications for design and statistical analysis of drug trials, with, of course, strong echoes in practical therapeutics.

ACKNOWLEDGEMENTS: The author has had useful discussions on key points in this paper with Carl C. Peck, Lewis B. Sheiner, and Gerhard Levy.

REFERENCES

1. Harter JG, Peck CC. Chronobiology: suggestions for integrating it into drug development. Ann NY Acad Sci 1991;618:563-571.
2. Cramer JA. Microelectronic systems for monitoring and enhancing patient compliance with medication regimens. Drugs 1995;49:321-327.
3. Kastrissios H, Blaschke TF. Medication compliance as a feature in drug development. Ann Rev Pharmacol Toxicol 1997;37:451-475.
4. Urquhart J. The electronic medication event monitor - lessons for pharmacotherapy. Clin Pharmacokinet 1997;32:345-356.
5. Guillebaud J. Any questions. Brit Med J 1993;307:617.
6. Johnson BF, Whelton A. A study design for comparing the effects of missing daily doses of antihypertensive drugs. Am J Ther 1994;1:260-264.
7. Vaur L, Dutrey-Dupagne C, Boussac J. Differential effects of a missed dose of trandolapril and enalapril on blood pressure control in hypertensive patients. J Cardiovasc Pharmacol 1995;26:127-131.
8. Leenen FHH, Fourney A, Notman G, Tanner J. Persistence of anti-hypertensive effect after 'missed doses' of calcium antagonist with long (amlodipine) vs short (diltiazem) elimination half-life. Br J Clin Pharmacol 1996;41,83-88.
9. Hernandez-Hernandez R, Armas de Hernandez MJ, Armas-Padilla MC, Carvajal AR, Guerrero-Pajuelo J. The effects of missing a dose of enalapril versus amlodipine on ambulatory blood pressure. Blood Pressure Monitoring 1996;1:1121-1126.
10. Rosenbaum JF, Fava M, Hoog SL, Ascroft RC, Krebs WB. Selective serotonin reuptake inhibitor discontinuation syndrome: a randomized clinical trial. Biol Psychiatry 1998;44:77-87.
11. Levy G. A pharmacokinetic perspective on medicament noncompliance. Clin Pharmacol Ther 1993;54:242-244.
12. PRILOSEC (omeprazole). In: Physicians' Desk Reference. Montvale (NJ): Medical Economics Co., 1998;528-532.

13. Urquhart J. Pharmacodynamics of variable patient compliance: implications for pharmaceutical value. Adv Drug Delivery Revs (in press).
14. Yates FE, Brennan RD, Urquhart J. Application of control systems theory to physiology. Adrenal glucocorticoid control system. Fed Proc 1969;28:71-83.
15. Pullar T, Kumar S, Tindall H, Feely M. Time to stop counting the tablets? Clin Pharmacol Ther 1989;46:163-8.
16. Urquhart J, Chevalley C. Impact of unrecognized dosing errors on the cost and effectiveness of pharmaceuticals. Drug Inform J 1998;22:363-378.
17. Urquhart J. Can drug delivery systems deliver value in the new pharmaceutical marketplace? Brit J Clin Pharmacol 1997;44:413-419.
18. Rangno RE, Langlois S. Comparison of withdrawal phenomena after propranolol, metoprolol, and pindolol. Am Heart J 1982;104:473-478.
19. Psaty BM, Koepsell TD, Wagner EH, LoGerfo JP, Inui TS. The relative risk of incident coronary heart disease associated with recently stopping the use of beta blockers. JAMA 1990;263:1653-1657.
20. Anon. Long-term use of beta blockers: the need for sustained compliance. WHO Drug Information 1990;4:52-53.
21. Veterans Administration Cooperative Study Group on Hypertensive Agents. Effects of treatment on morbidity in hypertension. Results in patients with diastolic blood pressure averaging 115 through 129 mm Hg. JAMA 1967;202:1028-1034.
22. Veterans Administration Cooperative Study Group on Hypertensive Agents. Effects of treatment on morbidity in hypertension. II. Results in patients with diastolic blood pressure averaging 90 through 114 mm Hg. JAMA 1970;213,1143-1152.
23. Cox D. Discussion: Limburg Compliance Symposium. Stat Med 1998;17:387-389.

<u>Discussion</u>: Variable patient compliance as a source of variability in drug response

M. Lader:

I was involved in writing for a patient group recently and the person who ran this group said I must not use the word "compliance", I must use the word "concordance". Have you encountered this opinion?

J. Urquhart:

Some see in the term 'compliance' an authoritarian doctor-patient relationship, but 'compliance' is the term under which published papers in this field are indexed by the Index Medicus, regardless of the term used by the authors, e.g. adherence. The document you cite [Marinker M, (for the Working Party). From compliance to concordance: achieving shared goals in medicine taking. London: Royal Pharmaceutical Society, 1997], emphasized patient 'empowerment' as a means to help patients achieve satisfactory treatment. This theory is challenged by the prevalence of poor compliance among physicians who self-prescribe. As my paper notes, ambulatory pharmacotherapy has a beginning (acceptance) a middle (drug regiment execution), and an end discontinuation of the treatment regimen). For successful treatment, the patient has to accept, execute, and then at the proper time, discontinue treatment. Treatment can fail at any phase, so "adherence" can be a useful blanket term, with "nonadherence" implying non-acceptance, early discontinuation, or poor execution of the prescribed regimen. To study, however, the pharmacometric consequences of actual dosing patterns, we need a defined parameter for deviations of actual from prescribed dosing patterns. For that, 'compliance with the prescribed drug regimen' is apt. If 'concordance' adds anything but novelty, it escapes me.

L. Aarons:

I would like to ask you to comment a bit more about the quality of electronic monitoring data, from the perspective that what is being measured is the removal of the lid, or whatever, of the bottle.

J. Urquhart:

Certainly a patient intent on creating a false dosing record can open and close the containers, and not take the medicine. But he has to do it on schedule because everything is time-stamped and it is not possible to change the timing. If people manipulate the package and do not take the medicine, then the data are worse than I have shown you, not better. Occasionally an issue with electronic monitoring of is oral dosage forms arises with patients who are set on using a dose organiser. They do not want to use one of these cup-type packages for one drug in their multi-drug regimen. If you have a patient who is adamant about using an organizer, my suggestion is to let him do so and classify him or her *a priori* as a full complier. Some day there will be an electronically monitored multi-dose organiser. With eye-drop medicines, the monitor records time and date when you take the cap off and turn the bottle upside down. That again is difficult to falsify. The people who have worked with the method are convinced that it is a substantially reliable measurement of exposure and the best currently available. If you try so to use chemical marker methods, you encounter problems with pharmacokinetic variance. One of the best methods is Morgan Feely's phenobarbitone method, which is surprisingly good considering that from a single measurement on 1 day you can obtain a reliable aggregate view of drug intake over the last 10-14 days. But it does not tell you when doses were taken, and I think the timing information is really the critical finding, because of drug holidays. If you look at the drug holiday from a pharmacometric point of view, it is quite worrying because it opens up a whole new set of adverse reaction possibilities.

I.P. Hall:
I was wondering if you had any data on what the effects of electronic drug monitoring are on compliance. Despite having some sort of electronic monitoring, people could say they are taking the medication when they are not.

J. Urquhart:
Joyce Cramer has looked at this by randomising patients between being informed and not being informed (Cramer JA *et at.*, Epilepsia, 1990) and found no difference. In general, if you do not stress the issue, whether patients are informed or not does not have any discernible effect. A very striking point is soon to be published by Hans Brunner's hypertension group in Lausanne. They have studied patients who have gone through the four-step care scheme with no response to multiple doses and drugs, and then have been sent to the University Clinic for a work-up for drug resistant hypertension, which means renal angiograms, and pheocromocytoma tests, etc. Initially, the patients are put on a basic thiazide plus β-blocker regimen for 60 days with electronic monitoring, and explained in detail the procedure and the reasons for this study. In the first 32 patients, 14 of them returned with a record of good compliance and were normo-tensive for the first time in a whole series of treatment strategies. This is a powerful step forward in this field, and I think we will see more cases like this. To return to the step-care scheme, if, for example step 1 to step 2 consists of a change of a 20 cents a day treatment cost to a 2 $ treatment cost, it is worth spending 15 cents a day for approximately a month to see whether the patients are taking their medication. If you can keep a few people at the 20 cent a day level and not have to pay the 2 $, it makes economic sense. However, it is only over the last 2 years that this approach has now become practical.

I.P. Hall:
I suppose that electronic drug monitoring works well for diseases where you have got a clearly defined end-point. It is less good in the field I work in, asthma, where you are largely dependent upon patients' subjective reporting of symptoms, unless you believe all their peak flow records, which is subject to the same problem as medication recording is.

J. Urquhart:
Some problems with anti-depressant treatment should also be considered. For example, what happens when drug dosing suddenly stops. About a year ago, Lilly sponsored a study in which they randomised people between sertraline, paroxetine, and fluoxetine, treated them for about 8 or 10 weeks, and then did a placebo substitution for 7 days. There was a very striking clinical deterioration in the paroxetine group, the drug that has the shortest half-life of the three. Whether it was caused by rebound effects or just return of the depression is not clear. This deterioration was a hitherto unknown aspect of that mode of treatment, and it is in a grey area where it is hard to make measurements. Nevertheless, one can still see that these problems.

N. Benowitz:

In those drugs with not very good efficacy, compliance may not be an important issue. But there may be toxicity, for example in the case of non-steroidal anti-inflammatory drugs. Are there studies about the relationship between compliance and drug toxicity, independently of efficacy?

J. Urquhart:

I mentioned there was just some sort of hit-or-miss issues. For example, in an hypertension trial there was a patient who after a week of taking isradipine according to the schedule, suddenly took six doses within a relatively short time and then took nothing for the next week. He decided to stop the treatment because of a terrible reaction of nausea, dizziness and feeling bad. But when one sees those patterns of underdosing not always there is some drug-related reason, because you can also see the same patterns when you look at placebo compliance. The thing that drives the regimen execution goes back to the kinds of routines people have in their lives. If they are in a chronic dosing situation and they have reasonably good routines, they can fix the dosing behaviour so that it is triggered by some recurring routine in your life (tooth-brushing, walking the dog, watering the plants, etc.). Then you will be a pretty good complier as long as things do not fall apart. I have a stockbroker in New York who has glaucoma, and he said to me at one point his big problem was taking his midday dose. I said to him, well, what do you do at lunch? And he said well my wife packs a paper bag with a couple of sandwiches. I said, next time you get your prescription filled, get a couple of extra bottles of the medicine and have her pack the medicine in the lunch bag so when you dump your lunch out, there is the medicine and then you can take it. He was thunderstruck by the originality of the notion that you would have more than one medicine container. And a couple of months later he said: it really works. I have solved the problem, except on the occasional day when the market is really crazy and then he never gets around to opening the lunch bag, so he does not get the medicine, but that does not happen very often. So I think, when you look at those patterns, and if you have in your mind's eye the slide I showed with similar compliance patterns in three very disparate disease conditions, it suggests that those are not responses to treatment situations so much as they are reflections of the way people organise their lives.

If you have an individual patient without very good routines in their life, then you have to question what is best to do. If the treatment requires punctuality for continuity of drug action in order to get a therapeutic benefit, and if interruptions in drug action are hazardous, then I do not think you should give the patient the medicine. There are some circumstances where drug actions are such as to modulate dosing behaviour. If your patient receives a bolus dose of furosemide every morning, the brisk diuresis that ensues prevent his doing anything else in the next several hours. Perhaps he is taking four or five other medicines, he may take those but decide to delay the diuretic. A deferred dose is outside the normal routine and is a dose more likely to be missed, which can risk the problem of salt and water accumulation.

C. Martínez:

Would you conclude that if you do real-life studies and look at compliance, that we would get an under-estimate of the risk of drugs?

J. Urquhart:

Yes. Let's take the case of the selective COX-2 inhibitors. If you are going to do a clinical programme, you want to be able to show your selective COX-2 inhibitors devoid of the usual kind of gastrointestinal side-effects. That question is answerable in about one third of the people you bring in a randomised controlled trial, without some kind of compliance selection, because it is only in a third of the patients you are going to have unrelenting exposure. There is another hypothesis that another third tests: What is the effect of off-again on-again dosing? It may be with GI bleeding, which is still mysterious, that on and off dosing may be some kind of a special trigger. Maybe not. But there is one way to tell, there is a natural experiment going on out there all the time that you can look at, but you have to do the compliance monitoring to know which patients are doing it and when. And then while it is an observational study, subject to biases and so on, there is one nice check in this, which is, that causality flows downhill in time, it only goes in one direction. If you see the drug holiday and then you see the problem, that is a nice temporal association. But it means you have got to time the occurrence of clinical events correctly, and that is not always the easiest thing to do.

C. Martínez:

But in general, we could then say that the type A reactions, those that are dose-dependent, would be under-estimated?.

J. Urquhart:

If you say unrelenting exposure is needed to elicit this particular adverse effect, and you have three thirds of your patients, in only one third of whom there is unrelenting exposure, then you under-estimate by a factor of three. But underestimating risk by a factor of three is not a major sin.

C. Martínez:

If you take GI bleeds, it is a lot.

J. Urquhart:

It depends who you listen to. If you get excited about these little tiny relative risk differences, then it does matter. But I have another rule of thumb, called the rule of fives, which is if the relative risk is not bigger than five or if it is not one of the top five causes of death, I just do not pay any attention to it.

C. Martínez:

Then you did not listen to my presentation.

G.T. Tucker:

I just wondered whether we could recognise a non-compliant phenotype, or even a gene for non-compliance, perhaps?

J. Urquhart:

The behaviourists have looked for predictors, but nobody has found reliable methods to measure personality traits of compliance. In countries where doctors as a routine do home visits, they get a very much clearer view.

D.A. Smith:

Does it make sense to reduce the number of pills, and are combination products helpful in improving compliance?

J. Urquhart:

One issue is the number of pills you take at a time, and the other is how many doses a day. The number of doses per day issue is up in the air at the moment. Pretty much everybody who has looked at it has seen that if you just look at the percentage of prescribed doses taken, you get a little higher percentage with a once-a-day than you do with a twice-a-day regimen. But it is a small difference. But then, if you start looking at the timing, there are some studies that indicate that, with once-a-day dosing, you tend to get more egregiously long lapses in dosing with the once-a-day than with twice. It may happen that, from a marketing point of view, we must have a once-a-day product, because otherwise we cannot sell it, and the formulators go and torture the product until they squeak it past the 24th hour. Then you put a very unforgiving product in the market. That is fine, but if you then depend on outcome studies to sell the product in the long run, you are going to lose, because if you put an unforgiving product in the market, you are going to get poor outcomes later, because you are going to have that many more gaps in treatment; if continuity of drug action is essential for good outcome, then you are not going to get good outcomes.

D.A. Smith:

I was specifically not asking on once-a-day or twice-a-day. If you took a β-blocker and a diuretic, it is two pills, and you replaced it with a combination in one pill, does that aid compliance?

J. Urquhart:

Joyce Cramer looked at this in a big epilepsy study (Cramer JA *et al.*, Epilepsia, 1995) where people took one, two, three, up to four different medicines synchronously. Basically, if they take one, they take them all, almost invariably.

M. Reidenberg:

A couple of decades ago, the group at McMaster's (Haynes RB, *et al.* In Sackett DL, eds. Compliance in Health Care, Baltimore, Johns Hopkins U. Press, 1979) claimed that what would influence compliance was the patient's knowledge of the severity of the illness and the degree of efficacy of the treatment.

J. Urquhart:

Never did there come from that group a strong voice for reliable measurement. All those measurements were based on methods in which the patient could easily censor evidence for omitted doses, and when you have methods like that, you are doomed. I think most of the conclusions drawn were specious. I think that what we have in hand now is we have got methodology that allows you to do real management.

M. Reidenberg:

Their outcome measure was fall in blood pressure in patients with hypertension.

J. Urquhart:

Using the drug response as an end-point is a difficult and awkward manoeuvre. What we should look at is the dosing record, what I call management methods and I think it is the best we have.

M. Kinirons:

Can you comment on the role of educational aids to assist in the initiation? I have this perception that if you spend some time with a patient and you give them some leaflet, you aid in compliance. Is that true or false?

J. Urquhart:

Information and compliance are qualitatively very different. For securing the patient's acceptance of treatment, you need all the help you can get, for you have to convince the patient in some way or another that the disease is real and that there are real methods of treatment. In day to day execution of the regimen, however, information does not, *per se* compete well with priority in a busy schedule. So advanced knowledge about drugs and their mechanisms of action and the rationale for their use does not guarantee punctual execution of the drug regimen.

E.M. Sellers:

A variety of sociologic studies would suggest that along some social value axes and health belief axes, women are different from men. For example, about 35% of women state a much higher degree of risk aversion than do men. I am wondering, with respect to health behaviours around compliance, whether there is any data that would suggest that there are differences between men and women either on average, or whether there are sub-groups of individuals. The sociologic data would predict that the perception of adverse reactions, or perhaps even the actual occurrence of them, might have greater saliency in women. Is there any evidence to support this at all?

J. Urquhart:

The risk aversion and the question of adverse reactions relates more to discontinuation than it does to a daily debate about whether to take the medicine. As far as the execution issue goes, the person who is done more of this than anyone else is Joyce Cramer at Yale. She just throws up her hands and says, there is nothing that you can look at. The only predictor of compliance is compliance. In other words, if you have measured it in the patient, it is a good predictor of what is going to happen subsequently. But male/female, old/young people, it all tends to come out about the same, with such a wide range of values that do not mean anything.

Variability in Human Drug Response
G.T. Tucker, Editor

Placebo Response

Malcolm Lader

Institute of Psychiatry, London, U.K.

ABSTRACT

The placebo is defined in medicine as an inactive substance or preparation given to satisfy the patient's symbolic need for drug therapy, and used in controlled studies to determine the efficacy of medicinal substances. In clinical trials it is used as a way of separating the therapeutic effects intrinsic in the pharmacological properties of the active substance from the non-specific effects attendant on giving a medication. Such placebo effects can be quite substantial as is seen in the literature on antidepressants. It is easy to confuse a placebo response with natural remission, in a condition in which natural fluctuations occur.

In practical terms the placebo should resemble the active treatment as closely as possible. This also allows an estimate to be made of the adverse reactions associated with the active compound. Occasionally the unwanted effects of an active drug can unblind the investigator and patient so that "active" placebos may be needed. Placebos are perfectly ethical in clinical trials as they enable a true measure of efficacy to be obtained.

The placebo response is not a fixed entity but depends on many factors including the patient, the doctor, the doctor-patient relationship, and factors in society.

Key words: placebo, ethics, natural remission, placebo responders.

Correspondence: Prof. Malcom H. Lader, Institute of Psychiatry, Department of Psychiatry, Section of Clinical Psychopharmacology (MRC), De Crespigny Park, Danmark Hill, London SE5 8AF, U.U., Tel: +44-171-703-5411, Fax: +44-171-252-5437

INTRODUCTION

Mindful that this is a symposium on variability in drug response, I shall be somewhat selective about the areas of placebo response to be discussed. There is a large literature on the placebo, both as a control in clinical trials and as a therapy in its own right. It is also only part of the wider issue of non-specific aspects of treatment [1,2]. In the former capacity the properties of the placebo were discussed in great detail from the 1950's onwards, and when the whole concept of the controlled clinical trial was introduced, first in the United Kingdom and then more widely.

I will draw attention to two main areas of relevance to this meeting. Firstly, there is the contrast between the concept of placebo as the inner control in which case the response is required to be as small as possible and placebo as an active therapy when it is hoped that the response will be large and clinically significant [3]. The second area that I shall focus on is the confounding of placebo response i.e. apparent therapeutic improvement following the administration of dummy medication and spontaneous remission i.e. an improvement in the illness for which the placebo has been administered. I will use the topic of antidepressant medication to illustrate these various points.

DEFINITION

The word placebo goes back for centuries [4]. It means 'I shall please', the first-person singular future tense of the Latin verb placere, meaning 'to please' [5]. The word entered the English language in about the 12th century as the name commonly given to the Vespers for the Dead. A century or two later, the term placebo began to take on secular constructs but was predominantly used in an unflattering manner indicative of opprobrium. For example, there is a character named that in Chaucer's Canterbury Tales who was a servile sycophant. Another reference is to professional mourners hired as substitutes for members of the family to sing placebos at the bier of the deceased.

The first definition in medicine appeared in 1785 in Motherby's New Medical Dictionary where it was defined as 'a common place method or medicine'. In the next edition 10 years later, the description also included the words 'calculated to amuse for a time, rather than for any other purpose'. Then the implication was added that the placebo is both inert and harmless, devoid of effect. This is often taken as the popular definition although placebos can both induce harm and can certainly produce worthwhile therapeutic effects. A well-known dictionary (Dorland) includes the definition: an inactive substance or preparation given to satisfy the patient's symbolic need for drug therapy, and used in controlled studies to determine the efficacy of medicinal substances.

PLACEBO IN CLINICAL TRIALS

The most widely used research context for placebo is in clinical trials [6]. In this technology, a therapeutic procedure is evaluated in terms of its 'true' efficacy. This is taken to mean that the medication may have therapeutic effects intrinsic in its pharmacological properties. The use of the placebo is to separate by subtraction so called 'non-specific factors' which can produce a therapeutic improvement and yet are not intrinsic or characteristic of the therapeutic procedure tried [6]. In the simplest statistical terms, a linear equation is constructed comprising the mean value for the sample plus an element related to the placebo effect plus an element related to the specific therapeutic effect of the test agent or procedure plus a factor relating to error. The placebo is assumed to have the same elements except for the characteristic therapeutic effects. By subtraction, therefore, the efficacy of the test procedure or agent can be established. Of course, there are many assumptions in the model, not least of which is that it is a linear model with no interaction between the various elements. In particular, it is assumed that the therapeutic effect adds to the placebo effect and yet this is by no means a self-evident assumption (Figure 1).

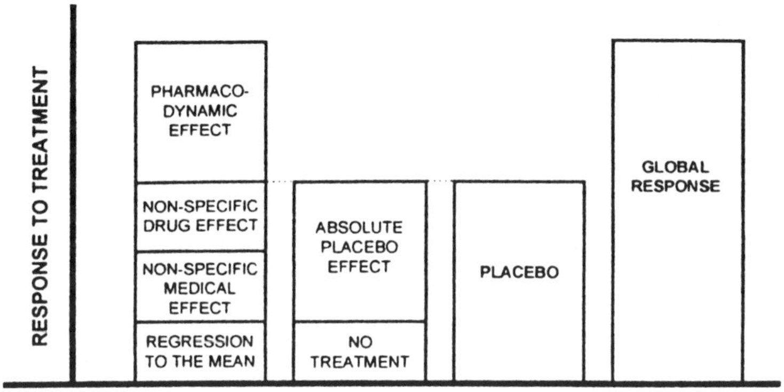

Figure 1. The placebo effect in the overall response to a treatment. The global response is the pharmacodynamic effect plus the placebo effect, which is itself the result of the 'absolute placebo effect' and the effect of regression to the mean. The absolute placebo effect includes the non-specific effect of the drug and the non-specific effect of the medical act. The effects presented in the figure are arbitrary and do not represent any specific drug.
(Reproduced with permission from Garcia-Alonso *et al.* 1988 [14])

Placebos are used in clinical trials whenever this is ethically justifiable; this is generally speaking when either the condition to be treated is fairly trivial and certainly not life threatening or when there is no established treatment for the condition. In this way patient is not deprived of potential benefit. However, wherever possible, in particular within the regulatory context, placebo is to be preferred as it gives the opportunity to measure the true intrinsic therapeutic effect of the test agent. If a presumed active drug is used as comparison, a failure to differentiate it from the test agent may mean that both agents are effective, both agents are ineffective, or that the test system was insensitive.

One problem in such clinical trials is the fact that an effect attributable to placebo can often be quite substantial. This can be evidenced in two ways. Firstly, there may be an improvement across all subjects showing up as a mean effect. An example is an improvement in Hamilton depression scores with an antidepressant. However, the placebo group may also improve across time. The second way is to look at people attaining a certain criteria of response say, 50% diminution in a rating scale or an operational outcome such as discharge from hospital. However, the number of placebo patients meeting this criterion can be quite substantial. In most antidepressant trials it can be 35-50% and even higher in trials of anxiolytics or of psychotherapeutic procedures. The problem with the placebo response is most acute where the efficacy of the test procedure is incomplete, either due to only partial efficacy or to the inclusion in the sample of patients who do not respond to the treatment for whatever reason. Often, however, the reason for treatment – unresponsiveness is never discovered. For example, it is well established that only about 70% of schizophrenic patients treated with the older typical antipsychotic drugs show a response. The characteristics of non-response, apart from compliance problems, is quite unclear. Pharmacokinetic factors seem inadequate to explain the difference.

Consequent upon this the efficacy of a compound may have a fairly narrow window in which to be detected. Typically, with a placebo response at 35% and a drug response of 70%, efficacy can usually be established within fairly large-scale trials. However, if the placebo response rate moves up to 50%, it is almost impossible to establish efficacy in a formal comparison.

Placebo response versus natural remission

This topic is surprisingly neglected, few commentators having discussed it in any detail. However, the usual design of the double blind placebo controlled study does not differentiate between these two factors. To do this a no treatment arm needs to be included. This is not common although there has been a relatively large number of psychotherapy trials, which have a no treatment group, usually, a "wait-list" group that is later randomised into treatment.

The reason why this is important relates to the natural history of diseases and the methods of determination of patients coming to treatment. Many conditions are chronic and fluctuating or they may be relapsing conditions with natural remissions. The patient tends to come to notice or for treatment when his condition has worsened either due to spontaneous fluctuations in severity (i.e. we don't know why) or to some extraneous factors such as nutrition, stress etc. With a naturally fluctuating condition then regression to the mean is likely to be manifest as an improvement in the condition [8] (Figure 2). Only in some conditions is it likely that

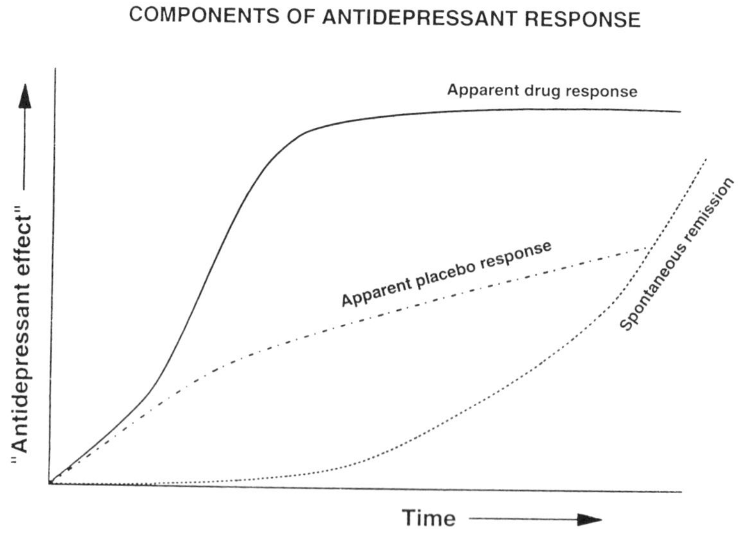

Figure 2.

the condition will progress to include increasing severity, morbidity and even death. In many disorders the severity will tend to lessen as time goes on. This means that a proportion, sometimes a substantial proportion, of what appears to be a placebo response is in fact a natural remission and is not related to the administration of medication. A sophisticated discussion regarding drug-placebo differences in onset of response concluded that antidepressant drugs may convert a percentage of non-responders (to placebo) to responders [9].

In statistical terms in clinical trials this natural remission is not a real problem because it should apply equally to both active treatment and placebo groups, providing true random allocation to treatment has been effected. However, it is a problem in trying to estimate the placebo response.

SOME PRACTICAL CONSIDERATIONS

Placebos in clinical trials should be as sufficiently closely matched to the active treatment that it is impossible for both the patient and the doctor to distinguish between them. There are anecdotal stories about placebos differing in some subtle way from the active medication and one can be sure that if there is some way of distinguishing then patients with infinite ingenuity will find those ways. Therefore, the colour, size, weight etc of placebo in a controlled trial is fixed by the formulation parameters of the active treatment (Table 1).

Table 1.
Minimal specifications to manufacturers of capsules or tablets to be used in a comparative trial

1. To match perfectly* for:	2. To match as closely as possible for:
(a) Shape	(a) Taste on licking
(b) Size	(b) Taste on chewing
(c) *Surface* colour	(c) *Internal* colour
(d) *Surface* texture	(d) *Internal* texture
(e) Weight	(e) Smell
	(f) Specific gravity

3. To bear no external distinguishing signs, and to be put up in containers free of identifying marks. The containers for each treatment should be packed in separate boxes labelled with the identity of their contents.

* Samples must be indistinguishable to a panel of four judges.
(From Joyce, 1968)

(Reproduced with permission from Joyce CRB, 1982 [6]

The placebo concept should be included in all areas of therapeutic endeavour. It has been used in surgery where sham operations may be performed consisting of anaesthesia and incision of the skin. Foods or complete diets that look alike but differ in their composition can be used in dietetics. In acupuncture placebo points can be used which are not related to the traditional acupuncture points. In electroconvulsive therapy a series of studies was carried out which used anaesthesia, muscle relaxation, positioning of the electrodes but no actual shock. And, of course, it can be used in psychotherapy in some form [10].

The need for placebos to be indistinguishable from active treatment is because of the tendency for placebos to be regarded as being in some sense weaker or less credible or applied in a less enthusiastic manner than therapies believed to have intrinsic activity. At a minimum the placebo controls should be equivalent on major recognised common factors which might include expectancy of improvement, credibility of rationale, credibility of the actual procedures meeting the demand for improvement and the attention, enthusiasm, effort and perceived belief in treatment procedures and commitment to client improvement in the therapist him /or herself. As will be mentioned later, these factors are important in maximising placebo response but also maximising response to active medication as well.

ADVERSE REACTIONS

Although placebos are incorporated into comparative studies in order to control primarily for efficacy issues, they are also invaluable in providing a controlled database for unwanted effects and safety aspects. In that controlled environment, the differential elicitation of unwanted effects can be carried out and significances sought between the incidence and prevalence of such unwanted effects in the placebo and active treatment groups. The placebo may appear to give rise to such adverse effects (”nocebo” effects) [11] for four main reasons.

1. The placebo may not itself be totally inactive. For example, colouring matter on a capsule has been known to induce allergic or hypersensitivity reactions.
2. The illness itself may develop or even worsen and this is attributed to adverse effects of the medication.
3. The attempt to withdraw the medication may be followed by apparent discontinuation effects and this is well known to happen with long-term administration of placebos as well.
4. The method of administration may itself have some adverse effects even though the drug to be administered or the procedure to be given itself has no intrinsic dangers.
5. Previous administration of a similar but active preparation may have caused adverse effects [12].

Despite all of this a comparison between placebo and active drug groups provides the most accurate estimate of the adverse effects of the active medication. However, as the database for such clinical trials rarely exceeds 2000 patients per group, only relatively common adverse effects can be quantified in this way. Beyond that, one must rely on the inaccurate and often rather suspect methods such as spontaneous reporting and post marketing surveillance.

A complicating factor in drug-placebo comparisons with antidepressants is the unblinding of both patients and investigator by the detection of adverse effects of the antidepressant. The use, of so-called “active” placebos to mimic side effects of medication has been advocated as a solution [13].

ETHICS OF PLACEBO STUDIES [6]

The problem of placebos in clinical trials relates to the therapeutic studies only. In non-therapeutic studies, administration of the active medication when there is no therapeutic reason pre-empts any considerations that the placebo might be unethical. Indeed, it could be argued that failure to incorporate a placebo when one is exposing a non-patient to some tests, drug or procedure is itself unethical. With clinical trials, however, the need for a placebo requires careful consideration and may indeed vary from institution to institution [14]. In my own hospital, quite severely ill patients are referred to us, as a post graduate centre, and the use of placebo is less frequently justified than in primary care settings. The other factor to take into account is how well established the efficacy of a comparative study procedure is, not merely in the literature but within the context of the setting in which the study is to be carried out. If the investigators with their patients and selection procedures in that institution have consistent effects for a comparative substance then the use of the placebo is less necessary. The use of very low doses of a drug as a placebo is an unsatisfactory solution to this problem as it is still a placebo. In my experience, patients are surprisingly willing to accept that they may be given a dummy medication and do understand that a response may still be forthcoming to that "sugar pill".

THE PLACEBO RESPONSE

The problem of differentiating this from natural remission has been described earlier. The question of the time cause of the placebo response is usually that it shows a similar pattern to that of active medication. This may be somewhat belated compared with the active medication. The question of the further outcome in patients who have responded to placebo has been little addressed but there is some evidence, at least with antidepressant medication that the placebo response may not persist, particularly in the more chronically ill patients. This does seem to be reasonable. In other words, if natural remission takes place then the condition does not recur but if it is a chronic condition then the placebo response (wears off). A major question concerns the factors that govern placebo response and whether these are the same as those that govern response to an active medication. Firstly, of course, it should not be possible for the patient to determine whether or not they have taken an active medication. This is the goal of the double blind controlled trial but this can be vitiated by the obvious subjective effects of some medications. Secondly, the placebo response may not be sustained [15] (Figure 3).

The factors that govern the response to placebo are as follows:

The patient – there are important correlations between patient personality traits such as introversion/extraversion and "neuroticism" and drug response. The personality dimensions can influence response to active medication and can also influence quite profoundly response to placebos. The personality dimension that has been emphasised is suggestibility although in the present day usage of untried medications, the term gullibility might be more appropriate. The response of otherwise quite sensible people to claims for therapeutic efficacy of compounds which are unlikely to be active beggars belief. I do not want to get embroiled in whole question of homeopathic medicine but the pharmacology and rationale of such treatments is so obscure that one is forced to conclude that it is one of the most powerful sets of placebo responses available.

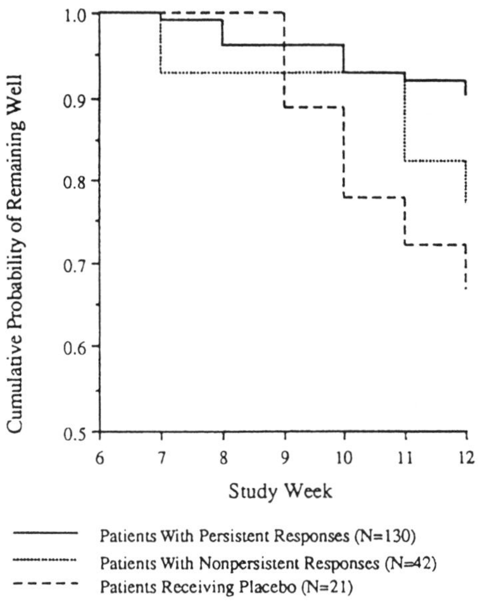

Figure 3. Cumulative probability of remaining well during study weeks 7-12 for patients with persistent and nonpersistent responses to drug treatment and for all patients receiving placebo (Reproduced with permission from Quitkin *et al.* 1993 [15])

Placebo responders among depressed patients include those who were apparently reacting to events or to life circumstances, those more recently becoming depressed and the less ill as assessed by standard rating scales [16] (Table 2).

The features in patients include motivation, expectation and experience but there is no clear type of individual who will respond to medication, rather response is individual, situation, complaint, and therapist influenced. This is so even for an interpersonal transaction such as psychotherapy [17]. Thus a patient may respond to all medication in one context, to another in another context, and be unresponsive in third context. It is also important to acknowledge the necessity for good information and it is also almost impossible to underestimate the ignorance that the average man in the street entertains concerning his or her bodily processes and their amenability to modification by therapy.

The doctor – the doctor's training, experience, susceptibility to suggestion himself, his scepticism and knowledge about medication will all influence the placebo response. Some workers suggested that the effects of sedatives on patients depend on the personality type of the physician, particularly whether or not he was authoritarian in urging the patient to show response. His enthusiasm for the treatment is also important and therapists' expectations often predict outcome. The use of alternative medication together with standard procedures may also increase by an interactional placebo effect.

Table 2.
Variables that differentiate placebo responders from nonresponders

	Responders	Nonresponders
Clinical and diagnostic variables		
Endogenous subtype	Nonendogenous	Endogenous
Length of illness[1]	Shorter	Longer
Abusive disorders[2]	Present	Absent
Beck depression inventory items		
Reduced ability to work (no. 15)	None to slight	Marked
Worsened appearance (no. 14)	None to slight	Marked

1. Length of illness is defined as time in months since the first episode of depression
2. Abusive disorders refer to a history of alcohol or drug abuse
(Reproduced with permission from Fairchild *et al.* 1986 [16])

Doctor – patient relationship.
The relationship between the doctor and the patient is important in deciding whether a placebo response can occur. Some physicians are dictatorial, others are much more amenable to discussion with the patient of their needs and expectations, so called "concordance". Some doctors are better at communicating with their patients and are sensitive to the patients' psychosocial situation. The quality of communication is more important than quantity. It is also increasingly evident that patients need written material to take away with them as the anxiety and stress associated with a consultation militate against the proper assimilation of information regarding treatment. This is usually effected by information leaflets and so on.

Societal factors
The attitude of society to patients and doctors continuously alters [18]. We have recently seen a phase of anti-science together with anti-medicine. This is compounded by the necessity now in Western societies to ration health care for a variety of reasons not relevant here. Accordingly, society is exploring alternative methods of therapy, particularly those which are cheaper or which appear to carry few if any unwanted effects [19]. That the efficacy of many of these procedures is untried seems to escape the notice of Society, the media and politicians. The placebo effects which are intrinsic in this response have received very little attention. Group effects are also important, responses depending upon what other treatments are given in a group [20].

THE DRUG

In clinical trials placebo must match the active drug in all respects except the inclusion of the active constituent. However, with placebo response, a whole variety of factors may come into play. The size, shape, colour of the tablets or capsule, and the taste of the liquid formulation are all very important. In some countries injections have a much more powerful placebo effect than do oral medications. Children believe large tablets are more powerful than small ones because they contain more drug, whereas adults tend to think that small tablets must be more potent. There is even an anecdotal report that one anxious patient reported that his minor tranquilliser, formulated as a two coloured capsule, worked better if he swallowed it green end first!

EXCLUSION OF THE PLACEBO RESPONDERS

One practical implication of the placebo response is the widespread practice of trying to remove placebo responders from clinical trials. It is customary, particularly with chronic conditions, to have a "wash-out" period during which the patient can be recruited, various tests such as liver function test carried out and any current medication stopped and washed out of the system. This is obviously acceptable providing that any potential withdrawal reaction is either detected or the time frame is such that it will have concluded by the time that the trial proper starts.

However, it is often the practice to administer a placebo, single blind, during the week or two before the commencement of the trial proper. The patient is assessed before and after this period and if a response has occurred, defined in some specific way, that patient is then excluded from the study. Statistically, this results in an enriched sample and will bias the study in favour of the active medication, as the placebo responders will have been selected out. The use of this enrichment procedure is justified where it is essential to establish as soon as possible, i.e. in phase II trials that a putative therapeutic agent is in fact active. However, in later studies the efficacy of the active medication will be exaggerated and certainly when the medication is licensed and released, disappointment may be an inevitable outcome of this practical use.

PLACEBO MECHANISM

It might be thought that this section is redundant. After all, placebo will have an effect through a variety of non-specific factors but it is hard to envisage any specific mechanisms that would be common or could be common to all therapeutic procedures. Nevertheless, there have been some interesting approaches to searching for such common factors. An example is the use of naloxone in attempts to block the analgesic effect of placebo procedures which are believed to be releasing endorphins. Other mechanisms could be invoked, such as the production of other neurotransmitters like GABA to induce sedation and 5-HT to elevate mood. The development of antagonists and the use of more focused induction techniques for mood are an obvious way forward in this respect.

CONCLUSIONS

Placebo reactions need future further study and analysis in order to optimise not only their usage in selected areas, but also to optimise the use of active medications which incorporate a placebo response as an element. The wise physician uses his skills and personality to maximise the impact of the placebo effects in his therapeutic endeavours. The careful medical scientist goes to great pains to control the placebo response in order to evaluate the therapeutic effects as precisely as possible of his curative techniques such as medications.

REFERENCES

1. Turner JL, Gallimore R, Fox-Henning C. An annotated bibliography of placebo research. (Journal Supplement Abstract Service) Washington, DC: Amer Psych Assoc 1980.
2. Shepherd M, Sartorius N (eds.) Non-Specific Aspects of Treatment. Toronto: Hans Huber, 1989.
3. Grünbaum A. The placebo concept in medicine and psychiatry. Psychol Med 1986; 16:19-38.
4. Shapiro AK. A contribution to a history of the placebo effect. Behav Sci 1960;5:109-135.
5. Shapiro AK. Semantics of the placebo. Psychiat Quart 1968;653-696.
6. Joyce CRB. Placebos and other comparative treatments. Br J Clin Pharmac 1982;13:313-318.
7. Critelli JW, Neumann KF. The placebo. Amer Psychol 1984;39:32-39.
8. McDonald CJ, Mazzuca SA, Mc Cabe GP How much of the placebo 'effect' is really statistical regression? Stat Med 1983;2:417-426.
9. Stassen H H, Angst J. Delayed onset of action of antidepressants. CNS Drugs 1998;3:177-184.
10. Suedfeld P. The subtractive expectancy placebo procedure: a measure of non-specific factors in behavioural interventions. Behav Res Ther 1984;22:159-164.
11. Morgan PP. Ten words to adopt for 1986. Can Med Ass J 1985;133:1193.
12. Modestin J. Psychological components of psychopharmacological side effects. Bull Menninger Clinic 1985;49:29-36.
13. Moncrieff J, Wessely S, Hardy R. Meta-analysis of trials comparing antidepressants with active placebos. Br J Psychiat 1998;172:227-231.
14. Garcia-Alonso F, Guallar E, Bakke O.M. Use and abuse of placebo in phase III trials. Eur J Clin Pharmac 1998;54:101-105.
15. Quitkin FM *et al.* Further advice that a placebo response to antidepressants can be identified. Am J Psychiat 1993;150:566-570.
16. Fairchild CJ at al. Which depressions respond to placebo. Psychiat Res 1986;18:217-226.
17. Frank JD. Therapeutic components of psychotherapy. J Nerv Ment Dis 1974;159:325-342.
18. Glyn JR, Heymann TD. Factors that influence patients in Sri Lanka in their choice between Ayurvedic and Western medicine. Br Med J 1985;291:470-472.

19. Coakley DV, McKenna GW .Safety of faith healing. Lancet 1986;I:444.
20. Nowlis V, Nowlis HH. Office of Naval Research Tech Rep Proj NR 1953:144-060:5400.

Discussion: Placebo response

A. Breckenridge:

I assume that even within psychiatric disease, there is a hierarchy of conditions where the placebo response may be more obvious than others. For example, I would imagine that in anxiety and depression you would get a bigger placebo response than in schizophrenia. Is that correct?

M. Lader:

That is not necessarily true. One of the conditions which had a very gratifyingly low placebo response was obsessive-compulsive disorder. As the medications for treating it became available, and more patients were being treated, the placebo response rate went up. But the placebo response is more related to severity than the actual diagnosis of the condition, and it is also related to the natural fluctuation in the illness. Psychiatric conditions are notorious for their fluctuation; and for the fact that people come to notice, not just because of worsening of the severity, but because of social factors as well.

M.M. Reidenberg:

In the development process of a new drug, one would try to select patients whose history is such that you will show the biggest difference from the placebo to get the drug registered. Then one is also selecting patients that are progressively less representative of the total population with the disease. And the difference between the efficacy in the clinical trials and the efficacy in the real world will get bigger as we learn more about placebo response, and whatever the condition is one is developing the drug for. Are there ways that we ought to handle this, so as not to exaggerate the potential benefit of a drug as we use it?

M. Lader:

The most obvious way is the exclusion of the placebo responders. Very often a study will have a placebo run-in period of one to two weeks. Any patient who improves by 20-40% on the rating scale is then excluded from randomisation. If the placebo responders are taken out, the sample is enriched with an artificial high measure of the effectiveness. The other particular problem in psychiatry is the co-morbidity. In anxiety disorders, there is something like 60-70% co-morbidity of disorders with social phobia. If these people are excluded, a measure of the drug efficacy in a 'pure' population is obtained, whereas in practice co-morbidity is the norm. I would like to see realistic studies (I do not mean natural history studies, and just giving the drug out) that recruit patients who have got co-morbidity. I think that probably just reflects the inchoate nature of psychiatric classification.

E.A. Kalso:

We have been looking at the effectiveness of anti-depressants in the chronic pain syndrome, and the amount of adverse events with the placebo is quite striking. The chronic pain syndrome is seen as a somatising syndrome. I was wondering whether our patients are especially prone to being strong placebo responders, and whether you are aware of any studies where a symptom check-list, for example, had been used in order to predict placebo responders.

M. Lader:

When a patient is in pain, depression is a very important adjunct, and a depressed patient will complain more severely of pain. It is unclear why they should particularly respond to placebo, but certainly within depressed patients who are not in pain, there is a high placebo response rate.

E.A. Kalso:

We have also seen that other adverse effects, which have nothing to do with depression or pain, are very frequent in the placebo group.

M. Lader:

It is probably something to do with the sensitisation of the patient's bodily symptoms. They become introspective, they pick a bodily change very easily. Panic disorder patients do the same, and therefore any spontaneous physical feeling will be magnified into a complaint.

E.A. Kalso:

Should we use the placebo also in the clinic, in order to find out in which patients we should use the real drug, and in which the placebo does the same?

M. Lader:

It would depend on the condition and on the particular patient. If a patient is believed to be over-responding to their minimal symptoms, then it might be worth trying the placebo. But I would only do it with the permission of the patient. There is occasionally a place for it. With the sort of patients I see, they have had placebos, usually it is a low dose of a drug given by the primary care practitioner.

J. Urquhart:

This discussion on placebo response, reminds me of what was a seminal court case in the history of American drug regulation in 1909. A drug company made an anti-cancer drug and made elaborate claims on the label for its efficacy. The then new FDA moved against him for mislabelling. It went up to the U.S. Supreme Court and Justice Oliver Wendell Holmes junior, who was a great American jurist, ruled for the majority and said that "As everyone knows, drug efficacy is a question of opinion, not of scientific fact. Therefore the claims on the label were protected by the First Amendment protection for freedom of speech". When you get into all these intricacies, if we should exclude placebo responders and so on, I wonder if Justice Holmes was not right.

M. Lader:

When I was on the UK regulatory authority, one of the great problems we had to address was homeopathy. Is the homeopathic remedy really a remedy or is it just an extremely elaborate, well-structured placebo response?

Variability in Human Drug Response
G.T. Tucker, Editor

Pharmacogenetic basis of variation in drug dependence

Edward M. Sellers, Myroslava K. Romach and Rachel F. Tyndale

Departments of Pharmacology, Medicine and Psychiatry, University of Toronto; and Centre for Addiction and Mental Health, Toronto, Canada.

ABSTRACT

Pharmacogenetic variations in the patterns of metabolism among individuals can importantly modulate the risk of drug dependence. Cytochrome P450 drug metabolizing enzymes (CYPs), can "activate" drugs of abuse (e.g. codeine to morphine) or deactivate drugs (e.g. nicotine to cotinine). Some CYPs are polymorphic, that is, there are gene mutations which result in no active enzyme (null mutations). Individuals with two null mutations appear in the population as phenotypic "poor metabolizers".

Using *in vitro* studies, we have identified drugs of abuse that are substrates of the polymorphic enzymes CYP2D6, CYP2A6 and CYP2C19. In human experimental studies, we have shown that CYP phenotype and genotype affect abuse liability for CYP2D6 metabolized drugs of abuse. In addition, we inhibited CYP2D6 and decreased individuals' risk of dependence experimentally and in treating codeine dependence.

In epidemiologic studies CYP2D6 and CYP2A6 null mutations protect individuals from becoming codeine and tobacco dependent, respectively. With respect to CYP2A6, heterozygote individuals, if they become smokers, smoke about 25% fewer cigarettes because of their slower nicotine metabolism. Since normally occurring mutations in CYP alleles decrease the risk of dependence, pharmacologic modification of CYP activity has the potential to prevent and treat drug dependence.

Key words: CYP2A6, CYP2D6, CYP2C19, behaviour, tobacco.

Correspondence: Dr. Edward M. Sellers, Department of Pharmacology, Room 4334, Medical Sciences Building, University of Toronto, 1 King's College Circle, Toronto, Ontario M5S 1A8, Canada, Tel: +1-416-323-7552, Fax: +1-416-323-7553, Email: e.sellers@utoronto.ca

Funding acknowledgement: This chapter and the research described were supported by the NIDA grant DA06889, MRC grant MT-14719, the University of Toronto, the intramural grants program of the Addiction Research Foundation of Ontario, and Nicogen Inc.

DRUG DEPENDENCE AS A MODEL OF BEHAVIOUR

Drug dependence is the consequence of the interaction of the drug, the individual and the environment. With respect to the drug, it must serve as a reinforcer by increasing the probability that once taken the drug will be taken again. Drugs that are reinforcers can have this action by having positive rewarding effects (e.g. subjective euphoria) or by removing punishing or unpleasant experiences (e.g. alleviating depression during the "crash" from cocaine). Drugs which have aversive properties are less likely to be abused unless tolerance to the unpleasant effects occurs. Other features of the drug, which are important, include the rate of absorption and entry into the brain, lipid solubility and pattern of metabolism. For some drugs of abuse the parent drug is principally responsible for the drugs reinforcing properties (e.g. cocaine, nicotine, and amphetamines) while for others the metabolites are most important (e.g. codeine conversion to morphine).

Even though drug dependence is complex, its study is quite straightforward since precise and well-validated measures of the behaviour exist. Extensive methodology exist for quantitating the frequency of drug taking (an excellent measure of the strength of the reinforcer), the objective and subjective consequences of drug use, the physiologic effects of drug and the socio-economic effects of drug abuse. For this reason drug dependence provides an unusually precise model with which to determine the consequences of variations in drug disposition on behaviour.

THE CYTOCHROME P450 POLYMORPHISMS

Cytochromes (CYP) P450 (P450s) are enzymes involved in the oxidative metabolism of a wide array of endogenous and exogenous molecules, including steroids, plant metabolites, prostaglandins, biogenic amines, drugs and chemical carcinogens. This broad spectrum of reactions is due to multiple P450 isozymes, with differing but overlapping substrate specificities. The mammalian P450 super-family consists of at least 12 families and over 400 individual genes. Genetic variants of P450 have been discovered because of atypical clinical responses in individuals who were shown subsequently to have a reduced ability to metabolize a drug. These phenotypically different individuals (also called poor metabolizers [PMs]) have been the basis of identifying the genetic basis of the variants and denoting pharmacogenetic polymorphisms. Those with enzyme activity are termed extensive metabolizers (EMs). The phenotype of individuals is determined along with the activity of CYPs using a sub-clinical dose of a probe drug such as dextromethorphan (CYP2D6), omeprazole (CYP2C19) or coumarin (CYP2A6). The genotype of the individual is determined with allele specific polymerase chain reaction amplification assays developed for the detection of specific mutations in the CYP gene.

In addition, to the most commonly occurring or normal ("wild type") allele, for most CYPs, allele variants have been identified that result in the gene producing an inactive enzyme (null mutation) or an enzyme with lower or even higher activity. As a result in any population combinations of homozygote wild type and null mutations exist along with the heterozygotes for all allele variants. With respect to nomenclature the wild type is denoted as the *1 allele and subsequent allele variants are denoted as *2, *3, *4, etc. based on their order of discovery.

For CYPs with null mutations the frequency-distribution of the logarithm of the ratio of parent drug to metabolite may be bimodal with varying percentages of the population comprising the upper mode with low activity (PMs). The frequency of the PM phenotype and allele frequencies shows considerable inter-ethnic variation [1].

IMPACT OF PHARMACOGENETIC POLYMORPHISMS ON DEPENDENCE RISK

Because these cytochrome are involved in the metabolism of drugs of abuse it is likely that differences in patterns of metabolism among individuals and across ethnic group will importantly affect the risk of drug abuse and dependence (e.g. CYP2D6 codeine, hydrocodone, p-methoxyamphetamine, amphetamine) or inhibitors (e.g. (-)-cocaine, pentazocine; CYP2A6 nicotine; CYP2C19 diazepam and other benzodiazepines). The consequences of absent or inhibited CYP activity for any particular drug will depend on the relative activity of the parent drug and its various metabolites. In some cases, the pharmacology of the metabolite is qualitatively similar to the parent; in other cases, the pharmacology is different (e.g. dextromethorphan to dextrorphan); more usually, it is not properly understood. In addition, some CYPs occur within the CNS. Their role in the brain is unknown, but potential formation of active drug metabolites at their site of action makes the presence of them potentially of great functional significance. A computer simulation study of inter-regional differences in CNS drug metabolism has provided a model which could account, in part, for large inter-subject variability in the pharmacodynamic effects of psychoactive drugs [2].

CYP deficient individuals should have a much decreased probability of abusing a drug converted to an active metabolite capable of maintaining drug-taking behaviour (e.g. codeine, oxycodone, hydrocodone, dextromethorphan). In EMs, the probability of dependence is increased, and proportionate to their genotype (homozygous versus heterozygous) and absolute CYP activity. Conversely, PMs should experience greater risk of abuse or of toxicity to a drug which is inactivated by a CYP and EMs a lesser risk. The clinical consequence of this could be either an increased risk or decreased risk of dependence depending on the relative punishing as versus reinforcing drug properties.

CYTOCHROME P450 2D6

Several drugs of abuse, codeine [3], hydrocodone, oxycodone [4], dextromethorphan [5], and p-methoxyamphetamine [6] are known to be metabolized by this enzyme.

i) **Amphetamines**

Deficiency in the p-hydroxylation of amphetamine was one of the observations that led to the discovery of the CYP2D6 polymorphism [7,8]. A single oral administration of the radiolabelled enantiomers of amphetamine to three volunteers with subsequent analysis of urine indicated that about 5% of (+)-amphetamine was converted to p-hydroxyamphetamine in two subjects but to a much less extent in a subject who was later found to have CYP2D6 deficiency [7,8].

The central nervous system stimulant p-methoxyamphetamine (PMA) is extremely O-demethylated by CYP2D6 to form 4-hydroxyamphetamine [6,9]. In the early 1970's, PMA was associated with a number of idiosyncratic deaths in Canada [10]. A cardinal feature of these deaths was increased blood pressure, arrhythmias and hyperthermia. The lack of relationship to dose suggests that the individuals who died may have been CYPD6 (PMs). These clinical data and *in vitro* studies [11] suggest that CYP2D6 activity and individual genotype may contribute to amphetamine dependence risk and toxicity.

ii) **Dextromethorphan**

Dextromethorphan has the opposite steric configuration to codeine and morphine, is devoid of analgesic effects but is as potent an antitussive as codeine. It is the most commonly used antitussive world-wide. Systematic studies concerning its abuse liability are few. In the earliest report [12] no abuse liability was found with oral doses up to 100 mg. However, there are many case reports of dextromethorphan abuse and endemic use principally among young people [13]. Monkeys and rats can be trained to self administer dextromethorphan (with difficulty) but will do so more easily for its active metabolite dextrorphan. They will also recognize dextrorphan in particular as a discriminative stimuli and will generalize from and to phencyclidine [14] suggesting dextromethorphan abuse potential is due to its metabolite dextrorphan. Dextromethorphan is metabolized to its active metabolite dextrorphan by CYP2D6. Variations in the activity of the enzyme results in different kinetics and pharmacologic effects in EM and PM individuals [15,16]. EM individuals produce almost 40-fold more dextrorphan than PMs. In 4 EM and 2 PM normal volunteers given 3.0 mg/kg of dextromethorphan p.o. the effects of dextromethorphan are very different [16]. EMs show more euphoria and high effects and less sedation and dysphoria. As a result PM, individuals are probably protected from becoming dextromethorphan abusers by having greater punishing effects of the drug (sedation and dysphoria) and fewer pleasant effects (high and euphoria).

iii) **Codeine**

From a public health perspective, the misuse and abuse of opiate containing prescription medications is a poorly understood and largely unaddressed issue. Prescription analgesics including opioids (e.g. codeine, oxycodone, and hydrocodone) alone and in combination (e.g. 222®, Tylenol #3®) are extensively used worldwide and are always within the major classes of drugs prescribed in all countries.

Codeine is converted to morphine by CYP2D6. Morphine is at least 10-fold more potent than codeine as an analgesic and is responsible for the clinical efficacy of codeine and probably the side effects. In human experimental studies we have shown that CYP activity is a major determinant of codeine abuse liability [17]. In an epidemiologic study, the PM phenotype and genotype were absent among codeine dependent individuals compared to never dependent and dependent on other drugs of abuse comparison groups [18]. In addition, very high CYP2D6 activity was also not found among codeine dependent individuals suggesting that very extensive conversion to morphine (and its attendant side effects) might also protect against dependence.

CYTOCHROME P450 2A6

Recently a genetic polymorphism for CYP2A6 has been established PMs (lacking CYP2A6 activity) excrete less than 0.1% of the coumarin probe drug as 7-hydroxycoumarin [19,20].

Due to the recent identification of this polymorphism, the numbers of people who have been phenotyped/genotyped is small, however it appears that the allele frequency varies among ethnic groups.

i) **Nicotine Metabolism and Smoking Behaviour**

Nicotine is the primary compound present in tobacco that is responsible for establishing and maintaining tobacco dependence; dependent smokers adjust their smoking behaviour to maintain peripheral and central nicotine levels [21]. Evidence includes increased smoking behaviour if nicotine content in cigarettes is decreased, increased smoking if nicotine excretion is increased by urine acidification, decreased smoking with concurrent intravenous or patch IC [22]. Approximately 50% of initiation of smoking dependence is genetically influenced, while persistence of smoking and amount smoked have approximately a 70% genetic contribution. In humans, approximately 70% of nicotine is metabolized by inactivation to cotinine. We, and others, recently identified the genetically polymorphic CYP2A6 enzyme as the enzyme responsible for the majority of the metabolic conversion of nicotine to cotinine [23,24]. There is considerable interindividual variability in hepatic CYP2A6 function due predominantly to genetic variation in the *CYP2A6* gene locus. Three *CYP2A6* alleles have been identified: wild-type (*CYP2A6**1), and two defective null alleles (*CYP2A6**2 and *CYP2A6**3) [20]. Individuals with the *CYP2A6*2/ CYP2A6*3* and *CYP2A6*3/ CYP2A6*3* genotype have no CYP2A6-mediated metabolism.

Individuals with impaired nicotine metabolism (carriers of a defective *CYP2A6* allele[s]) would be protected from becoming tobacco-dependent. When learning to smoke individuals often find the nicotine unpleasant (e.g. causing dizziness or nausea). In individuals where nicotine metabolism was decreased, due to defects in the *CYP2A6* gene, the aversive effects might last longer or reach higher levels. Tobacco dependent (DSM-IV criteria) only, alcohol and tobacco dependent (DSM-IV criteria), and never-tobacco dependent groups were genotyped for *CYP2A6*. Twenty percent of the non-smoking population were carriers of defective *CYP2A6* alleles. In contrast to the non-smokers, in the dependent-smokers with or without alcohol dependence, only 12% of the individuals had *CYP2A6* defective alleles (20.1% [n = 213] versus 11.7% [n = 317], $p < 0.01$, χ-square; Odds Ratio = 1.9, 95% Confidence Intervals 1.2 - 3.2). This data provides evidence that impaired nicotine metabolism due to defective *CYP2A6* alleles is protective against becoming tobacco-dependent [25].

Within the tobacco-dependent group, those who had one defective and one active *CYP2A6* gene copy smoked significantly fewer cigarettes per day and per week than smokers without impaired nicotine metabolism ([carriers of two *CYP2A6* active alleles] 129 versus 159 cigarettes/week, t-test $p < 0.02$). These data show that heterozygosity in a single gene, the *CYP2A6* gene, significantly decreases both initiation of dependence and the drug-taking behaviour.

CYTOCHROME P450 2C19

The metabolism of mephenytoin and omeprazole are biomodal in the population, the deficiency is inherited at a single gene locus of CYP2C19. This CYP metabolizes many clinically used drugs including benzodiazepines. Ethnic differences in the PM frequency occur.

Three deficient variants from the active form of (*2, *3 and *4) have been identified; neither gene variant produces a functional CYP2C19 protein.

i) **Diazepam and Flunitrazepam Abuse**

Diazepam, is an established and important drug of abuse among opiate addicts, poly-drug abusers (including those with alcoholism), and young abusers worldwide especially in Asia [26]. However, flunitrazepam is the benzodiazepine with the highest abuse liability (followed by diazepam and is reported worldwide as the benzodiazepine most widely abused by opioid abusers [27]. Flunitrazepam is not marketed in the U.S. or Canada but is a growing and endemically abused drug in parts of the U.S. Two abuse liability experimental study of snorted flunitrazepam have shown increases in liking with increased doses of flunitrazepam. Subjective ratings and liking were highly correlated with flunitrazepam plasma levels [28]. Heroin users surveyed [27] reported using flunitrazepam only orally before 1990, but by 1994 36% of users reported injecting it i.v., usually in combination with heroin, allegedly to augment and prolong the subjective effects of heroin. Similarly, the fact that flunitrazepam tablets can be ground up and inhaled raises concern about toxicity and abuse. Heroin users or methadone patients have ranked flunitrazepam first in preference among benzodiazepines.

The mean clearance of diazepam and desmethyldiazepam is slower (about 40%) in the CYP2C19 PMs but there was considerable variability among individuals [29]. Inter-racial differences are likely due to concurrent differences in CYP2C19 and CYP3A. The higher frequency of 2C19 mutated gene in Asians and overrepresentation of heterozygous among Asian extensive metabolizers is one of the possible explanations for the observed differences both in clearance and subjective effects of diazepam. Omeprazole inhibits diazepam CYP2C19-mediated clearance and slows its elimination in Caucasian CYP2C19 EM [30]. Omeprazole (40 mg/ day for 21 days) decreased diazepam clearance by 28 ± 14.4 % and decreased desmethyldiazepam AUC by 42.4 ± 17% in Caucasians, which was significantly more than in Chinese (20% and 25% changes) [31].

The few studies of flunitrazepam metabolism have shown metabolism to desmethyl-flunitrazepam, 7-amino-flunitrazepam, 3-hydroxy-flunitrazepam and other aminobenzophenones. The compound mainly responsible for the hypnotic effect is thought to be the parent compound [32]; however, the N-desmethyl-metabolite also has affinity for the $GABA_A$ receptor complex [33]. Two studies have identified catalytic outliers who produced little or no N-desmethyl, consistent with CYP2C19 deficiency; one was an American Indian [32,34].

We now have preliminary evidence that genotype profoundly influences the objective and subjective effects of flunitrazepam in Chinese healthy volunteers. Two Chinese PMs and one EM subjects were administered flunitrazepam (1 mg, orally) after 8 h fasting period. Objective and subjective effects were then measured before and 0.5, 1, 2, 3, 4, 6 and 9 hours after flunitrazepam administration. Results showed that the PMs have significantly decreased psychomotor performance than the EMs. Also, sedation, elation and "spacey" and other subjective effects associated with benzodiazepine toxicity and abuse (e.g. drug liking, good effects, etc.) were significantly higher in PM compared to EM [35].

CONCLUSIONS

These studies establish that pharmacogenetic variations in drug metabolism have important behavioural consequences altering the risk of drug abuse and dependence. In addition, since these enzymes can be inhibited there are important implications with respect to the development of new and needed prevention and treatment approaches to this major public health problems.

REFERENCES

1. Sellers EM, Otton SV, Tyndale RF. The potential role of the cytochrome P450 2D6 pharmacogenetic polymorphism in drug abuse. In: Rapaka RS, Chiang N, Martin BR (eds.) Pharmacokinetics, metabolism, and pharmaceutics of drugs of abuse. NIDA Research Monograph #173. Rockville: U.S. Department of Health and Human Services, 1997;6-26.
2. Britto M, Wedlund PJ. Cytochrome P-450 in the brain. Potential evolutionary and therapeutic relevance of localization of drug-metabolizing enzymes. Drug Metab Dispos 1992;20:446-450.
3. Chen ZR, Somogyi AA, Bochner F. Polymorphic O-demethylation of codeine. Lancet 1988;2:914-915.
4. Otton SV, Schadel M, Cheung SW, Kaplan HL, Busto UE, Sellers EM. CYP2D6 phenotype determines the metabolic conversion of hydrocodone to hydromorphone. Clin Pharmacol Ther 1993;54:463-472.
5. Schmid B, Bircher J, Preisig R, Kupfer A. Polymorphic dextromethorphan metabolism: Co-segregation of oxidative O-demethylation with debrisoquine hydroxylation. Clin Pharmacol Ther 1985;38:618-624.
6. Kitchen I, Tremblay J, Andres J, Dring LG, Idle JR, Smith RL, Williams RT. Interindividual and interspecies variation in the metabolism of the hallucinogen 4-methoxyamphetamine. Xenobiotica 1979;9:397-404.
7. Dring LG, Smith RL, Williams RT. The metabolic fate of amphetamine in man and other species. Biochem J 1970;116:425-435.
8. Smith RL. Introduction: Human genetic variations in oxidative drug metabolism. Xenobiotica 1986;16:361-365.
9. Wu D, Otton SV, Inaba T, Kalow W, Sellers EM. Interactions of amphetamine analogs with human liver CYP2D6. Biochem Pharmacol 1997;53:1605-1612.
10. Sellers EM, Martin PR, Roy ML, Sellers EA. Amphetamines. In: Lomax P, Schonbaum, E, (eds.) Modern pharmacology-toxicology, 16 - Body temperature: Regulation, drug effects and therapeutic implications. New York: Marcel Dekker, Inc., 1979;461-498.
11. Wu D, Otton SV, Kalow W, Sellers EM. Effects of route of administration on dextromethorphan pharmacokinetics and behavioral response in the rat. J Pharmacol Exp Ther 1995;274:1431-1437.
12. Isbell H, Fraser HF. Actions and addiction liabilities of Dromoran derivaties in man. J Pharmacol Exp Ther 1953;107:524-530.
13. McElwee NE, Veltri JC. International abuse of dextromethorphan (DM) products: 1985 to 1988 statewide data. Vet Human Toxicol 1990;32:355.

14. Holtzman SG. Phencyclidine-like discriminative effects of opioids in the rat. J Pharmacol Exp Ther 1980;214:614-619.
15. Schadel M, Wu D, Otton SV, Kalow W, Sellers EM. Pharmacokinetics of dextromethorphan and metabolites in humans: Influence of the CYP2D6 phenotype and quinidine inhibition. J Clin Psychopharmacol 1995;15:263-269.
16. Zawertailo LA, Gomez-Mancilla B, Kaplan HL, Tyndale RF, Sellers EM. Psychotropic effects of dextromethorphan are altered by the CYP2D6 polymorphism: A pilot study. J Clin Psychopharmacol 1998;18:332-337.
17. Kathiramalainathan K, Kaplan HL, Busto UE, Romach MK, Tyndale RF, Sellers EM. Inhibition of cytochrome P450 2D6 modifies codeine metabolism and abuse liability. Abstracts of XIth International Symposium on Microsomes and Drug Oxidations (Los Angeles, California) 1996;239.
18. Tyndale RF, Droll KP, Sellers EM. Genetically deficient CYP2D6 metabolism provides protection against oral opiate dependence. Pharmacogenetics 1997;7:375-379.
19. Rautio A, Holger K, Kojo A, Salmela E, Pelkonen O. Interindividual variability of coumarin 7-hydroxylation in healthy volunteers. Pharmacogenetics 1992;2:227-233.
20. Fernandez-Salguero P, Hoffman SM, Cholerton S, Mohrenweiser H, Raunio H, Rautio A, Pelkonen O, Huang JD, Evans WE, Idle JR, Gonzalez FJ. A genetic polymorphism in coumarin 7-hydroxylation: Sequence of the human CYP2A genes and identification of variant CYP2A6 alleles. Am J Hum Genet 1995;57:651-660.
21. McMorrow MJ, Foxx RM. Nicotine's role in smoking: An analysis of nicotine regulation. Psychol Bull 1983;93:302-327.
22. Benowitz NL. Pharmacologic aspects of cigarette smoking and nicotine addiction. New Engl J Med 1988;319:1318-1329.
23. Nakajima M, Yamamoto T, Nunoya K, Yokoi T, Nagashima K, Inoue K, Funae Y, Shimada N, Kamataki T, Kuroiwa Y. Role of human cytochrome P4502A6 in C-oxidation of nicotine. Drug Metab Dispos 1996;11:1212-1217.
24. Messina ES, Tyndale RF, Sellers EM. A major role for CYP2A6 in nicotine C-oxidation by human liver microsomes. J Pharmacol Exp Ther 1997;283:1608-1614.
25. Pianezza ML, Sellers EM, Tyndale RF. Nicotine metabolism defect reduces smoking. Nature, 1998;393(6687):750.
26. Sellers EM, Ciraulo DA, DuPont RL, Griffiths RR, Kosten TR, Romach MK, Woody GE. Alprazolam and benzodiazepine withdrawal. J Clin Psychiatry 1993;54(10,Suppl.): 64-75.
27. San L, Tato J, Torrens M, Castillo C, Farré M, Camí J. Flunitrazepam consumption among heroin addicts admitted for inpatient dextoxification. Drug Alcohol Depend 1993;32:281-286.
28. Bond A, Seijas D, Dawling S, Lader M. Systemic absorption and abuse liability of snorted flunitrazepam. Addiction 1994;89:821-830.
29. Bertilsson L, Henthorn TK, Sanz E, Tybring G, Säwe J, Villen T. Importance of genetic factors in the regulation of diazepam metabolism: Relationship to *S*-mephenytoin, but not debrisoquin, hydroxylation phenotype. Clin Pharmacol Ther 1989;45:348-355.
30. Ishizaki T, Sohn D-R, Kobayashi K, Kobayashi K, Chiba K, Lee KH, Shin S-G, Andersson T, Regårdh CG, Lou YC, Zhang Y, *et al.* Interethnic differences in omeprazole metabolism in the two *S*-mephenytoin hydroxylation phenotypes studied in Caucasians and Orientals. Ther Drug Monit 1994;16:214-215.

31. Caraco Y, Tateishi T, Wood AJ. Interethnic difference in omeprazole's inhibition of diazepam metabolism. Clin Pharmacol Ther 1995;58:62-72.
32. Wickstrøm E, Amrein R, Haefelfinger P, Hartmann D. Pharmacokinetic and clinical observations on prolonged administration of flunitrazepam. Eur J Clin Pharmacol 1980;17:189-196.
33. Garattini S, Mussini E, Randall LO (eds.). The benzodiazepines. Monographs of the Mario Negri Institute for Pharmacological Research. New York: Raven Press, 1973.
34. Boxenbaum HG, Posmanter HN, Macasieb T, Geitner KA, Weinfeld RE, Moore JD, Darragh A, O'Kelly DA, Weissman L, Kaplan SA. Pharmacokinetics of flunitrazepam following single- and multiple-dose oral administration to healthy human subjects. J Pharmacokinet Biopharm 1978;6:283-293.
36. Kilicarslan T, Li N-Y, Busto U, Tyndale RF, Sellers EM. Flunitrazepam: Polymorphic metabolism by CYP2C19. Clin Pharmacol Ther 1998;63:218.

Discussion: Pharmacokinetic basis of variation in drug dependence

H.K. Kroemer:
Do you know whether there is a regulation of CYP2A6 by nicotine?

E.M. Sellers:
Although CYP2A6 is in a general a regulated enzyme, it does not appear to be regulated by nicotine in any important way.

H.K. Kroemer:
Is there any evidence about the extrahepatic expression of CYP2A6?

E.M. Sellers:
CYP2A6 is found in the lung and also in some other tissues like in the brain, although in quite small amounts. But where it is found it is very close to the mapping of the nicotinic receptors. It is different to the other cytochromes, whose distribution seems to be unrelated to anything we can figure out. At least, in this case, we can have some hypothesis about the relationship in the brain.

G.T. Tucker:
You probably won't answer this question, but I wonder which compound you have patented as an inhibitor of CYP2A6?

E.M. Sellers:
You are quite right, I am not able to answer that question.

A. Breckenrigde:
There are not a lot of acceptable compounds which might fulfil these criteria. Is that right?

E.M. Sellers:
I said there were not many substrates. There might be potent inhibitors, not necessary chemical inhibitors, which could alter the CYP2A6 expression by different mechanisms.

U. Klotz:
If your hypothesis on nicotine is right, then addiction to smoking should be much less in the Asian population. Did you look at some interethnic differences, or are there any epidemiological data?

E.M. Sellers:
We have not looked at this directly. An important issue related to this question is that counting cigarettes is not really the best way to quantitate smoking behaviour. It is necessary to use more precise measures of smoking behaviour and exposure to smoke. The same would be true with, for example, the exposure to carcinogenic compounds and their activation. Related to these issues, the Japanese population are an interesting because they, and particularly males, smoke a lot. Up to 60% of males are regular smokers. However, Japanese

have among the lowest incidence of lung cancer. This is an interesting kind of dichotomy, so there may be other factors such as the environmental contribution.

U. Klotz:

In the very small opioid dependent group of 83 patients, you did not see any poor metaboliser. According to a recent publication (Chen *et al.*, Br J Clin Pharmacol 1997) in a group of healthy volunteers participating in clinical studies, the poor metaboliser frequency was 1.6%. So with n = 83 you might be just within the confidence interval of spontaneous variation.

E.M. Sellers:

That is a possibility. These results need to be replicated by larger studies. Another factor we found quite important here was that our control populations have a lower frequency of the PM phenotype, from 3.5 to 4%. In different countries you see this. It requires very careful assessment of drug-dependence criteria and other drug abuse.

I.P. Hall:

On the nicotine story, can you just go over the difference between heterozygotes and homozygotes? What I need reassuring is that there is good functional evidence that the heterozygote genotype has a major functional effect.

E.M. Sellers:

In *in vitro* studies, when a bank of 31 genotyped livers were studied, the relationship of the CYP2A6 content to nicotine metabolism was highly correlated (r=0.96), therefore very little else appears to be contributing in the *in vitro* model system.

I.P. Hall:

If you take heterozygote smokers, matched for smoking exposure, they have got higher nicotine levels. Is that correct?

E.M. Sellers:

Yes, they do.

Role of phenotyping and genotyping in the measurement of variability in human drug response

Julio Benítez

Department of Pharmacology and Psychiatry, Medical School, University of Extremadura, Badajoz, Spain

ABSTRACT

Among the causes of variability in human drug response, interindividual variation in enzymes, receptors and transporters play an important role. Best known are the interindividual differences in drug metabolism, caused by genetic-environmental interactions, especially for those drugs mainly metabolised by genetically polymorphic enzymes. The population was divided in extensive (EM) and slow, or so called poor metabolisers (PM). Side effects with normal doses were to be expected in PM patients treated with drugs metabolised by the polymorphic enzymes and perhaps lack of therapeutic effect in the faster EMs. Several drugs suffering polymorphic metabolism were withdrawn and the pharmaceutical industry usually decided not to develop drugs suffering polymorphic metabolism. However, most of the drugs metabolised in the body suffer interindividual differences in metabolism but that does not necessarily mean that clinically significant problems are always to be expected. On the other hand, the fast development of pheno and genotyping methodologies make it feasible to predict kinetics, and in many cases drug response, early in drug development and therefore prevent clinical problems in healthy volunteers or patients. The recent mibefradil case in the US could be an interesting example for consequences of not considering this issue at the right moment.

Key words: Pharmacogenetics, genetic polymorphisms, enzymes, drug effects.

Correspondence: Prof. Julio Benítez, Department of Pharmacology and Psychiatry, Medical School, University of Extremadura, 06071 Badajoz, Spain, Tel: +34-924-28-9458, Fax: +34-924-27-11-00, Email: jbenitez@unex.es

INTRODUCTION

Among the causes of variability in human drug response interindividual variation in human genes coding for enzymes, receptors and transporters could play an important role. Besides, dynamic interactions are known to occur between genetic and environmental factors causing large interindividual variations in drug response. Since the discovery of genetic polymorphism in the metabolism of isoniazid in the early 60s (now known to be mediated by N-acetyl transferase 2 or NAT2) and even more after a similar discovery for debrisoquine in the 70s

(CYP2D6), and other cytochrome isoenzymes thereafter, some of the causes for interindividual differences in drug response were identified. As it often happens, too simplistic conclusions were reached at the beginning. So the population was divided in extensive (EM) and slow or so called poor metabolisers (PM) and side effects with normal doses were to be expected in PM patients treated with drugs metabolised by the polymorphic enzymes. Likewise, lack of therapeutic effect in the faster EM was expected. Several drugs suffering polymorphic metabolism were withdrawn and the pharmaceutical industry was well advised not to develop drugs suffering polymorphic metabolism. However, most of the drugs metabolised in the body suffer interindividual differences in metabolism but that does not necessarily mean that clinically significant problems are to be expected in all of them. Those drugs, which have important active metabolites and/or several equally important metabolic pathways, mediated by different enzymes and/or have a high therapeutic index, will very rarely cause clinically significant problems because of differences in metabolic capacity.

Recent availability of pheno and genotyping methodology is making possible to prevent or diminish many of these problems, both in drug development and in actual clinical practice. *In vitro* studies are now carried out for most new drugs under development to find out its main metabolic pathways and the enzymes involved. This way some side effects and drug interactions with potential clinical significance can be predicted. Rapid development of newer methodologies, such as DNA sequencing, will make feasible in the near future to extend this knowledge to most drugs metabolised in the body. However, correlation between geno and phenotype and actual drug effects should not be forgotten if we really want to get the best safety and efficacy in treatment to most patients [Kalow, 1989].

ENZYMES POTENTIALLY IMPORTANT IN DRUG METABOLISM IN MAN

In table 1 main liver enzymes known to be involved in drug metabolism in man are shown. More will appear in the near future but we will concentrate on those already studied in man. All the enzymes shown belong to the cytochrome P-450 system, with the exception of NAT2. The arylamine N-acetyltransferase (NAT-2) polymorphism causes impaired drug metabolism in about half of the white population [Agúndez, 1994],[Agúndez, 1996],[Carrillo, 1994]. However, most of the drugs so far known to be metabolised by this enzyme have either a high therapeutic index, or they are not so commonly used. Therefore, NAT2 has had more implications from the toxicological point of view and for carcinogenic mechanisms [Agúndez, 1995],[Agúndez, 1996],[Agúndez, 1996],[Martínez, 1995]. Drug-metabolizing enzymes encoded by the cytochrome P450 genes, are noted for their high degree of interspecies and intraspecies variability [González, 1990]. Cytochrome P-450 comprises several enzymes but we will consider here only those so far found to be potentially important in for drug metabolism in man.

CYP1A2

Phenotyping methods for this enzyme have been developed and tested in different populations by the group of Kalow [Kalow, 1991],[Tang, 1994],[Tang, 1996] and several others [Fuhr, 1996]. Caffeine is the probe more frequently used for CYP1A2 phenotyping [Carrillo, 1996]. The metabolic profile of caffeine biotransformation by CYP1A2 averages around 80% for paraxanthine, 11% for theobromine and 5% for theophylline formation [Gu, 1992]. So far, no genotyping method is available for CYP1A2 and it is an enzyme with very important environmental influence. Caffeine, smoking and several drugs can modify significantly CYP1A2 phenotype. The atypical antipsychotic drug clozapine, as well as many other psychotropic drugs are metabolised by CYP1A2 to a major extent [Bertilson, 1994]. Moreover, changes in the habitual caffeine intake alter the metabolism of clozapine in schizophrenic patients [Carrillo, 1998].

Table 1.
Main liver enzymes known to be involved in drug metabolism in man

Enzyme	Usual probe	Genetic polymorphism	Typing methods available
CYP1A2	Caffeine	?	Phenotype
CYP2C9	Diclofenac	Yes	Pheno/Genotype
CYP2C18	Tolbutamide	Yes	Pheno/Genotype
CYP2C19	S-mephenytoin	Yes	Pheno/Genotype
CYP2D6	Debrisoquine	Yes	Pheno/Genotype
CYP2E1	Chlorzoxazone	Yes	Pheno/Genotype
CYP3A4	Midazolam	?	Phenotype
NAT2	Caffeine	Yes	Pheno/Genotype

CYP2C

Four members of this subfamily have been identified so far in humans: CYP2C8, CYP2C9, CYP2C18, and CYP2C19. CYP2C9 and CYP2C19 are much better characterised than CYP2C8 and CYP2C18 in man. CYP2C9 is important in the metabolism of certain therapeutically used drugs including the anticoagulant drug warfarin and a number of nonsteroidal antiinflammatory drugs. A number of allelic variants of CYP2C9 exist in humans, but the effects of these allelic variants on metabolism *in vivo* remain to be determined. Diclofenac is being used as a probe for CYP2C9 phenotyping, although some discrepancies have been found between geno and phenotype [Klose, 1998],[Yamazaki, 1998].

A well-characterised genetic polymorphism occurs in CYP2C19, which is associated with the metabolism of the anticonvulsant drug mephenytoin. In population studies, individuals can be segregated into extensive and poor metabolizers of mephenytoin. Poor metabolizers are unable to 4'- hydroxylate the S-enantiomer of mephenytoin. There are marked interethnic variations in the frequency of the poor metabolizer phenotype, which represents 1 to 5% of Caucasians. Mephenytoin is the most frequently used probe for CYP2C19 phenotyping [Goldstein, 1994],[Stubbins, 1996].

CYP2D6

The debrisoquine hydroxylase (CYP2D6) catalyzes the oxidative metabolism of more than 40 different clinically important drugs. The CYP2D6 gene is highly polymorphic. Defect alleles, causing the poor metabolizer phenotype, and also alleles with duplicated or multiduplicated active genes, causing ultrarapid metabolism, have been described. It is clearly the most thoroughly studied drug metabolic polymorphism so far. From 5% to 10% of Caucasians designated as poor metabolizers (PMs) of the debrisoquine/sparteine polymorphism have a severely impaired capacity to metabolize several therapeutically used drugs [Alván, 1990],[Benítez, 1988]. Debrisoquine [Lennard, 1990], followed by dextromethorphan [Henthorn, 1989] and sparteine [Eichelbaum, 1979] are the most frequently used probes for CYP2D6 phenotyping. The gene controlling CYP2D6 is located on the long arm of chromosome 22 [Gaedigk, 1991],[González, 1991],[Linder, 1997]. Ultrarapid metabolism of debrisoquine has been shown in 1% to 30% in several populations [Johansson, 1993],[Akullu, 1996],[Agúndez, 1995]. Several methods for genotyping have been developed [Dahl, 1995],[Johansson, 1996],[Agúndez, 1994]

CYP2E1

Ethanol-inducible CYP2E1 is an enzyme of interest because it metabolizes several procarcinogens and solvents to reactive metabolites. CYP2E1 has also been implicated in alcohol liver disease because of its contribution to oxidative stress. However, not many drugs have been found to be metabolized by CYP2E1 so far [Tateishi, 1997]. Chlorzoxazone is being used for CYP2E1 phenotyping [Bachmann, 1996],[Lucas, 1996],[Burckart, 1998]. Previously, polymorphic alleles with mutations in introns and in the 5'-flanking regulatory region have been described, and their presence has been related to the incidence of alcohol liver disease and lung cancer. Genotyping studies in man have shown that the CYP2E1 gene is functionally surprisingly well conserved compared with other cytochrome P450 enzymes active in drug metabolism, which suggests an important endogenous function in humans [Hu, 1997].

CYP3A

CYP3A isoforms are responsible for the biotransformation of a wide variety of exogenous chemicals and endogenous steroids in human tissues. Two members of the CYP3A subfamily display developmentally regulated expression in the liver; CYP3A7 is expressed in the fetal liver, whereas CYP3A4 is the major cytochrome P-450 isoform present in the adult liver. CYP3A4 expression is transcriptionally activated during the first week after birth and is accompanied by a simultaneous decrease of CYP3A7 expression, in such a way that the overall CYP3A protein content remains nearly constant [Lacroix, 1997].

Cytochrome P-450 enzymes of the CYP3A gene subfamily account for up to 30% of the total cytochrome P-450 present in the adult human liver and for the majority of cytochrome P-450 in the human small bowel [Shimada, 1994]. Many *in vitro* and *in vivo* drug interactions have been reported at the CYP3A site. There are pronounced patient differences caused by genetic and environmental factors in the metabolism of CYP3A substrates. Midazolam has been suggested as probe for CYP3A4 phenotyping [Carrillo, 1998]. CYP3A isoforms are also expressed outside the liver and this could have implications, both for the initiation of pulmonary carcinogenesis by agents that require metabolic activation, such as tobacco-derived polycyclic aromatic hydrocarbons and perhaps for local metabolism of topical drugs. CYP3A5 is the predominant CYP3A form in human lung and CYP3A4 is expressed in about 20% of individuals, but considerable variation of pulmonary expression occurs in both CYPs between individuals [Anttila, 1997].

CONCLUSIONS

Several enzymes of the cytochrome P-450 system have been found to be causing clinically significant variability in human drug response. Among them CYP1A2, CYP2C9, CYP2D6 and CYP3A4 are perhaps the most important. Pheno and/or genotyping all the possibly involved relevant enzymes should be a must for phase I clinical trials and very useful in certain cases in phase II and III clinical trials for new drugs under development. More basic research in man with regard to genetic-environmental interactions in drug metabolism, as well as that related to drug receptors and transporters, is urgently needed. This will be the only way to avoid toxicity and increase efficacy during drug development as well as to facilitate molecule selection. Although methods for phenotyping and genotyping exist for most relevant enzymes, better possibilities are foreseen in the near future that will make it possible to predict with more accuracy drug metabolism and response.

REFERENCES

· Agúndez JA, Martínez C, Olivera M, Ledesma MC, Ladero JM, Benítez J. Molecular analysis of the arylamine N-acetyltransferase polymorphism in a Spanish population. Clin Pharmacol Ther 1994;56:202-9.

· Agúndez JA, Martínez C, Ledesma MC, Ladona MG, Ladero JM, Benítez J. Genetic basis for differences in debrisoquin polymorphism between a Spanish and other white populations. Clin Pharmacol Ther 1994;55:412-7.

· Agúndez JA, Ladero JM, Olivera M, Abildua R, Román JM, Benítez J. Genetic analysis of the arylamine N-acetyltransferase polymorphism in breast cancer patients. Oncology 1995;52:7-11.

· Agúndez JA, Ledesma MC, Ladero JM, Benítez J. Prevalence of CYP2D6 gene duplication and its repercussion on the oxidative phenotype in a white population. Clin Pharmacol Ther 1995;57:265-9.

· Agúndez JA, Olivera M, Martínez C, Ladero JM, Benítez J. Identification and prevalence study of 17 allelic variants of the human NAT2 gene in a white population. Pharmacogenetics 1996;6:423-8.

· Agúndez JA, Menaya JG, Tejeda R, Lago F, Chávez M, Benítez J. Genetic analysis of the NAT2 and CYP2D6 polymorphisms in white patients with non-insulin-dependent diabetes mellitus. Pharmacogenetics 1996;6:465-72.

· Agúndez JA, Olivera M, Ladero JM, *et al.* Increased risk for hepatocellular carcinoma in NAT2-slow acetylators and CYP2D6-rapid metabolizers. Pharmacogenetics 1996;6:501-12.

· Akullu E, Persson I, Bertilsson L, Johansson I, Rodrigues F, Ingelman-Sundberg M. Frequent distribution of ultrarapid metabolizers of debrisoquine in an ethiopian population carrying duplicated and multiduplicated functional CYP2D6 alleles. J Pharmacol Exp Ther 1996;278:441-6.

· Alván G, Bechtel P, Iselius L, Gundert RU. Hydroxylation polymorphisms of debrisoquine and mephenytoin in European populations. Eur J Clin Pharmacol 1990;39:533-7.

· Anttila S, Hukkanen J, Hakkola J, *et al.* Expression and localization of CYP3A4 and CYP3A5 in human lung. Am J Respir Cell Mol Biol 1997;16:242-9.

· Bachmann K, Sarver JG. Chlorzoxazone as a single sample probe of hepatic CYP2E1 activity in humans. Pharmacology 1996;52:169-77.
· Benítez J, Llerena A, Cobaleda J. Debrisoquin oxidation polymorphism in a Spanish population. Clin Pharmacol Ther 1988;44:74-7.
· Bertilsson L, Carrillo JA, Dahl ML, *et al.* Clozapine disposition covaries with CYP1A2 activity determined by a caffeine test. Br J Clin Pharmacol 1994;38:471-3.
· Burckart GJ, Frye RF, Kelly P, *et al.* Induction of CYP2E1 activity in liver transplant patients as measured by chlorzoxazone 6-hydroxylation. Clin Pharmacol Ther 1998;63:296-302.
· Carrillo JA, Benítez J. Caffeine metabolism in a healthy Spanish population: N-acetylator phenotype and oxidation pathways. Clin Pharmacol Ther 1994;55:293-304.
· Carrillo JA, Benítez J. CYP1A2 activity, gender and smoking, as variables influencing the toxicity of caffeine. Br J Clin Pharmacol 1996;41:605-8.
· Carrillo JA, Ramos SI, Agúndez JA, Martinez C, Benítez J. Analysis of midazolam and metabolites in plasma by high-performance liquid chromatography: probe of CYP3A. Ther Drug Monit 1998;20:319-24.
· Carrillo JA, Herraiz AG, Ramos SI, Benítez J. Effects of caffeine withdrawal from the diet on the metabolism of clozapine in schizophrenic patients [In Process Citation]. J Clin Psychopharmacol 1998;18:311-6.
· Dahl ML, Johansson I, Bertilsson L, Ingelman-Sundberg M, Sjoqvist F. Ultrarapid hydroxylation of debrisoquine in a Swedish population. Analysis of the molecular genetic basis. J Pharmacol Exp Ther 1995;274:516-20.
· Eichelbaum M, Spanbrucker N, Steincke B, Dengler HJ. Defective oxidation of sparteine in man. A new pharmacogenetic defect. Eur J Clin Pharmacol 1979;16:183-187.
· Fuhr U, Rost KL, Engelhardt R, *et al.* Evaluation of caffeine as a test drug for CYP1A2, NAT2 and CYP2E1 phenotyping in man by *in vivo* versus *in vitro* correlations. Pharmacogenetics 1996;6:159-76.
· Gaedigk A, Blum M, Gaedigk R, Eichelbaum M, Meyer UA. Deletion of the entire cytochrome P450 CYP2D6 gene as a cause of impaired drug metabolism in poor metabolizers of the debrisoquine/sparteine polymorphism. Am J Hum Genet 1991;48:943-50.
· Goldstein JA, de Morais SM. Biochemistry and molecular biology of the human CYP2C subfamily. Pharmacogenetics 1994;4:285-99.
· González FJ, Nebert DW. Evolution of the P450 gene superfamily: animal-plant 'warfare', molecular drive and human genetic differences in drug oxidation. Trends Genet 1990;6:182-6.
· González FJ, Meyer UA. Molecular genetics of the debrisoquin-sparteine polymorphism. Clin Pharmacol Ther 1991;50:233-8.
· Gu L, González FJ, Kalow W, Tang BK. Biotransformation of caffeine, paraxanthine, theobromine and theophylline by cDNA-expressed human CYP1A2 and CYP2E1. Pharmacogenetics 1992;2:73-7.
· Henthorn TK, Benítez J, Avram MJ, *et al.* Assessment of the debrisoquin and dextromethorphan phenotyping tests by gaussian mixture distributions analysis. Clin Pharmacol Ther 1989;45:328-33.
· Hu Y, Oscarson M, Johansson I, *et al.* Genetic polymorphism of human CYP2E1: characterization of two variant alleles. Mol Pharmacol 1997;51:370-6.
· Johansson I, Lundqvist E, Bertilsson L, Dahl ML, Sjoqvist F, Ingelman-Sundberg M. Inherited amplification of an active gene in the cytochrome P450 CYP2D locus as a cause of

ultrarapid metabolism of debrisoquine [see comments]. Proc Natl Acad Sci U S A 1993;90:11825-9.
· Johansson I, Lundqvist E, Dahl ML, Ingelman-Sundberg M. PCR-based genotyping for duplicated and deleted CYP2D6 genes. Pharmacogenetics 1996;6:351-5.
· Kalow W. Genetic polymorphism in drug oxidation. Psychopharmacol Ser 1989;7:148-62.
· Kalow W, Tang BK. Use of caffeine metabolite ratios to explore CYP1A2 and xanthine oxidase activities. Clin Pharmacol Ther 1991;50:508-519.
· Klose TS, Ibeanu GC, Ghanayem BI, *et al.* Identification of residues 286 and 289 as critical for conferring substrate specificity of human CYP2C9 for diclofenac and ibuprofen [In Process Citation]. Arch Biochem Biophys 1998;357:240-8.
· Lacroix D, Sonnier M, Moncion A, Cheron G, Cresteil T. Expression of CYP3A in the human liver--evidence that the shift between CYP3A7 and CYP3A4 occurs immediately after birth. Eur J Biochem 1997;247:625-34.
· Lennard MS. Genetic polymorphism of sparteine/debrisoquine oxidation: a reappraisal. Pharmacol Toxicol 1990;67:273-83.
· Linder MW, Prough RA, Valdes R, Jr. Pharmacogenetics: a laboratory tool for optimizing therapeutic efficiency. Clin Chem 1997;43:254-66.
· Lucas D, Menez JF, Berthou F. Chlorzoxazone: an *in vitro* and *in vivo* substrate probe for liver CYP2E1. Methods Enzymol 1996;272:115-23.
· Martínez C, Agúndez JA, Olivera M, Martín R, Ladero JM, Benítez J. Lung cancer and mutations at the polymorphic NAT2 gene locus. Pharmacogenetics 1995;5:207-14.
· Shimada T, Yamazaki H, Mimura M, Inui Y, Guengerich FP. Interindividual variations in human liver cytochrome P-450 enzymes involved in the oxidation of drugs, carcinogens and toxic chemicals: studies with liver microsomes of 30 Japanese and 30 Caucasians. J Pharmacol Exp Ther 1994;270:414-23.
· Stubbins MJ, Harries LW, Smith G, Tarbit MH, Wolf CR. Genetic analysis of the human cytochrome P450 CYP2C9 locus. Pharmacogenetics 1996;6:429-39.
· Tang BK, Zhou Y, Kadar D, Kalow W. Caffeine as a probe for CYP1A2 activity: potential influence of renal factors on urinary phenotypic trait measurements. Pharmacogenetics 1994;4:117-24.
· Tang BK, Kalow W. Assays for CYP1A2 by testing *in vivo* metabolism of caffeine in humans. Methods Enzymol 1996;272:124-31.
· Tateishi T, Watanabe M, Nakura H, *et al.* Halothane inhalation inhibits the metabolism of chlorzoxazone, a substrate for CYP2E1, in rabbits. Anesth Analg 1997;85:199-203.
· Yamazaki H, Inoue K, Chiba K, *et al.* Comparative studies on the catalytic roles of cytochrome P450 2C9 and its Cys- and Leu-variants in the oxidation of warfarin, flurbiprofen, and diclofenac by human liver microsomes. Biochem Pharmacol 1998;56:243-51.

Discussion: Role of phenotyping and genotyping in the measurement of variability in human drug response

"Due to problems with the recording of this presentation, reproduction of the discussion was not possible. The Esteve Foundation apologises to the author and discussants."

Variability in Human Drug Response
G.T. Tucker, Editor

Population Modelling

Leon Aarons

School of Pharmacy and Pharmaceutical Sciences, University of Manchester, Manchester, U.K.

ABSTRACT

Frequently dosing recommendations that emerge from a clinical drug development program are found inappropriate and when individual dose adjustment is needed, the recommendations provided may not be informative enough to allow the adjustment to be undertaken in an optimal manner. Frequently, and particularly in the later stages of drug development, only relatively sparse observational concentration and effect data are available. Recently developed statistical methods offer the possibility of gaining integrated information on pharmacokinetics and response from such data, obtained directly in patients who are being treated with the drug under development. The methods allow the incorporation of data from patient groups which are often excluded from classically designed clinical trials and also the analysis of a variety of unbalanced designs that frequently arise in the evaluation of dose or concentration- efficacy and -safety profiles, which do not readily lend themselves to other forms of statistical analysis. The analysis of sparse observational data, which is called the population approach, has been implemented in phase III studies to obtain additional information about the PK/PD model. However, the primary purpose of phase III clinical trials generally is not PK/PD and consequently population PK/PD studies must be carefully interwoven with existing protocols.

Key words: drug development, pharmacokinetics, pharmacodynamics, sparse data.

Correspondence: Leon Aarons, School of Pharmacy and Pharmaceutical Sciences, University of Manchester, Manchester M13 9PL, U.K., Tel: +44-161-275-2357, Fax: +44-161-275-2396, Email: l.aarons@man.ac.uk

INTRODUCTION

Pharmacokinetics, from the literal Greek meaning of the name, is the study of drug movement in the body. More specifically it is the study of the processes of drug absorption, distribution and elimination and frequently the definition is extended to encompass the relationship between plasma concentration and pharmacological effect, which more correctly is described as pharmacodynamics. Traditionally, pharmacokinetic studies have involved intensive experimentation in small groups of subjects, often healthy volunteers, in which a relatively large number of blood samples are withdrawn following drug administration. The design and analysis of such experiments is well established [1].

However consider the following data on tobramycin obtained during routine therapeutic drug monitoring [2]. Data from 97 patients (45 female, 52 male) were collected. The duration of therapy in individual patients ranged from 14 to 520 hr. 322 concentrations were available for data analysis with between 1 and 9 per individual (median 2). Drug concentrations were measured usually 2 and 6 hr after the dose in patients with normal renal function, with additional measurements (12 and 24 hr after the dose) in patients with impaired renal function. The age of the patients ranged from 16 to 85 yr, weight ranged from 42 to 120 kg and creatinine clearance ranged from 10 to 160 $ml.min^{-1}$. There are several points worth noting about this data set. Whereas in "conventional" pharmacokinetic study designs exclusion criteria are used to make the study population as homogeneous as possible (at least within a block) the population from the tobramycin study is very heterogeneous. No attempt was made to balance subject variables such as age, weight and renal function. The optimum pharmacokinetic model for tobramycin is the standard two-compartment model which involves four parameters. One does not have to be a statistician to realize that with, in some cases, only one plasma concentration per individual it is not possible to determine all four parameters. This sort of data is often referred to as **sparse**. Clearly there is information in the data but it is not possible to extract this information by conventional means, that is by investigating the parameters of each individual. To make progress one has to forget about individual analysis, at least to start with, and concentrate on the central tendency of the whole data, that is to determine the population pharmacokinetics.

Population pharmacokinetics is the study into the pharmacokinetic similarity and differences between individuals from measurements of drug levels in biological fluids of subjects or patients arising from some population of interest [3]. In contrast to a traditional study a population pharmacokinetic study involves large numbers of patients with very heterogeneous characteristics. Study control is difficult: many studies involve outpatients and many centres are involved. The reason for adopting a population approach to pharmacokinetic studies is that it has become increasingly obvious that one should study the drug in the target population, which may be different from a normal population. For example, pharmacokinetics may be altered by pathophysiological factors such as renal disease. In addition, apart from estimating mean pharmacokinetic parameters it is important to both quantify and explain interindividual variability, information which is important for the design of dosage regimens and therapeutic drug monitoring.

TERMINOLOGY

Like all fields that bridge a number of disciplines, population pharmacokinetics is bedevilled by a mix of terminology and jargon. Some of the more common terms are defined here and, in the process, some aspects of data analysis are described.

Population pharmacokinetics. The study of the variability in plasma drug concentrations between individuals when standard dosage regimens are administered. Essentially the field deals with the exploration and quantification of trends in pharmacokinetic parameters as a function of patient characteristics: for example the dependency of renal clearance on renal function and volume of distribution on body size.

Interindividual variability. When applied to population pharmacokinetics, the average deviation of the drug concentration-time profile of an individual from the population mean.

This deviation may be explainable in terms of **covariates** such as renal function, age and weight.

Intraindividual variability. When applied to population pharmacokinetics, the residual variability in the drug concentration that is not explained by interindividual variability. The residual variability may be due to variability in the drug measurement, "biological" variability or to misspecifying either the pharmacokinetic model or the model describing the interindividual variability. These two sources of variability are contrasted in Figure 1.

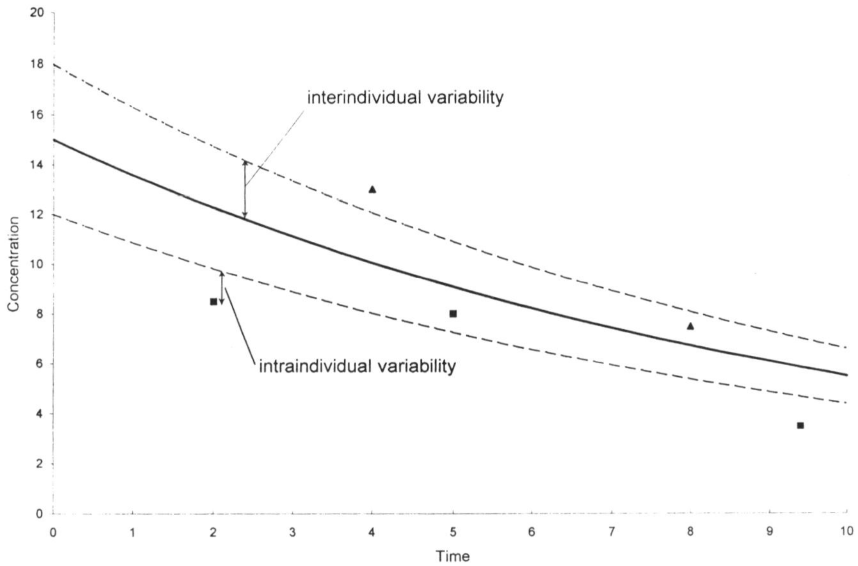

Figure 1. Sources of population pharmacokinetic variability. The solid line represents the "population mean" profile while the broken lines represent the individual profiles for subject j (data ▲) and subject k (data ■). The difference between an individual profile (at any time) and the mean profile is due to interindividual variability and the residual difference between the data and the individual profile is due to intraindividual variability.

Population pharmacokinetic model. The population pharmacokinetic model is a model that describes the drug concentration-time profiles of individuals within a population. It is comprised of two parts: a **structural model**, usually a conventional pharmacokinetic model, such as a one-compartment model, which may also involve covariates such as age and weight; and a **variance model**. It should be noted that the population pharmacokinetic model is not simply obtained by substituting the means of the pharmacokinetic parameters, obtained from fitting individual profiles, in the appropriate pharmacokinetic model.

Variance model. The variance model describes the difference between the drug concentration in an individual and that predicted by the structural model. The variance model may be a function of the pharmacokinetic parameters and covariates and in addition may involve other parameters. If the departure of an individual drug concentration from the population value is independent of concentration the variance model is said to be **additive**. On the other hand if the variance model is additive only after the structural model is log transformed, the variance model is said to be **multiplicative**.

Some examples. Consider a drug which can be described by a one-compartment pharmacokinetic model following iv administration, viz

$$C(t) = D/V{*}\exp[-CL/V{*}t]$$

where CL, the clearance, and V, the volume of distribution are the pharmacokinetic parameters. If in a population of patients receiving this drug the CL varies in proportion to renal function, as measured by creatinine clearance, CL_{Cr}, and the volume of distribution is proportional to body weight, then the pharmacokinetic model for the ith patient receiving a dose, D_i, would be

$$C(t) = D_i/(\theta_1{*}BWT_i){*}\exp[-(\theta_2{*}CL_{Cr})/\theta_1{*}BWT){*}t]$$

where θ_1 and θ_2 are the proportionality constants. The population pharmacokinetic model for the case where the inter- and intraindividual error terms are additive would be

$$C(t) = f(\theta_1,\theta_2,BWT,CL_{Cr},t)+\eta_i+\varepsilon_{ij}$$

where f is the concentration predicted by the model, η_i is the difference between the population prediction and the prediction for subject i and ε_{ij} is the residual departure of the predictions from the observations after accounting for interindividual effects. Normally the interindividual variability would be further partitioned into the contributions arising from the differences in pharmacokinetic parameters between individuals.

Nonlinear mixed effects model. A mixed effects model refers to a statistical model in which some characteristics are taken as fixed, that is known exactly, and others are assumed to be random. A nonlinear mixed effects model implies that the model is not a linear function of the parameters, which are to be determined from the data. Age and weight would be examples of fixed effects whereas inter- and intraindividual effects are random. The most widely known computer program in the area of population pharmacokinetics, **NONMEM** [4], implements a nonlinear mixed effect model (hence the name).

Bayesian analysis. If some population pharmacokinetic information is available from previous studies this **prior** information can be formally incorporated into the analysis of current data using Bayesian techniques [5].

COMPUTER SOFTWARE

The analysis of data arising from a mixed effects model is not a trivial matter and requires sophisticated computer software. A number of approaches have been suggested [4-7]. An expert meeting to discuss population pharmacokinetic/pharmacodynamic (PK/PD) software was held in Brussels in 1993 under the auspices of the European Co-operation in Science and Technology (COST), Medicine (B1) programme. The meeting developed from a successful conference (New Strategies in Drug Development and Clinical Evaluation: the Population Approach) held in Manchester in 1991 [8], also organized under the auspices of the COST B1 programme. The purpose of the Brussels meeting was to evaluate the present state of existing software and software under development; to specify the needs and wishes of potential users' of such software; and to integrate users' needs and software structures.

A full report of the proceedings of this meeting has been published [9]. The main message from the meeting was that the development of population software is an area of active interest. Already several very good packages are available and more are in development. There was general agreement that well validated, easy to use software was essential to the implementation of the population approach to drug development. The following is a summary of the important conclusions from the meeting.

- Software should be sufficiently user-friendly to allow an informed user to carry out population PK/PD analysis
- It is essential to be able to fully specify sparse data, including data arising from complex dosing histories
- Similarly it should be possible to specify pharmacokinetic and pharmacodynamic models in a completely flexible manner
- Good graphical diagnostics are essential for population analysis
- It is crucial that software is adequately supported and maintained.

DESIGN AND PERFORMANCE OF POPULATION PK/PD STUDIES

The subject of the design of PK/PD studies was the subject of another COST-B1 meeting [10]. The purpose of the design meeting was to discuss current experience in the design and performance of population PK/PD studies. The main conclusions arising from the meeting were:

- When participating in the design of a new study, the population approach group must be careful not to include sampling or data collection items that would compromise the main objectives of the clinical trial.
- It is particularly important to communicate the purpose of the population PK/PD analysis to the investigators and to convince them of the importance of accurate timing and documentation.
- Some prior knowledge of the PK and PD models and covariate relationships is necessary for the analysis of sparse phase III data.
- Subject numbers are often dictated by the main objective of the clinical trial. However computer simulation and optimal design measures may be useful to define sampling times.
- Population methods must be specified in the protocol. Although population PK/PD analysis is often exploratory, the data analysis strategy should be specified as fully as possible.

PHARMACOKINETIC SCREEN

The current interest in population pharmacokinetics was prompted by the concern that drugs, even drugs likely to be used in the elderly are not studied adequately in elderly patients and that as a consequence older patients are more likely than younger patients to suffer adverse drug reactions to drugs [11]. The FDA recommended that clinical trials should be conducted in target populations and the variability of the responses should be analyzed. During premarketing clinical trials, drugs should be subjected to a "pharmacokinetic screen". The spirit of the proposal was to look for unexpected phenomena and for large deviations in important features, such as side effects. Any finding should be followed up in subsequent, well-controlled trials. Sheiner and Benet [12] defined a number of ways in which this pharmacokinetic screen could be implemented.

1. A full pharmacokinetic study. This is the traditional approach of intensive sampling in a small number of subjects. As we have already remarked, this approach is not suitable for population pharmacokinetic studies.
2. Single trough screen. The number of subjects studied can be increased by reducing the number of samples taken per individual. The limit is one sample per individual and the obvious time to take this sample is just before a dose, that is a trough sample. Although such data can be analyzed by conventional ANOVA and the influence of covariates can be assessed, it provides limited pharmacokinetic information and does not allow the separation of intra- and interindividual variability.
3. Multiple trough screen. By taking more than one trough sample it is possible to partition intra- and interindividual variability, but such data still has limited pharmacokinetic information.
4. Full screen. If only a limited number samples can be taken for each individual than these samples should be spread throughout the dosing interval so that the data set viewed in its entirety maps out the concentration-time profile. Such designs allow the estimation of pharmacokinetic parameters and the separation of the different components of variability. The price that has to be paid is that sophisticated data analysis techniques have to be employed.

THE CURRENT SITUATION

The last ten years has seen an increased activity in the area of population pharmacokinetics [8,13]. This interest was initially driven by therapeutic drug monitoring (TDM) and the need to make sense out of limited data [14]. However the methodology has now been applied to a wider range of problems. In particular the pharmaceutical industry has become aware of the advantages of analyzing data gathered during Phase II and III clinical trials, and it is apparent that a growing number of pharmaceutical companies are either actively investigating or are very interested in the use of population approaches in drug development [15]. Several issues need to be resolved:

1. Lack of trained personnel and user friendly software. These two go hand in hand. It is clear that the analysis of population pharmacokinetic data can not be treated as a hobby.

Staff have to be dedicated to population analysis and these activities need to be integrated into the drug development process.

2. Quality of data. Since much of the data generated during Phase III clinical trials is in outpatients there is a real concern about compliance and hence the quality of that data. Any solution that attempts to improve the quality of such data will inevitably incur a cost.
3. Experimental design and power. Experience with population approaches during drug development is increasing. However, so far only small scale simulation studies have been performed to investigate the optimal experimental design for the estimation of population pharmacokinetic parameters. Similarly little is known about the ability of population based approaches to detect important differences between subpopulations, that is to detect subpopulations at risk.
4. Selection of patients. Patients should be representative of patients receiving the drug. Certain subpopulations at risk should be preassigned and there should be a sufficiently large spread in important covariates such as age, weight, renal function etc.
5. The attitude of regulatory authorities. Regulatory authorities are aware of the interest in the area of population pharmacokinetics [16,17] but there is some concern about the acceptability of the approach. Recently the FDA has produced some draft guidelines for population pharmacokinetic studies [18].

SUMMARY

One tends to be wary about adopting new approaches in an area which has well-established and validated methodology, particularly when there is little real experience with the new approach. The population approach is **not** a replacement for the conventional approach in drug development. Instead it is envisaged that the information from population analyses would complement and extend the information that is already being gathered. Indeed it is necessary to have a lot of baseline data on a drug - such as a good idea of the optimal pharmacokinetic model, an understanding of the metabolic pathways and some knowledge of the subpopulations that may have different pharmacokinetics - before embarking on a population study. This information would come from conventional studies.

Population pharmacokinetics should be viewed as a tool that can be used to extract meaningful information from clinical trial data that, up until now, has been largely discarded. The extra information available from such studies must increase the knowledge base of the drug and therefore must be worthwhile. However the cost/benefit ratio needs to be monitored. Above all there is an overwhelming need to study the pharmacokinetics of a drug in the target population as early as possible in a drug's development. It is unfortunate that the current controversy/debate has occurred since, on reflection, most scientists involved in drug development will realize that they are working towards the same goal.

In summary the following points need to be emphasized:

1. There are logistic and ethical problems involved in carrying out traditional intensive pharmacokinetic studies in large numbers of patients. Consequently only sparse data is likely to be available from such studies. These data have to be analysed in a statistically correct manner. To ignore the potential information in this data is both a waste of money

and is ethically unacceptable. A pharmacokinetic screen has been suggested as a means of implementing population pharmacokinetic studies.
2. Population based analyses should be viewed as exploratory in nature and therefore any unusual findings should be followed up by well controlled clinical trials. There is a risk of detecting false positives and therefore studies should be conducted in the light of the accumulated information and proceed in a sequential manner.
3. Although the nature of the drug development programme will not be radically altered by the advent of population based methodology there are expenses that will be incurred. Firstly a number of staff have to be dedicated to population analysis and these staff have to be trained. Secondly there is a need for quality data (one would argue that there is always a need for quality data). To ensure the quality of data gathered during Phase III clinical studies - compliance, dosing history and timing of samples - an extra level of monitoring may be necessary. Thirdly there is a cost for computing software and hardware. Interestingly enough, although much of the debate on population approaches centres around the computer programmes that are used, the costs of computing are much smaller than those of staff.
4. There are a number of studies that will, by their nature, only generate sparse data. These include studies in neonates, the acutely ill, field studies in the third world and frail elderly subjects.

REFERENCES

1. Gibaldi M, Perrier D. Pharmacokinetics. 2nd ed. New York: Marcel Dekker, 1982.
2. Aarons L, Vozeh S, Wenk M, Weiss Ph, Follath F. Population pharmacokinetics of tobramycin. Br J Clin Pharmacol 1989; 28:305-314.
3. Aarons L. Population pharmacokinetics: theory and practice. Br J Clin Pharmacol 1991; 32: 669-670.
4. Beal SL, Sheiner LB. Estimating population kinetics. CRC Crit Rev Biomed Eng 1982; 8: 195-222.
5. Racine-Poon A, Smith AFM. Population models. In: Berry DA (ed.) Statistical Methodology in the Pharmaceutical Sciences. New York: Marcel Dekker, Inc., 1990, 139-162.
6. Mallet A. A maximum likelihood estimation method for random coefficient regression models. Biometrika 1986; 73: 645-656.
7. Lindstrom MJ Bates DM. Nonlinear mixed effects models for repeated measures data. Biometrics 1990; 46: 673-687.
8. Rowland M, Aarons L (eds.). New Strategies in Drug Development and Clinical Evaluation: the Population Approach. Luxembourg: Commission of the European Communities, 1992.
9. Aarons L, Balant LP, Mentré F, Morselli PL, Rowland M, Steimer J-L, Vozeh S. Population approaches in drug development. Report on an expert meeting to discuss population pharmacokinetic/pharmacodynamic software. Eur J Clin Pharmacol 1994; 46: 389-391.

10. Aarons L, Balant LP, Mentré F, Morselli PL, Rowland M, Steimer J-L, Vozeh S. Practical experience and issues in designing and performing population pharmacokinetic/pharmacodynamic studies. Eur J Clin Pharmacol 1996; 49: 251-254.
11. Temple R. Food and Drug Administration's guidelines for clinical testing of drugs in the elderly. *Drug Information Journal* 1985; 19: 483-486.
12. Sheiner LB, Benet LZ. Premarketing observational studies of population pharmacokinetics of new drugs. Clin Pharmacol Ther 1985; 38: 481-487.
13. Aarons L, Balant LP, Danhof M, Gex-Fabry M, Gundert-Remy UA, Karlsson MO, Mentré F, Morselli PL, Rombout F, Rowland M, Steimer J-L, Vozeh S (eds.). The Population Approach: Measuring and Managing variability in Response, Concentration and Dose. Luxembourg: Commission of the European Community, 1997.
14. Sheiner LB Beal SL. Bayesian individualisation of pharmacokinetics: simple implementation and comparison with non-Bayesian methods. J Pharm Sci 1982; 71: 1344-1348.
15. Jochemsen R. Current experience of population pharmacokinetics within the pharmaceutical industry: an introduction. In: Rowland M, Aarons L (eds.) New Strategies in Drug Development and Clinical Evaluation: the Population Approach. Luxembourg: Commission of the European Communities, 1992, 127-130.
16. Gundert-Remy UA. Population approaches in pharmacokinetics and pharmacodynamics - views within regulatory agencies: Europe. In: Rowland M, Aarons L (eds.) New Strategies in Drug Development and Clinical Evaluation: the Population Approach. Luxembourg: Commission of the European Communities, 1992, 153-156.
17. Peck C. Population approach in pharmacokinetics and pharmacodynamics: FDA view. In: Rowland M, Aarons L (eds.) New Strategies in Drug Development and Clinical Evaluation: the Population Approach. Luxembourg: Commission of the European Communities, 1992, 157-168.
18. http://www.fda.gov/cder/guidance/1852pk.htm

Discussion: Population modelling

N. Benowitz:

I was very curious about the statement that the FDA objected to the use of this modelling technique, because it was not planned as part of the analysis. Is there any bias that you can see in not planning this technique in advance?

L. Aarons:

I think they simply pointed out that 17% of cases were retrospective, and I am not sure that was an objection. The biggest problem they have is when someone has done the experiment and then he has asked the statistician to analyse the results. In this situation, the statisticians were never involved with the design of the experiment, and the chances of them being able to get a useful result out of it is fairly negligible. And the same is true here, if you are going to apply the method retrospectively, and it has not been designed appropriately, then the danger is that you really are not going to get useful information out of it.

A. Breckenridge:

My understanding of the European drug regulation authorities is that they have no objection to the use of population kinetics, provided it is backed up with a package of conventional pharmacokinetics. Is that your understanding as well?

L. Aarons:

I cannot answer that directly, but I can give you my opinion. Population PK/PD was never meant to replace traditional methodology, although in the early days it was thought to. It is another tool but it is not a panacea, therefore there is a place for the traditional Phase I studies. Now, how far should you go? There are situations where, in fact, data are not being analysed because they cannot be analysed by traditional methods. Therefore it is a tool which can analyse that data anyway. There are people who go a little further than that, and say that it is actually unethical not to analyse that data, with the provisos we just mentioned about design and so forth.

T. Salmonson:

Generally speaking, I think the lack of knowledge within regulatory agencies is greater in Europe than in the U.S., when it comes to population pharmacokinetic aspects. Having said that, I know that some companies are questioning if the FDA still is as favourable to the approach today as it was a number of years ago. In Europe it is regarded to be something to be used together with the standard package, not replace, which perhaps can give us additional information. I think it is also fair to say that few agencies do have statisticians or kineticists that can actually access this data. We are quite proud in Sweden to have that knowledge. The population approach is becoming more and more interesting from a regulatory perspective, but it is very slowly maturing in Europe compared to the US.

J. Urquhart:

One of the things that is striking in the contrast between PK and PD is that when you get into the PD side, you have what I call hard non-linear areas, which their reflection is the dynamic asymmetries between on and off responses. You have some drugs like omeprazole that turn on quickly and go off very slowly, and others, like paroxetine, which go on very slowly and go off very rapidly. If you only have observations on the one side, you are in total darkness about what the other side is going to look like. There is a kind of a minimum data set that you have got to have, to be able to sketch out at least roughly the nature of those asymmetries, without which you are stuck when you come to making satisfactory models. You can do the PK side pretty nicely and project the time course of drug concentration, but you cannot project the damned actions because of the missing half of the sort of one-sided nature of PD's protocols, that leave you in the dark about off responses. I do not think there is any magic modelling technique that allows you to cut through that.

L. Aarons:

No, there is not. In fact, it comes back to the point about experimental design. With poor design you cannot get that information. So I agree entirely that if you do not have the data to allow you to do the appropriate modelling, then there is very little you can do, unless you have some prior information and can use Bayesian techniques to help you over the gaps in your data base. Perhaps it is also the reason I have got a problem with this term dose-dependent idiosyncratic responses, because I suspect they fall into this category you are talking about.

M.M. Reidenberg:

In doing just the PK work, it is my impression that the critical measurements are the time of drug administration, and then the time of sampling. You have shown that in the ICU 20% of cases had to be dropped. In other kinds of less rigorous settings, have there been studies on how accurate these recorded times are, and how much difference it makes with whatever degree of error is in the time recording?

L. Aarons:

It really does come back to recording accurately the dosing history and also the timing of the samples. I have not got any numbers that I can give you directly, but we are participating in a study to look at the impact of real compliance patterns, that is ones that actually have been measured in real settings, on the PK/PD analysis. So in the future we may have some answers for you.

Can we design drugs with low variability

Dennis Smith

Drug Metabolism, Pfizer Central Research, Ramsgate Road, Sandwich, Kent, U.K.

ABSTRACT

The reasons for inter-subject variability in dose response can reside within the pharmacokinetic (PK) or the pharmacodynamic phase (PD) of the classical PK/PD model. Thus concentrating solely on pharmacokinetics may not result in markedly reduced variation in response. However, some reasons for variability in the pharmacokinetic phase are additive and therefore should be targets for drug design. For instance, unreliable or erratic absorption can be overcome by correct physiochemical properties. Extremes of variation in clearance can be limited by avoiding metabolism by polymorphic cytochrome P-450, such as CYP2D6 and CYP2C19. However, clearance will always remain a large source of variability and has to be addressed by having sufficient selectivity for the target to avoid side effects. Patient compliance probably represents one of the largest reasons for variability in drug effect and design has to focus on medicines that have convenient twice or once a day dosage regimens, that are not complicated by food effects or concomitant administration with other drugs.

Key words: Pharmacodynamics, absorption, food, P450, polymorphism, compliance.

Correspondence: Dr. Dennis A. Smith, Department of Drug Metabolism, Central Research, Pfizer Limited, Sandwich, Kent CT13 9NJ, U.K., Tel: +44-1304-64-6343, Fax: +44-1304-65-6433, Email: Dennis_A_Smith@sandwich.pfizer.com

PHARMACOKINETIC VARIABILITY AND PHARMACODYNAMICS

When one considered the question "can we design drugs for low variability?" further clarification of what constitutes variability is needed. Variability can only really be considered from the point of view of dose and pharmacological effect. Attenuation of the variability in a single event in the cascade that follows the swallowing of an oral dose and observing the pharmacological effect of the drug may not have the desired outcome in an overall reduction in variability of dose response. Figure 1 illustrates a typical PK/PD model, dividing drug activity into the pharmacokinetic phase and the pharmacodynamic phase. The pharmacodynamic phase is further subdivided into the interaction with the drug receptor triggering post receptor events, eventually leading to actual drug effect. The impact of considering this model is that variability in the pharmacokinetic phase may not be the dominant factor in the overall variability of response [1]. To exert an effect drugs must occupy the receptor to differing degrees. For instance, many 7 trans-membrane spanning receptor/anatgonists (7-TM's, such as β-adrenoceptor antagonists, dopamine antoagonists, etc) require around 75% occupancy to trigger efficacy [2]. In contrast ACE inhibitors are often dosed to maximally (95-100%) inhibit the enzyme (occupy the receptor). With their high degree of selectivity, considerable attenuation of the effects of any variability in pharmacokinetics occurs with this "maximal" dosing strategy. Noticeably the actual effects on lowering blood pressure still shows variability even when the degree of ACE inhibition is constant. This variability is the result of post-receptor events referred to above.

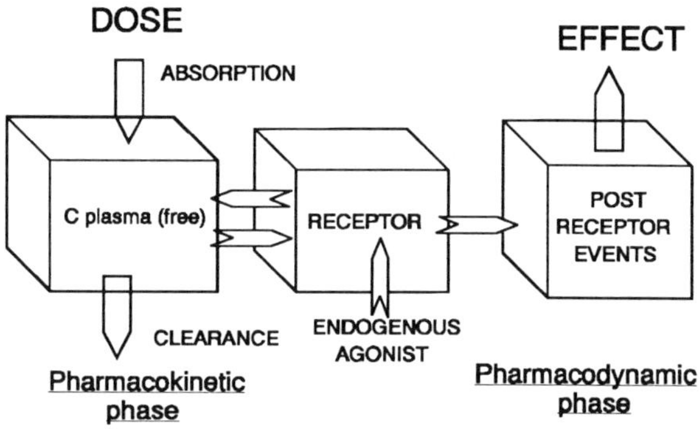

Figure 1. Pharmacokinetic/pharmacodynamic model linking administration of an oral dose of a drug and pharmacological effect.

For most drugs only a proportion of the target receptor is normally occupied for efficacy. Moreover drug concentration and effect can be modelled to provide sigmoidal or linear dose response relationships. Study of these relationships shows how variability in the pharmacokinetic phase can be exaggerated by the pharmacodynamic phase. Hill numbers, which refer to the steepness of dose response curves can range from 1 (Fenoterol, albuterol and noberastine), 2 (diazepam), 4-5 (midazolam, alfentanil, morphine and meperidine) to 20 (tocainide). The numbers are a summation of receptor occupancy, post receptor events, plus the actual effects observed, but do give an indication that pharmacokinetic variability is more critical to some pharmacological mechanisms than others.

It is clear that solving pharmacokinetic variability may not in itself rectify inter-individual variation. Nevertheless it is an appropriate target for some aspects of drug design as outlined below.

ABSORPTION, AN UNNECESSARY SOURCE OF VARIATION THAT IS AMENABLE TO DRUG DESIGN

It would seem a reasonable premise that variability is drug absorption is an unnecessary complication, regardless of the outcomes of the analysis above. In essence, drugs should have adequate aqueous solubility for dissolution of the compound to occur, followed by an ability to rapidly traverse the gastro-intestinal tract epithelium and enter the blood stream. Solubility is broadly inversely proportional to the number and type of lipophilic functions within the molecule and the tightness of the crystal packing of the molecule. Absorption across the gastro-intestinal tract normally involves the diffusion of the molecule through the apical and basolateral membranes of the cells lining the gastro-intestinal tract (transcellular absorption). To traverse this route the compound has to have sufficient lipophilicity to "dissolve" within the lipid core of the cells membranes. If a molecule has sufficient lipophilicity the large surface area of the microvillic means that absorption is rapid. Tight junctions formed by the proteins that act as the junction between cells, offer an aqueous channel (pore) for (paracellular) absorption. These pores are estimated to be a size of 3-10A and represent only 0.01% of the total absorptive surface area. Thus whilst available for small molecules, the aqueous pore paracellular pathway is an inefficient route. Moreover, adequate pores for drug absorption are only present in the upper gastro-intestinal tract, thus creating an "absorption window".

A number of drugs have very low aqueous solubility, mainly due to very high lipophilicity, but also due to lack of ionisable centre, and also the tight crystal packing referred to above. These drugs are erratically and incompletely absorbed due to this inability to dissolve in the gastro-intestinal tract following oral administration. Examples of low solubility, dissolution limited drugs include danazole [3], griseofulvin [4], halofantrine [5], ketoconzaole [6], nitrofurantoin [7], phenytoin [8] and trianterene [9]. Poor dissolution is responsible for both intra- and inter-patient variability.

Low or negligible lipophilicity compounds which rely on the paracellular aqueous pore pathway include atenolol, nadolol, pirenzipine, and ranitidine [2]. These compounds range in absorption from 51-13%, and are all simple, low molecular weight structures (266-351) as is necessary for acceptable absorption by this mechanism [10]. Whilst not highly variable per se, the incomplete absorption renders the mechanism particularly influenced by motility effects due to the "absorption window [11]".

Food is a complicating factor in drug absorption but its effects are largely limited to the above types of drugs, those either of very low lipophilicity, or those of very low aqueous solubility. Due to increased secretion of acid, bile, etc., the dissolution of poorly soluble drugs can be considerably increased (e.g. halofantrine, 1200% increase) [5]. In comparison food can reduce the absorption of low lipophilicity drugs due to effects on motility and shorter residence of the dose in the upper gastro-intestinal tract (e.g. atenolol, 20% reduction). The effect of food to increase the variability of absorption is shown schematically in Figure 2. To overcome these problems compounds in the "mid-ground" of the lipophilicity (log $D_{7.4}$ 0-2.0) offer the best chance for the optimal balance of properties to ensure rapid dissolution and subsequent efficient and complete transcellular absorption. Similarly such compounds are unlikely to show complications due to food, other than a delayed Tmax due to lengthened

Fluconazole is an example of a drug design programme aimed at producing an antifungal agent [2] with superior pharmacokinetics to the first orally active azole antifungal drug. ketoconazole (Figure 3). Ketoconazole is cleared primarily by hepatic metabolism and is difficult to formulate to obtain consistent absorption, due to poor aqueous solubility due to its high lipophilicity log P>5. Fluconazole is the least lipophilic (log P 0.5) member of a series of metabolically stable bis-triazoles. This ideal physicochemical profile gives fluconazole rapid dissolution and complete transcellular absorption. This complete absorption is not affected by food, achlorhydria, etc.

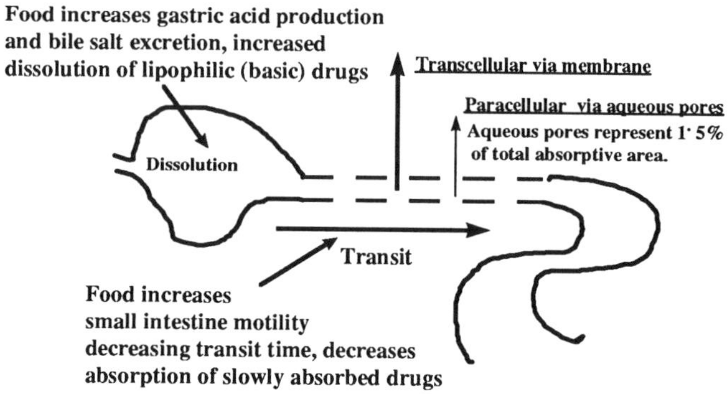

Figure 2. Schematic illustrating effect of food on the absorption of drugs of high and low lipophilicity

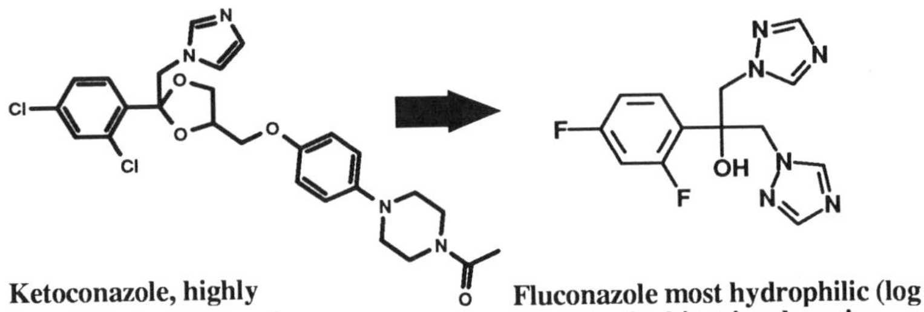

Figure 3. Fluconazole, an example of a drug discovery programme incorporating excellent absorption properties as part of the structure activity relationships.

CLEARANCE AND DESIGNING DRUGS TO LIMIT VARIATION

Given complete absorption, then the major sources of variation in the pharmacokinetic phase must reside in metabolic clearance, including first pass effects, and renal clearance. Minimal variation should be encountered with a drug that is 100% absorbed by the transcellular route and undergoes clearance by passive glomerular filtration (GF). Fluconazole is a rare example of such a drug. Base-line variation for such a compound is indicated by studies in healthy males [13]. In one such study (n=10), create clearance as an indicator of GF was 115 ml/min (90-140 ml/min) whilst fluconazole plasma clearance was 20 ml/min (15-23 ml/min). In such a study there is therefore a 1.5 fold range in fluconazole clearance values, directly reflecting a similar variation in GFR. In larger populations of patients [14] GFR varies more widely in patient populations. In a study in AIDS patients receiving fluconazole, GFR varied 4-fold from 36-138 ml/min, resulting in greater variation in fluconazole clearance [14]. Moreover, lower fluconazole values were also associated with lower CD4 cell counts. These studies indicate that variability in the pharmacokinetic phase is intrinsic in any drug and that the degree of variation is likely to increase from healthy volunteers to the wider patient population. Perhaps equally important, a large part of the variation is predictable from GFR measurements allowing dosage adjustment.

An examination of Pfizer compounds [15] undergoing early clinical studies and also going on to wider clinical studies indicated variation from 1.5 to 4.5 in Cl/F for 12 out of 15 drugs cleared by a variety of mechanisms. Lowest variation was seen for renally or partially renally cleared compounds, whilst higher variation was seen for those relying on metabolism. Compounds with wide variation (5-100 fold) were cleared by the polymorphic cytochrome P-450 isoenzymes CYP2D6 and CYP2C19. Where data was available, wider variation was encountered as a greater number of patients were studied

The substrate structure requirements of both these polymorphic isoforms is understood, particularly CYP2D6, and it is possible to include this knowledge in a drug design programme. For instance, the compound with 100 fold variation, UK-84,149(16, Figure 4), was identified by selective microsomal inhibition experiments as a CYP2D6 substrate. "First in man" studies included volunteers phenotyped and genotyped for CYP2D6 polymorphism and the results are shown in Figure 4. The unacceptably high variation led to termination of

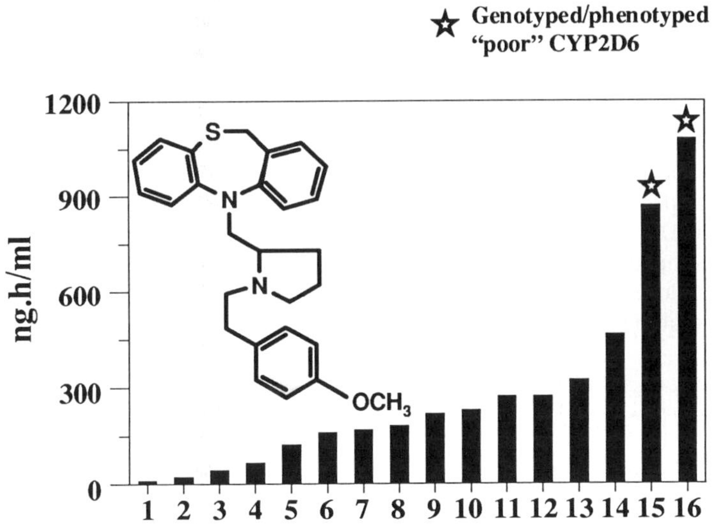

Figure 4. Variation in area under the plasma concentration time curve (AUC) following a single oral dose of UK-84,149, a compound metabolised by CYP2D6 (O-demethylation)

the development of the compound. Today protein homology and template overlay models exist that would have allowed the propensity for CYP2D6 metabolism for compounds of the UK-84,149 type to be predicted "in-silico" and the resultant structural features changed to avert metabolism by this isoenzyme. Alternatively, one could envisage that "population genotyping" would allow these variations to be predictable, in similar terms to GFR measurement.

In the wide patient population, variation in compounds metabolised by other P-450's is larger than expected. For instance, clozapine in small patient studies (n=16) shows a 6 fold variation [17] in CL/F (24.5, 11-63 L/H) and in larger studies (n=241) a 50 fold [18] variation (28.3, 5-250 L/H). Clozapine is metabolised by CYP3A4 and CYP1A2, isoenzymes [19] known to be variable, but involved in the metabolism of most basic lipophilic drugs. It seems difficult therefore that in terms of clearance to remove variation. The extremes can be removed by drug design, but "variation" will be present and needs to be accommodated in the selectivity, etc., of the compound.

REMOVING OTHER VARIABLES

Part of the extreme variability in the wide patient population is certainly the effects of patient compliance and concomitant medication. It seems prudent therefore that drugs should be designed that are convenient to take both by themselves and in combination. Thus pharmacokinetic properties should allow twice or preferably once a day administration. Drugs should be equally effective and tolerated when taken in the presence or absence of food. Whilst being a substrate for a P-450 enzyme is probably not avoidable (given the constraints of achieving activity, selectivity, absorption, etc.) the affinity for the system should be as low as possible. Thus the compound should not cause interactions either as a cytochrome P-450 inhibitor per se, or as an "efficient" substrate. Reduced affinity and greater metabolic stability go some way towards the pharmacokinetic properties for once a day therapy. Whilst not without exception metabolic stability and reduced affinity for P-450 enzymes such as CYP3A4 [2] can be gained by designing compounds in the "mid ground" of lipophilicity (log $D_{7.4}$ 0-2.0). Potent inhibition per se, can be limited by exclusion of unhindered pyridine, immidazole, or triazole functions. Duration of activity can also be enhanced by introduction of a basic group, to a neutral template, and its resultant effect on volume of distribution (2) as seen in examples such as amlodipine. Moreover such additions often bring extra benefit such as increased aqueous solubility.

CONCLUSION

Variation in dose response between patients is unavoidable. Pharmacokinetic variation can be limited but not avoided by careful drug design. Variation in the pharmacodynamic phase may in itself become attenuated as the full impact of genomics allows the sub-division of patients.

REFERENCES:

1. Levy G. Predicting effective drug concentrations for individual patients. Clin Pharm, 1998;34:323-333.
2. Smith, DA, Jones BC, Walker DK. Design of drugs involving the concepts of theories of drug metabolism and pharmacokinetics. Med Res Rev, 1996;16:243-266.
3. Badawy SF, Ghorab MM, Adeyeye CM. Characterization and bioavailability of danazol-hydroxypropyl β-cyclodextrin coprecipitates. Int J Pharm, 1996;128:45-54.
4. Hasegawa A, Kawamura R, Nakagawa H, Sugimoto I. Physical properties of solid dispersions of poorly water-soluble drugs with enteric coating agents. Chem Pharm Bull, 1995;33:3429-3435.
5. Humberstone AJ, Porter CJH, Charman WN. A physicochemical basis for the effect of food on the absolute oral bioavailability of Halofantrine. J Pharm Sci, 1996;85:525-529.
6. Baxter JG, Brass C, Schentag, JJ, Slaughter RL. Pharmacokinetics of ketoconazole administered intravenously to dogs and orally as tablet and solution to humans and dogs. J Pharm Sci, 1986:75:443-447.
7. Moolenaar F, Tromp TFJ, Huizinga T. Biopharmaceutical aspects of the absorption of orally administered nitrofurantoin. Pharm Weekbl 1976;111:1253-1264.
8. Varia SA, Schuller S, Sloan KB, Stella VJ. Phenytoin prodrugs. III: Water-soluble prodrugs for oral and/or parenteral use. J Pharm Sci, 1984;73:1068-1073.
9. Arias MJ, Gines JM, Moyano JR, Rabasco AM. The application of solid dispersion technique with D-mannitol to the improvement in oral absorption of triamterene. J Drug Target, 1994;2:45-51.
10. He YL, Murby S, Warhurst G, Gifford J, Walker D, Ayrton J, Eastmond R, Rowland M. Species differences in size discrimination in the paracellular pathway reflected by oral bioavailability of poly(ethylene glycol) and depeptides. J Pharm Sci, 1998;87:626-633.
11. Smith SE. Physiology of the gastrointestinal tract in relation to drug absorption. Int Pharm J, 1987;1:101-104.
12. Melander A, Stenberg P, Liedholm H, Schersten B, Waahlin-Boll E. Food-induced reduction in bioavailability of atenolol. Eur J Clin Pharmacol, 1979;16:327-330.
13. Tett SE, Moore, S, Ray J. Pharmacokinetics and bioavailability of fluconazole in two groups of males with human immuno deficiency virus (HIV) infection compared with those in a group of males without HIV infection. Antrimicrob Agents Chemother, 1995;39:1835-1841.
14. McLachlan AJ, Tett SE. Pharmacokinetics of fluconazole in people with HIV infection: a population analysis. J Clin Pharmacol, 1996;41:291-298.
15. MacIntyre F, Smith DA, Coates PE. Variability in human pharmacokinetics in volunteers studies and in the clinical situation. European conference on specificity and variability in Drug Metabolism, Besancon, 1995.
16. Wallis RM, Alker D, Burges RA, Cross PE, Greengrass PM, McIntyre P, Quinn P. UK-84,149: a novel gut-selective spasmolytic with calcium antagonist activity. Br J Pharmacol, 1994;112:574P
17. Choc MG, Hsuan F, Honigfeld G, Robinson WT, Ereshelsky L, Crismon ML, Salelad SR, Hirschavitz J, Wagner R. Single-vs multiple-dose pharmacokinetics of clozapine in psychiatric patients. Pharm Res, 1990;7:347-351.

18. Jerling M, Merle Y, Meritre F, Mallet A. Population pharmacokinetics of clozapine evaluated with the non parametric maximum likelihood method. Br J Clin Pharmacol, 1997;44:447-453
19. Eirmann B, Engel G, Johansson I, Zanger UM, Bertilsson. The involvement of CYP1A2 and CYP3A4 in the metabolism of clozapine. Br J Clin Pharmacol, 1997;44:439-446.

Discussion: Can we design drugs with low variability?

G.T. Tucker:

If I can just ask a question about eliminating CY2D6 substrates or inhibitors during drug development. How good are the active site models in terms of doing this? The topography of the binding area of the dopamine receptor, for example, is very similar to that of the active site of CYP2D6.

D.A. Smith:

If you are talking about the actual part the agonist binds, then definitely you have got aspartate salt bridges in both cases. When you are looking at adrenaline or dopamine, they are of a pretty similar size and they would fit into the CYP2D6 active site model. If you are trying to look for an agonist, then it is going to be very tough to get one. If you are looking for an antagonist, it does not have to bind into the agonist site with the same way. Then you are back to actually looking through high-throughput screening for other antagonists. So there is a chance you can actually get rid of that problem. The other thing is you can make antagonists that are not polymorphic, that we can actually do on certain occasions by blocking metabolism. One example, is going from metoprolol to betaxolol, which has actually used a substituent that is metabolically stable. The one compound is rapidly metabolised because it fits the model perfectly; the other has a metabolically stable substituent, that when it is actually bound it cannot be metabolised.

J. Benítez:

You said that one should try to escape from polymorphic enzymes, but you showed the case of clozapine with quite big individual variability and a lot of problems in clinical practice. Would not it be useful to look for drugs that could be metabolised by three or four different isoenzymes? So if one fails, the other one would take its place, and therefore there would be much less variability.

D.A. Smith:

It is clear there must be something extra in clozapine. I am not quite sure why it is so variable, because there is a difference when you look at different CYP3A4 substrates. The problem may be the way the data is collected. As soon as you go to sparse data, you only need someone who is not taking the drug to actually give you the low value. I think the idea of trying to get multiple metabolic routes in is an interesting one, particularly if you could perhaps use glucuronidation. That may actually damp down the variability. But the reason I was putting up the data is the recognition that variability is large rather than small with most metabolically cleared drugs. As I worked through it, I was looking for ways of getting rid of polymorphism, etc. But when one actually goes down and looks at the data, the variability is very large in all cases and we are stuck with that, and have to work through that one. Part of it, I think is getting really good selectivity in your compounds.

J. Benítez:

Did you check caffeine intake in those patients taking clozapine?

D.A. Smith:
That is a literature study and I do not know if they checked that.

U. Klotz:
Due to the lower variability if a drug is glucuronidated, one could do some drug design: if you have a handle on the molecule, like a hydroxyl group, you can improve the lipophilicity and affect the distribution volume. You might design a drug, forcing your molecule into glucuronidation pathway. On the other side, most of us are dedicated to drug metabolism, why not use more o less renally secreted drugs, where we get at least some standardisation by using creatinine clearance?

D.A. Smith:
I think the big problem there is absorption, of course, because you have to make them, in general, with low lipophilicity. Then you run into the problem of going via the paracellular absorption route, which limits you to very small molecules like atenolol, and you still have this marked reduction in bio-availability with food. Fluconazole is the pinnacle of that approach. Certainly, if it is a small molecule, it is attractive to go for the renal route if absorption problems can be overcome. Finally, it is always a balance you are looking at.

U. Klotz:
From a pharmaceutical point of view, I think the absorption can be handled by galenic tricks.

D.A. Smith:
There is no trick when you are in a poorly water-soluble compound. Once you are into a lipophilic one, you can come up with various formulations that will improve it. When people have looked for absorption enhancers of the paracellularly absorbed compounds, I am not aware there has been any advance at all in that area. There are compounds which ride this nicely, like fluconazole.

D.C. Brater:
I think no matter how much you try to custom-design things, you are not going to eliminate substantial variability. It seems that one of the themes we have here is that there is some lamenting that funding agencies do not embrace some of these concepts, and that sometimes industry and regulatory authorities do not embrace them. We cannot expect the practicing physician to pay attention to this variability in terms of how they deal with patients in the present climate of inattention. Perhaps we should discuss how we can attack this problem. Does it mean that we really need to think about a whole new different type of study, where we apply some of these concepts and conduct outcome studies? Does it mean we need to phenotype or genotype, or both, large numbers of patients and follow them prospectively over time to see if doing so has an important impact in caring for patients? It seems to me that such studies are a step that is going to be needed. After such studies, if you prove that this kind of information is helpful in terms of taking care of patients, we must then determine how we are going to get this information to practicing physicians. But they are being assaulted by all of the funding agencies and insurance companies to see patients in short periods of time. So we have to figure out ways in which we can get digestible packets of information to them,

using tools like computer information systems while they are actually taking care of the patient. If we think that all these issues are important, how are we going to convince other people that it is sufficiently important in terms of translating into patient care? We are kind of working in the trees here, and I just wonder if there is going to be an opportunity to talk about the forest, which I think is a bigger issue.

D.A. Smith:

There are few representatives from industry and from regulatory authorities in this meeting. It will have been very useful to have some of my clinical colleagues here, who actually can provide some comment as well through these issues. But I think that in general, most people feel the same way you have expressed.

G.T. Tucker:

I guess the key words are education, information and monitoring and how we implement them.

Variability in Human Drug Response
G.T. Tucker, Editor

Management of variability through dosage form design

Patrick du Souich, Ayman O.S. El-Kadi, Anne-Marie Bleau

Department of Pharmacology, School of Medicine, University of Montréal
Montréal, Québec, Canada

ABSTRACT

The repercussions of the formulation upon the variability of the pharmacological response are not uniform, so it is difficult to draw general conclusions. The variability of the response is greatly dependent upon the parameter assessed, the disease itself, the age and state of the patient, the drug and its dosage. The type of formulation, i.e. MRF bid or od, but not the brand influence the variability of the response. For drugs like theophylline, 5-aminosalicylic acid and budenoside a MRF reduces the variability of the response. On the other hand, for antihypertensive and antianginal drugs, such as verapamil, diltiazem, propranolol, and prazosin a MRF does not affect or decreases the variability of the response; however, nifedipine MRF increases the variability of parameters such as diastolic blood pressure, heart rate, time to elicit chest pain and total time of exercise. In addition, the formulation does not modify the variability of the response to opioid analgesics, NSAIDs, L-dopa, and diuretics (at steady state). Finally, a MRF increases the variability of undesired effects of benzodiazepines and of desired effects of procainamide and glipizide.

Key words: modified release formulations, pharmacodynamics, undesired effects, coefficient of variation, human.

Correspondence: Patrick du Souich, MD, PhD, Département de Pharmacologie, Faculté de Médecine, Université de Montréal, B.P. 6128, Succ. "Centre-ville", Montréal, Québec, Canada H3C 3J7, Tel: +1-514-343-6335, Fax: +1-514-343-2204, Email: dusouicp@ere.umontreal.CA

INTRODUCTION

Modified release oral formulations (MRF) are used not only to prolong the effect of a drug when it is rapidly eliminated, but also to modulate the pharmacological response of a drug. These goals are attained by changing the kinetics of absorption of the drug, by controlling the site of absorption, and by maintaining a steady effect. This review aims to evaluate the influence of a MRF on the variability of the response, desired and undesired, according to each of the objectives of a MRF. To minimize differences not due to the formulation, most of the literature discussed in this review includes articles where both the immediate release formulation (IRF) and the MRF were studied and compared in the same patients. All along the manuscript, variability will be assessed as the coefficient of variation (CV), calculated by dividing the standard deviation by the mean, and expressed as a percentage. We have assumed that a formulation-induced 30% or more difference in CV may have clinical repercussions, and this value has been used as threshold to accept a change in variability of the response. The difference in CV has been estimated with the following equation $(CV_{IRF} - CV_{MRF})/CV_{IRF}$.

MRF AIMED TO PROLONG THE DURATION OF THE EFFECT

In patients with uncomplicated asthma, average CV of the peak expiratory flow rate (PEFR) as a function of time following the intake of theophylline IRF is 85 ± 23% (± SD). The variability of the response to theophylline IRF is apparently not influenced by the severity of the disease, i.e. in patients with chronic obstructive lung disease (COLD), mean CV is 82 ± 48% [1]. When the CV of the PEFR is plotted as a function of time, it is apparent that the CV varies greatly soon after drug administration, variability that decreases to reach a minimum around 6 h, and increases later on (Figure 1).

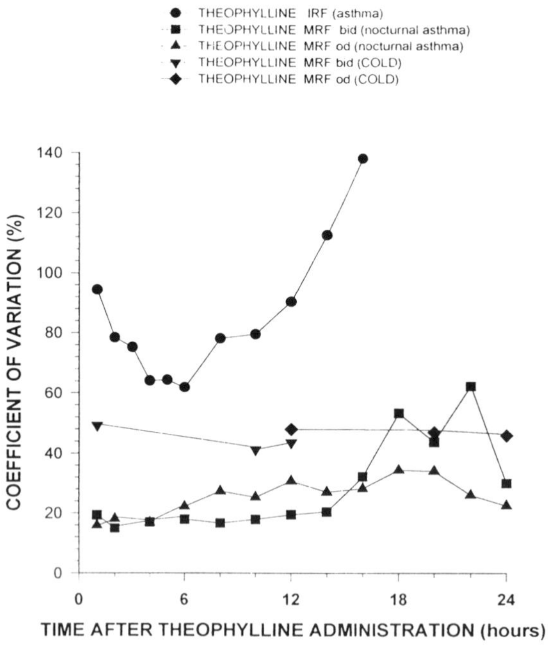

Figure 1. Coefficient of variation of the peak expiratory flow rate as a function of time of patients with uncomplicated asthma receiving theophylline IRF, in patients with nocturnal asthma taking theophylline MRF twice daily (bid) or once daily (od), and in patients with chronic obstructive lung disease (COLD) treated with theophylline MRF bid or od.

The use of a MRF of theophylline is justified because of the need to administer theophylline IRF four times a day and more importantly, to control nocturnal asthma. Originally, formulations allowed a twice-daily (MRF bid) administration of theophylline, and more recently once-daily formulations (MRF od) have been marketed. A double blind cross-over study, including patients with nocturnal asthma, compared the effect of theophylline MRF bid given at 8:00 and 20:00 h with theophylline MRF od given 20:00 h [2]; average CVs of PEFR are low for both formulations, i.e. 28 ± 16 and 25 ± 6%, respectively. Following the administration of theophylline MRF bid, the CV of the PEFR remains rather stable all along the day, however it increases during the night to reach at 2:00 a.m. values more than twice those observed during the day (Figure 1). On the other hand, the CV estimated with MRF od remains remarkably stable all along the day. In patients with reversible COLD, when Theo-Dur® MRF bid is compared with Uniphyl® MRF od, the average CVs of PEFR are of 45 ± 4 and 47 ± 1%, respectively, values that remain stable all along the day [3].

The CV of the PEFR assessed in patients given theophylline IRF is negatively associated with theophylline plasma concentrations (r = 0.793) (Figure 2). In fact, the CV of the PEFR

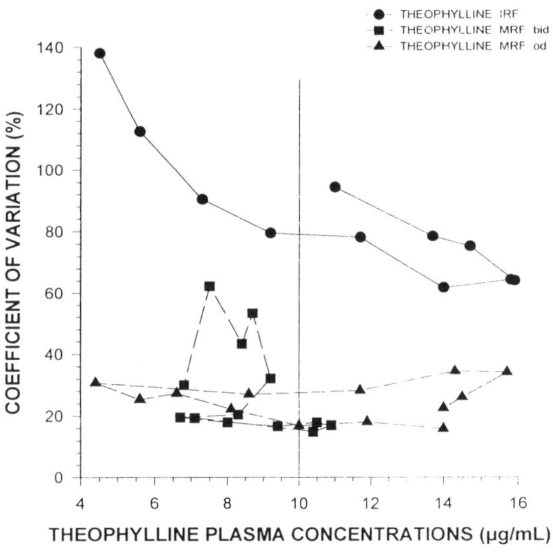

Figure 2. Coefficient of variation of the peak expiratory flow rate as a function of theophylline plasma concentrations in patients with uncomplicated asthma receiving theophylline IRF, and in patients with chronic obstructive lung disease (COLD) treated with theophylline MRF twice daily (bid) or once daily (od).

is rather stable above the theoretical minimal effective plasma concentration of 10 μg/mL, but increases below this threshold. In contrast, with theophylline MRF bid, the CV of PEFR shows an increase unrelated to the changes in theophylline plasma concentration. On the other hand, the CV of the PEFR in response to theophylline MRF od is independent of theophylline plasma concentrations [3].Despite differences in the design of the studies considered [1-3], the analysis of these reports suggests that by comparison to theophylline IRF, the use of a MRF reduces the CV of the pharmacological response of theophylline, the magnitude of the reduction being associated to the disease rather than the type of MRF (bid or od) or the brand.

In a double-blind, double-dummy, crossover study, patients received either 8 mg of salbutamol MRF bid or 4 mg in an IRF every 6 hours (q6h) for 2 weeks, and the effect of salbutamol was evaluated by documenting serial PEFR over a 12 h period. At steady state, average CVs of PEFR are 18 ± 3 and 17 ± 1% for the MRF and IRF, respectively. The variability in the response is not affected by the fluctuations in salbutamol plasma concentrations [4]. Moreover, the brand does not appear to influence the CV of PEFR, i.e. 21.1% v.s. 24.0% for Ethypharm Salbutamol SR® and Volmax®, respectively.

Opioid analgesics are frequently given in MRFs, since they are used over long periods in patients with cancer or other chronic pathologies. The CV of the analgesic response varies with the specific response taken into consideration, the intensity of pain, the dose used, and the cause of pain. In patients with stable cancer, the CV of the overall ordinal pain intensity score of morphine injected s.c. is around 50% [5], CV that increases by around 30% when the drug is administered by oral or rectal routes. With reference to the oral solution, the use of a MRF for oral or rectal routes do not change the CV [5-7]. The time of the day at which the response to morphine is evaluated does not influence the CV of the response [6].

The brand of morphine MRF does not influence the CV of the response. For instance, the CV of the response to MS Contin® MRF bid given to patients with stable cancer varies from 71 to 87%, compared to 70% for the solution of morphine [7-9]. The CV of the peak pain relief of Oramorph SR® MRF bid administered to patients undergoing an abdominal intervention is 54%, compared with 49% for MS Contin® MRF [10]. The CV is slightly higher when the response is evaluated in patients with advanced cancer, i.e. around 68% [6]. The CVs of the global pain index score (pain intensity score times the number of hours spent each day at that level of pain) assessed in patients with stable cancer are 21, 22 and 27% following the administration of the solution of morphine, MS Contin® MRF tablets, and M-Eslon® MRF capsules, respectively [11].

The CVs of the analgesic response to various opioid derivatives are similar. The CV of the antialgic response to oxycodone given in a solution q4h assessed by the mean pain relief with a visual analogue scale (VAS) is 88% [12]. In patients with stable cancer-related pain, when oxycodone MRF is compared to MS Contin® MRF the CV of the mean daily pain intensity is 63% vs 47%, respectively [13]. In patients with stable cancer pain given oxycodone MRF or hydromorphone MRF, the CVs of the categorical pain intensity are 40 v.s. 37%, respectively [14]. These examples show that the MRF of an opioid derivative given to patients with cancer, does not modify the variability of the analgesic response.

Concerning the variability of undesirable effects, such as nausea, it was shown in patients with advanced cancer-related pain, that the CVs of the VAS score of nausea induced by a solution of morphine or by MS Contin MRF given at doses ranging from 40 to 400 mg are 31 and 22%, respectively [15]. It is unclear whether the dose of morphine or the severity of the pain increase the CV of the VAS scores for nausea, i.e. in patients with chronic severe cancer-related pain receiving doses of 60 to 800 mg of morphine solution or MRF, the CVs are 230 and 280%, respectively [16]. On the other hand, in patients with stable cancer pain receiving 24 to 480 mg of morphine, the CV for the VAS score of nausea is 107% compared to 120% when the patients received 60 to 1200 mg of morphine MRF [6]. Similar variability is seen in patients with stable cancer pain receiving oxycodone or hydromorphone MRF, i.e. the CV for the VAS score of nausea is 104% [14].

With procainamide IRF, at average therapeutical plasma concentrations of 9.1 ± 3.4 μg/mL (± SD) abolishing about 40% of premature ventricular depolarizations (PVD) complexes, the CV of the decrease in PVD is 53% (Figure 3), value close to the CV of the incidence of PVD in absence of drug. At toxic plasma concentrations of procainamide of 22.8 8.5 μg/mL, when PVD are reduced by 97%, the CV increases to 105% [17]. Procainamide MRF given q6h (Procan SR®) or bid (Procanbid®) at a dose unable to reduce the PVD (1000 mg/day) does not change the CV of the incidence of PVD (Figure 3). However, at doses of 2000 and 4000 mg/day, able to reduce the incidence of PVD by 42 and 60% respectively, the CVs of the response increase to values ranging from 136 to 246% (Figure 3), and that despite rather stable procainamide plasma concentrations [18]. These results suggest that high doses of procainamide aimed to reduce maximally the incidence of PVD increase the CV of its response. Furthermore, a MRF increases the CV of the response possibly because it generates lower plasma concentrations of procainamide than the IRF.

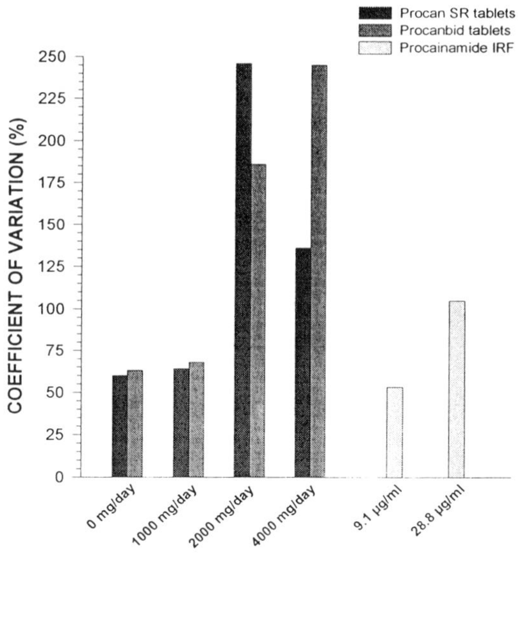

Figure 3. Influence of the daily dose of two MRFs of procainamide (Procan SR given q6h and Procanbid given twice daily) and of therapeutic and toxic plasma concentrations of procainamide given with an IRF on the coefficient of variation of the effect of procainamide on ventricular premature depolarization.

MRF AIMED TO IMPROVE THE SITE OF DRUG DELIVERY

In recent years, 5-aminosalicylic acid has been used as an enema whenever ulcerative colitis lesions are distal, and oral formulations are used for the disease localized proximally to the splenic flexure. The response to 1.5 g of rectal 5-aminosalicylic acid is rather variable, i.e. the CV of the activity index is 103% [19]. At low oral doses of 5-aminosalicylic acid given as a MRF (1 g/day) the CV of the activity index is similar to that observed with placebo, i.e. 71% v.s. 66. Increases in the oral dose of 5-aminosalicylic acid MRF enhance efficacy without major repercussions on the CV of the response, i.e. 78 and 83% for 2 and 4 g/day doses, respectively [20]. The CV of the response to low doses of oral 5-aminosalicylic acid MRF is smaller than the CV of the response to enema, probably because the drug is more closely and completely targeted to the inflammatory region.

Retention enemas of budenoside are used for the treatment of distal ulcerative colitis. Following 4 weeks of treatment with daily enemas containing 2.5 mg of budenoside, the CV of the disease activity index is 135% (Figure 4) [21]. On the other hand, the CVs of the response to maintenance treatments with 3 or 6 mg of oral budenoside MRF for periods up to 12 months are not affected by the dose used or the duration of treatment (Figure 4) [22]. In another study including 258 patients with ulcerative colitis treated with either placebo, 3, 9 or 25 mg of budenoside MRF for 8 weeks, the CVs of the Crohn's disease activity index are 38, 54, 57 and 65%, respectively, suggesting that the doses of budenoside and/or the severity of Crohn's disease increase the CV of the response [23]. As seen with 5-aminosalicylic acid, the response to budesonide enemas is more variable than when using oral budenoside MRF.

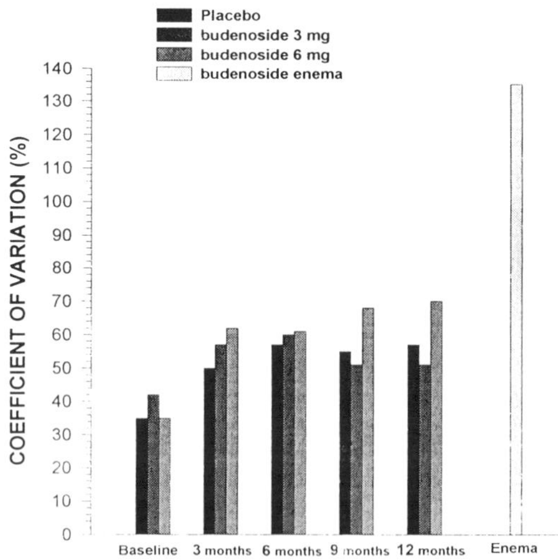

Figure 4. Effect of dose, duration of treatment and route of administration of budenoside MRF on enema on the coefficient of variation of Crohn's disease activity index.

MRF AIMED TO DECREASE THE RATE OF INPUT INTO THE BODY

The drug released from an IRF is rapidly absorbed into the body and as a consequence, the pharmacological response increases abruptly. In the case of drugs affecting cardiovascular homeostasis, the rapid increase in the response triggers reactions that may partially counterbalance the effect, i.e. vasoconstriction and antidiuretic effect with the use of antihypertensive medication and/or diuretics. Whenever the rate of input into the body is slowed by a MRF or an infusion, the efficiency of the drug is enhanced and the response is improved.

The MRF of furosemide increases its diuretic and natriuretic efficiency. The CV of the response to furosemide IRF depends upon the parameter assessed, i.e. the variability of the diuresis is lower than that of the natriuresis, chloruresis or kaliuresis (Figure 5). The CV of the effect of furosemide IRF does not decrease at steady state. On the other hand, after a single dose of furosemide MRF, the CV of the response is higher than that reported with furosemide IRF [24,25]; however, this difference tends to disappear when furosemide MRF is administered to steady state [24]. The CV of the diuretic, natriuretic, and chloruretic efficiency of furosemide MRF also tends to be higher than the CV of the efficiency of furosemide IRF [25].

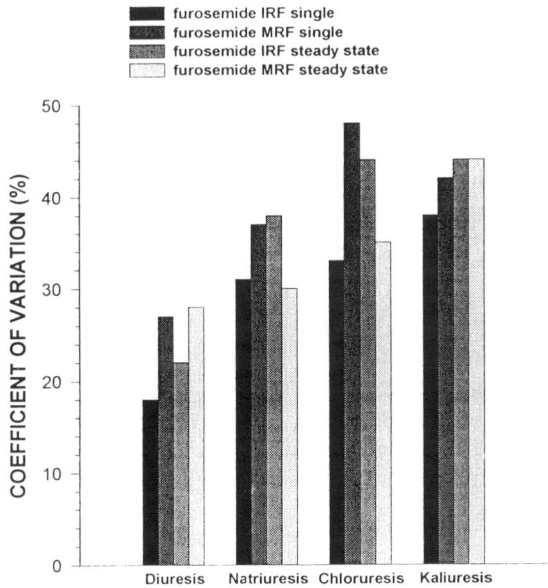

Figure 5. Repercussion of the formulation and the duration of treatment of furosemide on the coefficient of variation of the parameters assessing the response to the diuretic.

The influence of the formulation on the variability of the natriuretic and diuretic responses to diuretics in patients with cardiac, hepatic or renal pathology has not been documented. However, the effect of a continuous infusion of furosemide has been compared with the response to furosemide given as an i.v. bolus q8h to patients with congestive heart failure. Even if the diuretic and natriuretic efficiency of infused furosemide is greater than with the bolus, the CV of the diuresis is not affected by the form of administration [38 v.s. 30%, respectively), but the CV of the natriuresis is greater following the infusion of furosemide (85% v.s. 60%) [26]. Even if the infusion of bumetanide to patients with chronic renal insufficiency is more efficacious than the bolus, the variability of the response is not affected by the mode of administration. The CV of the diuresis (18%) is smaller than the CV of the natriuresis (27%), variability that is more than doubled when the natriuretic efficiency of bumetanide is taken into account, i.e. around 62% [27].

In healthy volunteers, at similar plasma concentrations, the infusion of nifedipine reduces diastolic blood pressure much more efficiently than does a bolus of nifedipine. Compared to the i.v. injection, the CV of the antihypertensive response of nifedipine is not changed by its infusion. On the other hand, the CV of the increase in heart rate is reduced by 33% with the infusion, probably secondary to diminished homeostatic responses as reflected by a smaller increase in heart rate [28]. When nifedipine is given orally as an IRF capsule or a MRF tablet, the CV of the decrease in diastolic blood pressure is greater than that observed using the i.v. route, but the formulation does not affect the variability. The CVs of heart rate and plasma noradrenaline concentration are higher with the MRF than with the IRF [29].

Used as an antihypertensive agent, in patients with moderate essential hypertention at doses ranging from 30 to 60 mg tid for 6 to 8 weeks, nifedipine IRF effectively reduces systolic and diastolic blood pressure with a rather uniform response. The position of the patient does not affect the CV of the effect of nifedipine on systolic blood pressure, i.e. 12.7% supine v.s. 14.5% upright [30,31]. However, the CV of supine systolic blood pressure is higher than the CV of diastolic blood pressure. On the other hand, compared to the supine position, the CV of diastolic pressure and of heart rate almost double in the upright position [31]. By reference to the IRF, nifedipine MRF 20 mg bid or 30 mg od do not modify the CV of systolic pressure, but increase the CVs of diastolic pressure and of heart rate (Figure 6) [32]. Doses of nifedipine up to 90 mg daily do not modify the CV of the response [33].

The CVs of systolic and diastolic pressure under nifedipine GITS (osmotic pump given od) are very similar to those reported with nifedipine CC (coat-core od), independently of the dose [34] or of the study [34,35], i.e. lower than 10%. The variability of the response is closely associated to the choice of the parameter selected to evaluate the response to nifedipine. When the response assessed is the change from baseline values, the CVs for the changes in systolic and diastolic pressures and for heart rate induced by nifedipine GITS are 80, 120 and 610%, respectively [36]. These values contrast with the figures of around 10% when the absolute value of blood pressure or of heart rate is taken into account. Compared to Caucasians with moderate hypertension, specific pathologic conditions like hypertensive crisis [37], and chronic renal insufficiency and long term dialysis [38] do not affect the CV of the response to nifedipine.

In patients with stable angina, the CV of the response to nifedipine IRF changes according to the parameter assessed, i.e. it is 44% for the duration of exercise to depress 1 mm the ST segment, 29% for the time required to present chest pain, and 18% for the total duration of the exercise. Compared with nifedipine IRF, nifedipine MRF bid increases the CVs of the time required to present chest pain and of exercise duration, although nifedipine MRF od augments only the CV of the total duration of exercise [39,40].

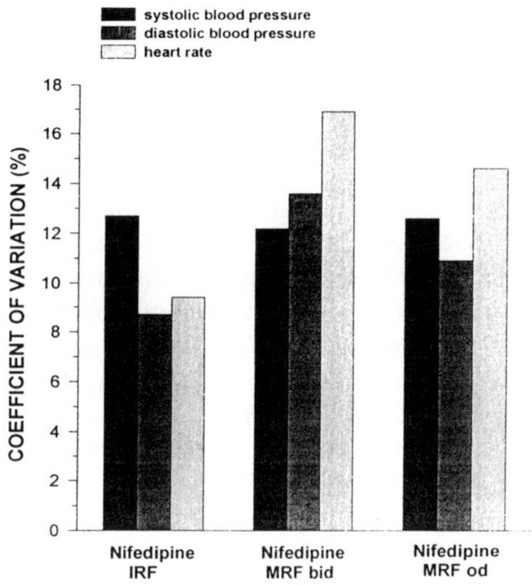

Figure 6. Repercussion of the formulation IRF and twice-daily (bid) or once daily (od) MRF of nifedipine on the coefficient of variation of blood pressure and heart rate.

In patients with mild to moderate hypertension, the repercussion of the formulation on the variability of the pharmacological response to daily doses of 240 or 480 mg of verapamil is minimal, i.e. at similar dosages, the CVs of the systolic and diastolic blood pressures, heart rate and PR interval are always in the range of 8 to 16% [41].

Diltiazem is extensively used as antihypertensive and as an antianginal agent. When diltiazem is given as an IRF at daily doses ranging from 180 to 360 mg to hypertensive patients, the CVs of supine or upright systolic and diastolic blood pressures are around 10% [42]. The use of diltiazem MRF bid does not change the CVs of systolic or diastolic blood pressure [43-46], but a MRF od decreases the CVs of upright systolic and diastolic blood pressure [47,48]. The CVs of heart rate are close to 16% with diltiazem IRF or MRF bid [42-46], and only 10% when MRF od is used [47,48]. The CVs of the effect of diltiazem MRF od on systolic or diastolic blood pressures remains unchanged as the daily dose is increased from 240 to 360 or 420 mg [47].

The CVs of the parameters assessing the effect of diltiazem on the treatment of stable exertional angina are four fold greater (33%) than the CV of the antihypertensive effect of diltiazem (8%). Contrasting with nifedipine, the CVs of the effect of diltiazem on the time to depress 1 mm the ST segment, the time to provoke chest pain and the effect on exercise duration are similar, i.e. around 30%. Compared to diltiazem IRF [49], diltiazem MRF bid [45,49] or MRF od [50,51] do not change the CV of these parameters. The dose of diltiazem

MRF bid (120 or 180 mg) [49] or od (180 or 300 mg), and the brand (Cardizem®, Tildiem® and Diltiazem SR Éthypharm®)[50-52] do not affect the variability of the response, nor does the duration of treatment (6 or 10 weeks) [45].

Compared to the IRF, prazosin MRF augments the antihypertensive response [53]. In patients with mild to moderate hypertension, at an average daily dose of 4 mg, by 12 weeks of treatment, the CVs of the response to prazosin IRF are 10 and 11% for the systolic and diastolic blood pressure, respectively [54]. On the other hand, following daily doses of 5 mg of prazosin MRF od, the CV of the systolic blood pressure is reduced to 4.8%, while the CV of the diastolic blood pressure is 11% [55].

In patients with essential hypertension, younger than 65 years given propranolol IRF bid, the CVs of the systolic and diastolic blood pressure and the heart rate range between 8 and 13%. The variability of the response is not affected by the administration of propranolol MRF od [56,57]. Neither the position of the body at which the blood pressure is measured (supine, sitting, or upright) nor the dose of propranolol affect the CV of the response [56,58]. In individuals subjected to an exercise on a bicycle ergometer to achieve a tachycardia greater than 100 beats/min, the CVs of the diastolic blood pressure and heart rate in response to propranolol MRF are lower than after propranolol IRF [57]. In elderly patients with hypertension, the CV of the response to propranolol IRF is less than half (around 4%) that measured in younger patients with essential hypertension (Figure 7), and propranolol MRF does not change the CV of systolic and diastolic blood pressure or of heart rate [59].

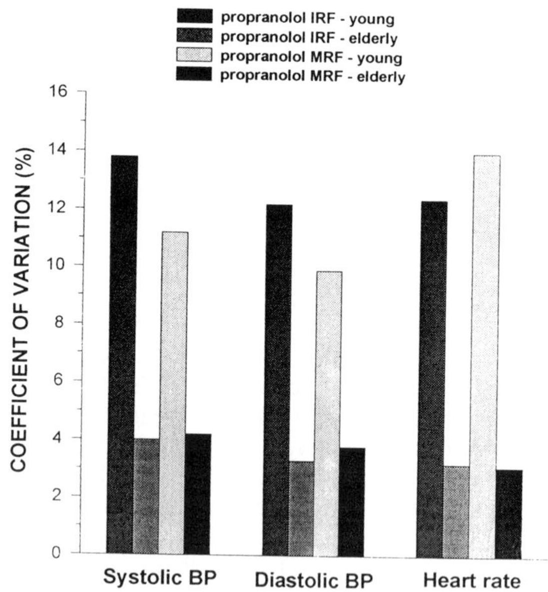

Figure 7. Influence of age of patients with essential hypertension treated with propranolol IRF and MRF on the coefficient of variation of the blood pressure and heart rate.

In patients with stable angina treated with daily doses of 160 mg of propranolol IRF, the CVs of exercise duration and time required to induce chest pain are 24 and 32% respectively. Doses of 80 or 160 mg propranolol MRF od do not affect the CV of exercise duration, but increases the CV of the time to induce chest pain by 55% [60-63], value that is decreased to 29% when the daily dose of propranolol MRF is increased to 320 mg [62].

In patients with essential tremor receiving propranolol IRF 80 mg q8h or propranolol MRF 240 mg od, at trough concentrations the CV of the magnitude of the tremor does not differ between formulations (251 v.s. 224%); at peak plasma concentrations, the CV decreases but it remains higher for the MRF (115 v.s. 168%). Concerning the CV of the tremor level, at trough concentrations it is lower with the MRF (193 v.s. 74%), and does not differ between formulations at peak plasma concentrations of propranolol (99 v.s. 97%). Increasing the daily dose of propranolol MRF to 320 mg does not modify the CV of the magnitude of the tremor or of the tremor level [64].

MRF AIMED TO DECREASE THE INCIDENCE OF UNDESIRED EFFECTS

Since 1980, when Hoftiezer *et al.* [65] reported that aspirin in an enteric-coated formulation prevented almost completely gastroduodenal mucosa damage, many non-steroidal anti-inflammatory drugs (NSAIDs) are marketed in a MRF. The CV of the effect of propionic [66-69] and acetic acid derivatives [70-72] in an IRF on spontaneous pain measured with a VAS ranges between 40 and 80% (Figure 8). The value of the CV depends upon the parameter

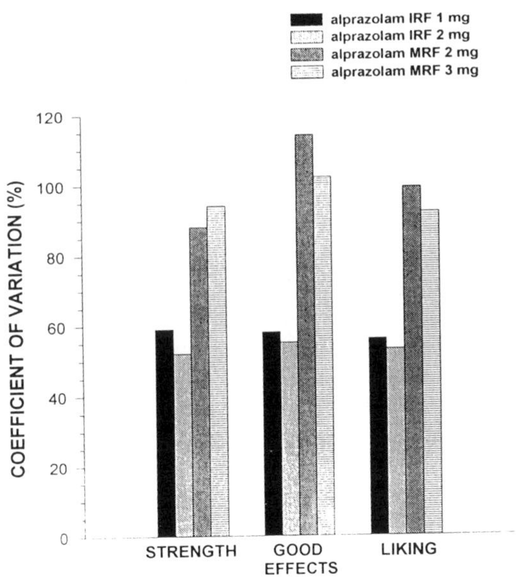

Figure 8. Effect of dose and formulation of alprazolam on the coefficient of variation of the parameters assessing abuse liability of alprazolam.

considered, i.e. 30% for pain on active motion, 17% for quality of sleep, and 14% for spine flexion [65]. The inter-drug variability in CV does not appear associated with the disease treated, i.e. osteoarthritis of several articulations [66,70], osteoarthitis of the knee [72], rheumatoid arthritis [68] or dental impaction pain [69], but rather to the method used to assess the effect of the NSAID on pain and on quality of life of the patient. Naproxen [67] or etodolac [72] response when assessed as the sum of the VAS of individual values of pain standing, walking, night and passive, or as an overall assessment allows CV estimates of 40%. A MRF of propionic acid and acetic acid derivatives does not change the CV of the response. In the case of ketoprofen, by reference to the IRF, the MRF reduces the CV of its effect on spontaneous pain by 50%, without affecting the CV of the measure of pain on active motion, quality of sleep and spine flexion [66].

The CV of the response to sulfonylureas such as glipizide IRF is associated to the parameter measured, to the response itself and to the time of drug utilization. For instance, in "responders" to ≤20 mg of glipizide IRF, at 10 weeks, 1.1 and 2.2 years, the CVs of fasting blood glucose (FBG) are 7, 12 and 23%, and the CVs of HbA_{1c} are 6, 10 and 10% respectively. In “non-responders”, at 10 weeks, 1.1 and 2.2 years, the CVs of FBG are 14, 21 and 31% and of HbA_{1c} 14, 15 and 10% respectively [73]. A MRF of glipizide has been released assuming that the incidence of hypoglycemic reactions will be reduced. Following daily doses of 5 to 60 mg of glipizide MRF for 15 weeks, the CVs of FBG and of HbA_{1c} average 31% and 19%, respectively, independently of the dose [74]. Ageing does not influence the CV of the effect on BFG of daily doses of 10 and 20 mg of glipizide MRF, although when FBG is estimated 24 hours (nadir) after drug intake, the CV increases to 41% [75]. Concerning another sulfonylurea, glibenglamide, the formulation did not affect the CVs of its antidiabetic effect, i.e. 15% and 13% for the IRF and MRF, respectively [76].

The variability in the response to the combination of L-dopa and carbidopa IRF (Sinemet®) is influenced by the parkinsonian sign assessed. The CVs of the Hoehn & Yahr stages and the Unified Parkinson's Disease Rating Scale (UPDRS) are 26 and 27%, respectively, while the CV of the Northwestern University Disability Scale (NUDS) is 39% [77]. MRFs of antiparkinsonian drugs are marketed to reduce undesired effects and to improve compliance. The CVs of the rating scales are not modified by the use of Sinemet CR® a MRF [77,78]. L-dopa combined with benserazide IRF (Madopar®) reduces the CVs of the Hoehn & Yahr stages and NUDS to 12 and 18%, respectively, but enhances the CV of the UPDRS to 51% [79]. Compared to Madopar®, the MRF (Madopar HBS®) does not modify the CVs of the rating scales assessed [79].

By comparison to plain diazepam tablets, diazepam MRFs provide anxiolytic effect with less side effects, may not cause an acute feeling of high, and reduce the development of “symptom-drug intake”. As depicted in table 1, with diazepam IRF the value of the CV is associated to the test conducted. The time the tests are conducted does not influence the CV, nor does the duration of treatment with diazepam (8 days), except for the CV of the digit symbol substitution test, which decreases on day 8, 3 h after drug administration. At days 1 and 8, the CV of the digit symbol substitution test is lower for diazepam MRF than for IRF at 1.5 h but not at 3 h. At day 1, the CV of the cumulative reaction time is greater with diazepam MRF than with IRF [80]. On day 8, 3 h after drug intake these differences tend to fade. No data is available to assess the influence of the formulation on the variability of the response to diazepam in patients. In patients with anxiety, the CVs of total scores for all symptoms increase from ≈34% to ≈63% and 92% with the duration of treatment with diazepam MRF, i.e. 0, 1 and 3 weeks, respectively [81].

Table 1.
Coefficient of variation of objective tests performed 1.5 and 3 hrs after the intake of 15 mg of IRF diazepam or of 20 mg of MRF diazepam by 9 healthy volunteers for 8 days

	DAY 1		DAY 8	
	1.5 h	3 h	1.5 h	3 h
Digit symbol substitution/3 min				
Diazepam IRF	15.7	19.7	12.8	10.6
Diazepam MRF	10.2	15.2	8.0	10.3
Tracking error severity				
Diazepam IRF	61	73	58	72
Diazepam MRF	58	65	73	68
Cumulative reaction time (sec.)				
Diazepam IRF	6.7	6.9	9.7	7.6
Diazepam MRF	10.8	14.5	9.4	7.7
Maddox wing (d)				
Diazepam IRF	66	58	64	66
Diazepam MRF	89	83	65	61

In patients with panic attacks, by the end of 6 weeks of treatment with alprazolam IRF the CVs of changes in the scores of the battery of tests assessed range between 6 and 13%. Alprazolam MRF is used for the treatment of panic disorders to avoid inter-dose anxiety as well as undesired sedation. In patients of identical characteristics and receiving the same doses of alprazolam MRF, the CV of the effect of alprazolam is smaller than 13% in one study [82], and ranges between 20 and 150% in another study [83]. Compared to alprazolam IRF, abuse liability is decreased by a MRF, however the MRF almost doubles the CV of the parameters assessing abuse liability, i.e. strength, good effects and liking (Figure 8) [84].

The influence of the formulation on the variability of the response to adinazolam depends upon the test evaluated. In healthy volunteers receiving a single doses of adinazolam, the CV of the mean number correct on word learning is 29% with the IRF and 20% with the MRF when plasma concentrations for both formulations are equal (at 6 h). The MRF does not influence the CV of the mean reaction time (≈20%), the mean number of intrusions on delayed recall (≈50%) and the nurse-rated sedation score (≈50%). However, the MRF increases the CVs of the mean number preserved on word learning (from 85 to 135%) and the mean number correct on delayed recall (from 110 to 160%) [85].

CONCLUSIONS

The repercussions of the formulation upon the variability of the pharmacological response are not uniform, so it is difficult to draw general conclusions. The variability of the response is greatly dependent upon the parameter assessed, the disease itself, the age and state of the patient, and the drug and its dosage. The type of formulation, i.e. MRF bid or od, but not the brand influence the variability of the response. For drugs like theophylline, 5-aminosalicylic acid and budenoside a MRF reduces the variability of the response, suggesting that proper targeting in time and/or place are important to an homogeneous response. On the other hand, the formulation does not modify the variability of the response to opioid analgesics, NSAIDs, L-dopa, and diuretics (at steady state). In addition, for antihypertensive and antianginal drugs, such as verapamil, diltiazem, propranolol, and prazosin a MRF does not affect or decreases the variability of the response; however, nifedipine MRF increases the variability of parameters such as diastolic blood pressure, heart rate, time to elicit chest pain and total time of exercise. The differences between calcium channel blockers are possibly associated to the preferential vasodilatation and lack of effect on heart conduction of nifedipine. The variability of sedative and abuse liability effects of benzodiazepines is in general increased by a MRF, possibly due to the marked reduction in the intensity of these undesired effects in some individuals. Finally, the MRF of drugs such as procainamide and glipizide enhances the variability of the desired response, and possibly multiple factors associated with the patient and the drug influence this effect, i.e. the mechanism of action of the arrhythmia, the dose, weight, diet, etc.

REFERENCES

1. Richer C, Mathieu M, Bah H, Thuillez C, Duroux P, Giudicelli JF. Theophylline kinetics and ventilatory flow in bronchial asthma and chronic airflow obstruction : influence of erythromycin. Clin Pharmacol Ther 1982;31:579-586.
2. Neuenkirchen H, Wilkens JH, Oellerich M, Sybrecht GW. Nocturnal asthma : effect of a once per day evening dose of sustained release theophylline. Eur J Respir Dis 1985;66:196-204.
3. Arkinstall WW, Atkins ME, Harrison D, Stewart JH. Once-daily sustained-release theophylline reduces diurnal variation in spirometry and symptomatology in adult asthmatics. Am Rev Respir Dis 1987;135:316-321.
4. Milroy R, Carter R, Carlyle D, Boyd G. Clinical and pharmacological study of a novel controlled release preparation of salbutamol. Br J Clin Pharmacol 1990;29:578-580.
5. Bruera E, Fainsinger R, Spachynski K, Babul N, Harsanyi Z, Darke AC. Clinical efficacy and safety of a novel controlled-release morphine suppository and subcutaneous morphine in cancer pain: a randomized evaluation. J Clin Oncol 1995;13: 1520-1527.
6. Finn JW, Walsh TD, Macdonald N, Bruera E, Krebs LU, Shepard KV. Placebo-blinded study of morphine sulfate sustained-release tablets and immediate-release morphine sulfate solution in outpatients with chronic pain due to advanced cancer. J Clin Oncol 1993;11:967-972.
7. Babul N, Provencher L, Laberge F, Harsanyi Z, Moulin D. Comparative efficacy and safety of controlled-release morphine suppositories and tablets in cancer pain. J Clin

Pharmacol 1998;38:74-81.
8. Cundiff D, McCarthy K, Savarese JJ, Kaiko R, Thomas G, Grandy R, Goldenheim P. Evaluation of a cancer pain model for the testing of long-acting analgesics. The effect of MS Contin in a double-blind, randomized crossover design. Cancer 1989;63:2355-2359.
9. Portenoy RK, Maldonado M, Fitzmartin R, Kaiko RF, Kanner R. Oral controlled-release morphine sulfate. Analgesic efficacy and side effects of a 100-mg tablet in cancer pain patients. Cancer 1989;63:2284-2288.
10. Bloomfield SS, Cissell GB, Mitchell J, Barden TP, Kaiko RF, Ftizmartin RD, Grandy RP, Komorowski J, Goldenheim PD. Analgesic efficacy and potency of two oral controlled-release morphine preparations. Clin Pharmacol Ther 1993;53:469-478.
11. Bernardi, M de, Bernardi F de, Colombo P. Randomised crossover comparison of the pharmacokinetic profiles of two sustained release morphine sulfate formulations in patients with cancer-related pain. Clin Drug Invest 1997;14 (Suppl 1):28-33.
12. Glare PA, Walsh TD. Dose-ranging study of oxycodone for chronic pain in advanced cancer. J Clin Oncol 1993;11:973-978.
13. Heiskanen T, Kalso E. Controlled-release oxycodone and morphine in cancer related patients. Pain 1997;73:37-45.
14. Hagen NA, Babul N. Comparative clinical efficacy and safety of a novel controlled-release oxycodone formulation and controlled-release hydromorphone in the treatment of cancer pain. Cancer 1997;79:1428-1437.
15. Hank GW, Twycross RG, Bliss JM. Controlled release morphine tablets: a double-blind trial in patients with advanced cancer. Anaesthesia 1987;42:840-844.
16. Arkisntall WW, Goughnour BR, White JA, Stewart JH. Control of severe pain with sustained-release morphine tablets v oral morphine solution. Can Med Ass J 1989;140: 653-661.
17. Myerburg RJ, Kessler KM, Kiem I, Pefkaros KC, Conde CA, Cooper D, Castellanos A. Relationship between plasma levels of procainamide, suppression of premature ventricular complexes and prevention of recurrent ventricular tachycardia. Circulation 1981;64:280-289.
18. Yang BB, Abel RB, Uprichard ACG, Smithers JA, Forgue ST. Pharmacokinetics and pharmacodynamic comparisons of twice daily and four times daily formulations of procainamide in patients with frequent ventricular premature depolarization. J Clin Pharmacol 1996;36:623-633.
19. Klotz U, Maier K, Fischer C, Heinkel K. Therapeutic efficacy of sulfasalazine and its metabolites in patients with ulcerative colitis and Crohn's disease. N Engl J Med 1980;303:1499-1502.
20. Hanauer S, Schwartz J, Robinson M, Roufail W, Arora S, Cello J, Safdi M, and the Pentasa Study Group. Mesalamine capsules for treatment of active ulcerative colitis: results of a controlled trial. Am J Gastroenterology 1993;88:1188-1197.
21. Danielson Å, Hellers G, Lyrenäs E, Löfberg R, Nilsson Å, Olsson O, Olsson S-Å, Persson T, Salde L, Naesdal J, Stenstam M, Willén R. A controlled randomized trial of budenoside versus prednisolone retention enemas in active distal ulcerative colitis. Scand j Gastroeterol 1987;22:987-992.
22. Greenberg GR, Feagan BG, Martin F, Sutherland LR, Thomson ABR, Williams CN, Nisson LG, Persson T, and the Canadian Inflammatory Bowel Disease Study Group. Oral budenoside as maintenance treatment for Crohn's disease: a placebo-controlled, dose-

ranging study. Gastroenterology 1996;110:45-51.
23. Greenberg GR, Feagan BG, Martin F, Sutherland LR, Thomson ABR, Williams CN, Nisson LG, Persson T, and the Canadian Inflammatory Bowel Disease Study Group. Oral budenoside for active Crohn's disease. N Engl J Med 1994;331:836-841.
24. Beerman B. Kinetics and dynamics of furosemide and slow-acting furosemide. Clin Pharmacol Ther 1982;32:584-591.
25. Alván G, Paintaud G, Eckernäs S-Å, Grahnén A. Discrepancy between bioavailability as estimated from urinary recovery of frusemide and total diuretic effect. Br J Clin Pharmacol 1992;34:47-52.
26. Dormans TP, Meyel JJ van, Gerlag PG, Tan Y, Russel FG, Smits P. Diuretic efficacy of high dose furosemide in severe heart failure: bolus injection versus continuous infusion. J Am Coll Cardiol 1996;28:376-382.
27. Rudy DW, Voelker JR, Greene PK, Esparza FA, Brater DC. Loop diuretics for chronic renal insufficiency: a continuous infusion is more efficacious than bolus therapy. Ann Int Med 1991;115:360-366.
28. Kleinbloesem CH, Brummelen P van, Danhof M, Faber H, Urquhart J, Breimer DD. Rate of increase in the plasma concentration of nifedipine as a major determinant of its hemodynamic effects in humans. Clin Pharmacol Ther 1987;41:26-30.
29. Kleinbloesem CH, Brummelen P van, Linde JA van de, Voogd PJ, Breimer DD. Nifedipine: kinetics and dynamics in healthy subjects. Clin Pharmacol Ther 1984;35: 742-749.
30. Marone C, Luisoli S, Bomio F, Beretta-Piccoli C, Bianchetti MG, Weidmann P. Pressor factors and cardiovascular pressor responsiveness after short-term antihypertensive therapy with the calcium antagonist nifedipine alone or combined with a diuretic. J Hypertension 1984;2 (Suppl 3):449-452.
31. Masotti G, Poggesi L, Castellani S, Morettini A, Galanti G, Scarti L. A study of the antihypertensive effect and some pharmacodynamic aspects of nifedipine in medium-term treatment. Int J Clin Pharm Res 1984;4:71-79.
32. Rahima-Maoz C, Grossman E, Nussinovitch N, Katz A, Rosenthal T. Nifedipine GITS replacing nifedipine SR: ambulatory blood pressure assessment of efficacy. Cardiology 1997;88 (Suppl 3):43-46.
33. Bonaduce D, Canonico V, Mazza F, Nicolino A, Ferrara N, Chiariello M, Condorelli M. Evaluation of the efficacy of slow-release nifedipine in systemic hypertension by ambulatory intraarterial blood pressure monitoring. J Cardiovasc Pharmacol 1985;7:145-151.
34. Gandhi AJ, Murphy CM, Zervopoulos PC, Evans RE, Carter BL, Bauman JL. Evaluation of two forms of sustained release nifedipine using 24 h ambulatory blood pressure monitoring. Am J Hypertens 1997;10:992-996.
35. Granberry MC, Gradner SF, Schneider EF, Carter IR. Comparison of two formulations of nifedipine during 24-hour ambulatory blood pressure monitoring. Pharmacotherapy 1996;16:932-936.
36. White WB, Black HR, Weber MA, Elliott WJ, Bryzinski B, Fakouhi TD. Comparison of effects of controlled onset extended release verapamil at bedtime and nifedipine gastrointestinal therapeutic system on arising and early morning blood pressure, heart rate, and the heart rate-blood pressure product. Am J Cardiol 1998;81:424-431.
37. Damasceno A, Sevene E, Patel S, Polónia J. Nifedipine-retard versus nifedipine capsules

for the therapy of hypertensive crisis in black patients. J Cardiovasc Pharmacol 1998;31:165-169.
38. Kusano E, Asano Y, Takeda K, Terao N, Hosoda S. Acute and chronic hypotensive effect of nifedipine and niludipine in hypertensive patients with chronic renal failure. Arzneim Forsch Drug Res 1984;34:624-629.
39. Crake T, Quyyumi AA, Wright C, Mockus L, Fox KM. Treatment of angina pectoris with nifedipine: a double blind comparison of nifedipine and slow-release nifedipine alone and in combination with atenolol. Br Heart J 1987;58:617-620.
40. Walker JM, Curry PVL, Bailey AE, Steare SE. A comparison of nifedipine once daily (Adalat LA), isosorbide mononitrate once daily, and isosorbide dinitrate twice daily in patients with chronic stable angina. Int J Cardiol 1996;53:117-126.
41. Fuenmayor NT, Faggin BM, Cubeddu LX. Comparative efficacy, safety and pharmacokinetics of verapamil SR vs verapamil IR in hypertensive patients. Drugs 1992;44 (Suppl 1):1-11.
42. Inouye IK, Massie BM, Benowitz N, Simpson P, Loge D. Antihypertensive therapy with diltiazem and comparison with hydrochlorothiazide. Am J Cardiol 1984;53:1588-1592.
43. Nikkilä MT, Inkovaara JA, Heikkinen JT, Olsson SOR. Antihypertensive effect of diltiazem in a slow-release formulation for mild to moderate essential hypertension. Am J Cardiol 1989;63:1227-1230.
44. Sridhara BS, Thomas P, Lahiri A, Raftery EB. Antihypertensive efficacy of twice daily controlled release diltiazem using 24 hour intra-arterial blood pressure monitoring. Eur J Clin Pharmacol 1994;46:427-430.
45. Kawanishi DT, Leman RB, Pratt CM, O'Rourke RA. Efficacy and safety of sustained-release diltiazem as replacement therapy for beta blockers and diuretics for stable angina pectoris and coexisting essential hypertension: a multicenter trial. Am J Cardiol 1987;60:29I-35I.
46. Pool PE, Massie BM, Venkataraman K, Hirsch AT, Samant DR, Seagren SC, Gaw J, Salel AF, Tubau JF. Diltiazem as monotherapy for systemic hypertension: a multicenter, randomized, placebo-controlled trial. Am J Cardiol 1986;57:212-217.
47. Nilsson P, Lindholm LH, Hedner T. The diltiazem different doses study. A dose –response study of once-daily diltiazem therapy for hypertension. J Cardiovesc Pharmacol 1996;27:469-475.
48. Dupont AG, Coupez JM, Jensen P, Coupez-Lopinot R, Schoors DF, Hermanns P, Nicolas M. Twenty-four hour ambulatory blood pressure profile of a new-slow release formulation of diltiazem in mild to moderate hypertension. Cardiovasc Drug Ther 1991;5:701-708.
49. Weiner DA, Cutler SS, Klein MD. Efficacy and safety of sustained-release diltiazem in stable angina pectoris. Am J Cardiol 1986;57:6-9.
50. Vliegen HW, Wall EE van der, Kragten JA, Holwerda NJ, Schenkel WM, Muijs van de Moer WM, Kate JBL ten, Mulder PGH, Bruschke AVG. Comparison of diltiazem standard formulation and diltiazem controlled release in patients with stable angina pectoris: a randomized, double-blind, cross-over, multicenter study. J Cardiovasc Pharmacol 1993;21:552-559.
51. Frances Y, Gagey S, Stalla-Bourdillon A. Twenty-four hour efficacy of two dose levels of a once daily sustained-release diltiazem formulation in stable angina: a placebo-controlled trial. Br J Clin Pharmacol 1995;39:277-282.
52. Debrégeas B, Duchier J. Efficacy and tolerability of once-daily sustained-release and

conventional diltiazem in patients with stable angina pectoris. Clin Drug Invest 1997;13:59-65.

53. Elliott HL, Vincent J, Meredith PA, Reid JL. Relationship between plasma prazosin concentration and alpha-antagonism in humans: comparison of conventional and rate-controlled (Oros) formulations. Clin Pharmacol Ther 1988;43:582-587.
54. Fukiyama K, Omae T, Iimura O, Koshinaga K, Yagi S, Inagaki Y, Ishii M, Kaneko Y, Yamada K, Ijichi H, Takeda T, Kuramochi M, Kokubu T, Ebihara A, Nakashima M. A double-blind comparative study of doxazosin and prazosin in the treatment of essential hypertension. Am Heart J 191:121:317-322.
55. Bourget P, Hernandez H, Edouard D, Lesne-Hulin A, Ribou F, Baton-Saint-Mleux C, Lelaidier C. Disposition of a new rate-controlled formulation of prazosin in the treatment of hypertension during pregnancy: transplacental passage of prazosin. Eur J Drug Metab Pharmacokin 1995;20:233-241.
56. Serlin MJ, Orme ML'E, MacIver M, Green GJ, Sibeon RG, Breckenridge AM. The pharmacodynamics and pharmacokinetics of conventional and long-acting propranolol in patients with moderate hypertension. Br J Clin Pharmacol 1983;15:519-527.
57. Rustin MHA, Coomes EN. Comparison of propranolol and propranolol LA in hypertension using 24-hr non-invasive blood pressure monitoring. Postgrad Med J 1983;59:770-774.
58. Carter BL, Gersema LM, Williams GO, Schabold K. Once-daily propranolol for hypertension: a comparison of regular-release, long-acting, and generic formulations. Pharmacother 1989;9:17-22.
59. Khan AU. Comparison of a long-acting form of propranolol and conventional propranolol in the treatment of hypertension in elderly patients. J Int Med Res 1987;15:128-133.
60. Kambara H, Kinoshita M, Hirota Y, Kadota K, Sawamura M, Saito T, Kawai C. Effect on exercise tolerance and pharmacokinetics of conventional and sustained release preparations of propranolol in patients with angina pectoris. Jap Cir J 1984;48:1066-1073.
61. Parker JO. Comparison of slow-release pindolol, standard pindolol and propranolol in angina pectoris. Am J Cardiol 1983;51:1062-1066.
62. Odemuyiwa O, Peart I, Alberts C, Hall RJC. Comparison of the effectiveness of slow-release propranolol (Inderal LA) 80, 160 and 320 mg orally daily in the treatment of angina pectoris. Br J Clin Pract1990;44:9-12.
63. Irving JB, Edwards RE. Double-blind comparison of long acting propranolol and sustained release metoprolol in the treatment of angina pectoris. Br J Clin Pract 1987;41:872-875.
64. Cleeves L, Findley LJ. Propranolol and propranolol LA in essential tremor: a double blind comparative study. J Neurol Neurosurg Psychiatry 1988;51:379-384.
65. Hoftiezer JW, Silvoso GR, Burks M, Ivey KJ. Comparison of the effects of regular and enteric-coated aspirin on gastroduodenal mucosa of man. Lancet 1980;I:609-612.
66. Marcolongo R, Rubegni M, Provvedi D, Giordano N, Frati E, Bruni G. A double-blind, interpatient comparison of plain and slow-release ketoprofen in osteoarthritis. Int J Clin Pharmacol Ther Toxicol 1984;22:377-381.
67. Kelly JG, Kinney CD, Devane JG, Mulligan S, Colgan BV. Pharmacokinetic properties and clinical efficacy of once-daily sustained release naproxen. Eur J Clin Pharmacol 1989;36:383-388.
68. Buchanan WW, Kean WF, St-Jean J, Gerecz-Simon E, Elie R. Clinical evaluation of a

sustained release compared to a standard formulation of tiaprofenic acid (Surgam®) in rheumatoid arthritis: a Canadian multicenter study. J Rheumatol 1991;18:1046-1054.
69. Cooper SA, Quinn PD, MacAfee K, Hersh EV, Sullivan D, Lamp C. Ibuprofen controlled-release formulation. A clinical trial in dental impaction pain. Oral Surg Oral Med Oral Pathol 1993;75:677-683.
70. Le Loët X, Dreiser RL, Le Gros V, Febvre N. Therapeutic equivalence of diclofenac sustained-released 75 mg tablets and diclofenac enteric-coated 50 mg tablets in the treatment of painful osteoarthritis. Int J Clin Pract 1997;51:389-393.
71. Briançon D. International experience with etodolac therapy for rheumatoid arthritis: an interim report of comparative efficacy. Clin Rheumatol 1989;8 (Suppl 1):63-72.
72. Porzio F. Meta-analysis of three double-blind comparative trials with sustained-release etodolac in the treatment of osteoarthritis of the knee. Rheumatol Int 1993;13:S19-S24.
73. Bitzén PO, Melander A, Scherstén B, Svensson M, Wåhlin-Boll E. Long-term effects of glipizide on insulin secretion and blood glucose control in patients with non-insulin-dependent diabetes mellitus. Eur J Clin Pharmacol 1992;42:77-83.
74. Simonson DC, Kourides IA, Feinglos M, Shamoon H, Fischette CT. Efficacy, safety, and dose-response characteristics of glipizide gastrointestinal therapeutic system on glycemic control and insulin secretion in NIDDM. Diacetes Care 1997;20:597-606.
75. Burge MR, Schmitz-Fiorentino K, Fischette C, Qualls CR, Schade DS. A prospective trial of risk factors for sulfonylurea-induced hypoglycemia in type 2 diabetes mellitus. JAMA 1998;279:137-143.
76. Ayanoglu G, Witte PU, Badian M. Bioavailability and pharmacodynamics of sustained release glibenglamide product (Deroctyl) in comparison to a standard tablet formulation (Euglucon, Daonil). Int J Clin Pharmacol Ther Toxicol 1983;21:479-482.
77. Feldman RG, Mosbach PA, Kelly MR, Thomas CA, Saint Hilaire MH. Double-blind comparison of standard Sinemet and Sinemet CR in patients with mild-to-moderate Parkinson's disease. Neurology 1989;39 (Suppl 2):96-101.
78. Wolters EC, Tesselaar HJM, International Sinemet CR Study Group. International (NL-UK) double-blind study of Sinemet CR and standard Sinemet (25/100) in 170 patients with fluctuating Parkinson's disease. J Neurol 1996;243:235-240.
79. Dupont E, Andersen A, Boas J, Boisen E, Borgmann R, Helgetveit AC, Kjaer MO, Kristensen TN, Mikkelsen B, Pakkenberg H, Presthus J, Stien R, Worm-Petersen J, Buch D. Sustained-release Madopar HBS® compared with standard Madopar® in the long-term treatment of *de novo* parkinsonian patients. Acta Neurol Scand 1996;93:14-20.
80. Mattila M. Acute and subacute effects of diazepam on human performance: comparison of plain tablet and controlled release capsule. Pharmacol Toxicol 1988;63:369-374.
81. Montandon A, Skreta M, Riggenbach H, Ward J. Comparison of controlled-release diazepam capsules and placebo in patients in general practice. Curr Med Res Opin 1986;19:10-16.
82. Pecknold J, Luthe L, Munjack D, Alexander P. A double-blind, placebo-controlled, multicenter study with alprazolam and extended-release alprazolam in the treatment of panic disorder. J Clin Psychopharmacol 1994;14:314-321.
83. Schweizer E, Patterson W, Rickels K, Rosenthal M. Double-blind, placebo-controlled study of a once-a-day, sustained-release preparation of alprazolam for the treatment of panic disorder. Am J Psychiatry 1993;150:1210-1215.
84. Mumford GK, Evans SM, Fleishaker JC, Griffiths RR. Alprazolam absorption kinetics

affects abuse liability. Clin Pharmacol Ther 1995;57:356-365.

85. Fleishaker JC, Sisson TA, Sramek JJ, Conrad J, Veroff AE, Cutler NR. Psychomotor and memory effects of two adinazolam formulations assessed by a computerized neuropsychological test battery. J Clin Pharmacol 1993;33:463-469.

<u>Discussion</u>: Management of variability through dosage form design

L. Aarons:

Could I make a plea to not use coefficient of variation as a measure of variability, in the sense that it is not a measure of variability. For example, you can have plus or minus one at the value of one, and you can have plus or minus one at the value of 100. At one it has got 100% variability, but at 100 it has got 1% variability. In both cases the variability is actually the same: It is plus or minus one at the bottom, and it is plus or minus one at the top. It actually depends on your reference, therefore it is not a measure of variability. I suspect some of the baselines were different here, so whereas the formulation may have had no effect on coefficient of variation, it presumably did have an effect on response. If you compare values at the same level of response, then the comparison is valid.

P. du Souich:

In theory you are correct. However, when considering the pharmacological response to two different formulations, the differences in the desired response cannot be important, otherwise the two formulations could not be considered as bioequivalents. Therefore, the mean values of the effect measured are usually rather close, what may vary is the variability around this mean. I believe that under such conditions the use of the coefficient of variability is not inadequate.

J. Urquhart:

There is another aspect to the nifedipine story that does not quite fit the formalism you have used. The reflex tachycardia approximately occurs in about 40% of patients who take nifedipine in a conventional dosage form. Back in the mid-80s several colleagues and I looked at the pharmacodynamics of this effect. It was evident from what we did that the trigger for reflex tachycardia is a high rate of increase of nifedipine concentrations. We suggested to give nifedipine in a constant rate released in oral dosage form as measure to avoid that major side-effect. That in fact was realised with an oral form of nifedipine in the clinical studies, and it opened up the use of nifedipine as an anti-hypertensive in the American market. It became the biggest-selling cardiovascular drug in history for five or six years until amlodipine came along and exceeded it. This is the biggest story in the whole drug delivery system arena, because the essential incidence of reflex tachycardia with that new dosage form, based on the published clinical data, is essentially zero. It is a real triumph, but a one-off thing because of the peculiarity of that drug and its funny pharmacodynamics.

P. du Souich:

It is important to differentiate desired from undesired response. Drugs to be marketed in a new formulation must be bioequivalent, i.e. it is always presumed that the response elicited by a certain dose is not affected by a formulation. However, when the formulation is changed to reduce a side effect, obviously the mean value of the measured side effect should be decreased. In the case of nifedipine, for the same dose, the desired effect, that is the antihypertensive effect obtained with the modified release formulation is similar to that elicited with the conventional formulation. Although the undesired effect, tachycardia, is reduced.

U. Klotz:

Concerning the example of budesonide and 5-aminosalicylic acid, both drugs are supposed to work topically, and depending on the site of the inflammation you take either the enemas or the modified-release oral preparation. The physician does not care about variation. Enemas are most effective in left-sided colitis, and modified-release preparations are more recommended for the small or upper large bowel. Thus, it always depends on the indication which one you take, because of the topical action.

P. du Souich:

However, in the same studies they did compare the enema and the modified-release formulation. Obviously, there is a bias because they gave both treatments to all the patients, and I agree with you that some of them probably were poorly treated.

N.L. Benowitz:

I am not sure that I understood some of the responses described for the coefficient of variation data from the calcium channel blocker studies. It was my impression that if you look at circadian variation, there is much more circadian variation with immediate release than sustained release calcium blockers. That is one of the theories at least for greater risk of adverse effects of immediate release calcium blockers in hypertensive patients, in terms of coronary events, sudden death, etc. Did you look at circadian variation in your analysis through the coefficients of variation?

P. du Souich:

No, what I am showing is in a group of patients with hypertension who have been treated with both drugs, is the variability of the hypotensive response.

N. Benowitz:

For hypertension the 24-hour response is really a key issue for variability. Were you looking at that, or were you looking at within-subject variations throughout the day?

P. du Souich:

No. They did not study the hypotensive response along the 24 hours, since here antihypertensive agents were usually given 2 or 3 times daily. So I do not include the possible influence of day-time or night-time variability. But the variability was anyway rather low. If again we accept this coefficient of variation as a measure of this variability, it was around 10% compared to 40% in angina, for instance, or much higher for other indications.

Variability in Human Drug Response
G.T. Tucker, Editor

Management of Variability – Regulatory Aspects

Tomas Salmonson and Janet R. Wade

Medical Products Agency, Uppsala, Sweden

ABSTRACT

The aim of this article is to give a very subjective, but regulatory perspective, on the issue of managing variability. It is recognised that the current health care environment favours a "one dose fits all" situation. However, everybody realises that the response in an individual patient to a given dose depends upon a unique combination of factors that can influence both the pharmacokinetics and pharmacodynamics of the drug. The major focus of the article has been placed on the more widely understood factors that influence pharmacokinetics and which can include, food effects, age effects, disease in the eliminating organ, etc. The impact of these factors on both inter- and intra-subject variability is discussed. It should be task of all regulatory agencies to encourage the drug developers to identify the factors that are of clinical relevance and so minimise their impact on inter- and intra-subject variability. Such knowledge could facilitate individualised treatment by recognising that each patient is unique. In this respect the Summary of Product Characteristics (SPC) could be used to a much greater extent to reward knowledge and penalise the opposite.

Key words: drug development, pharmacokinetics, drug label.

Correspondence: Dr. Tomas Salmonson, Medical Products Agency, P.O. Box 26, S-751 03 Uppsala, Sweden, Tel: +46-18-17-4600, Fax: +46-18-54-8566, Email: Tomas.Salmonson@mpa.se

INTRODUCTION

The clinical response to a drug in an individual patient depends upon a number of pharmacokinetic and pharmacodynamic variables. It is well recognised that there is both inter- and intra-individual variability in these variables. It would then seem logical that drug developers and the health care system, including regulatory agencies, would do their utmost to understand impact of the variable patient characteristics (such as age, gender and organ function) on and within the pharmacokinetic/pharmacodynamic relationship in order to minimise the variability therein. Such knowledge could facilitate individualised treatment by recognising that each patient is unique.

Today, unfortunately, the opposite situation is favoured in many cases. Any need for dose adjustment between different patient groups, or restrictions regarding the use of the drug (e.g. in relation to food) are perceived by many drug developers to be disadvantageous. A one dose fits all philosophy simplifies the use of the product and this is welcomed by a health care system under pressure. In other words, the health care system does not reward knowledge but rather ignorance. Regulatory agencies are to some extent also responsible for this dilemma by not better penalising companies that do not fully consider factors determining the clinical response in an individual patient. In this respect the Summary of Product Characteristics (SPC) could be used to a much greater degree to reward knowledge and penalise the opposite.

There are, however, reasons to be optimistic about a change in this situation in the future. Incorrect treatment with dose related adverse events or sub-therapeutic doses may be perceived to be, not only a clinical, but also a financial problem. In addition, recognition of some potential sources of variability, such as gender, are becoming politically as well as scientifically driven. As a result, guidelines are being developed within many areas such as drug metabolism, interactions, different age groups and decreased organ functions.

The aim of this paper is to discuss sources of variability in the pharmacokinetics of a drug and indicate how these can be managed from a regulatory point of view. This paper has chosen to focus on pharmacokinetic variability since there is a greater depth of knowledge as to the contributing causes, and so is the place where regulatory agencies today can have the most impact. This however, is only half of the story. Whilst it will not be discussed, is extremely important to bear in mind that variability in pharmacodynamic response to a given drug concentration also determines what magnitude of effect the drug will have. As has already been stated, the variability in pharmacokinetics and pharmacodynamics is comprised of both inter- and intra-subject components. In general, the regulatory agencies have a greater impact on managing inter-subject variability. There are fewer instances where regulatory agencies can impact on intra-subject variability and these will be pointed out.

SOURCES OF VARIABILITY – EXAMPLES

Compliance

This is a subject that is discussed elsewhere in this book and will not be considered in depth here, except to acknowledge that compliance, or lack of compliance, will contribute to both inter- and intra-subject variability in response to the drug. It is difficult to see how regulatory agencies could lessen this source of variability. The resolution of problems arising from inadequate compliance has to be dealt with through education of both prescriber and patient.

Absorption

Food is a well-known factor that can influence the absorption of drugs. In a small survey conducted at the Swedish Medical Products Agency (MPA) a few years ago, food was found to significantly influence the pharmacokinetic parameters in 79% of 33 new chemical entities assessed. Food can influence not only the drug substance itself, but also the dosage form, the behaviour of different theophylline slow-release formulations is an example of this. Consequently regulatory agencies require to know if an observed food effect is the result of an interaction with either the drug substance or the dosage form. Appropriate recommendations can then be made to the developer of the drug.

The uncertainty of food effects has been recognised by most drug developers and food interaction studies are often performed early in the clinical trial program. Nevertheless, at least two recent phase III programs have, partly or totally, probably failed because the effect of food was not fully considered in the design of the pivotal studies.

A recent example of the influence of food is illustrated in Figures 1 and 2. This drug is currently on its way into phase II. In the clinical trial protocol submitted to MPA two doses

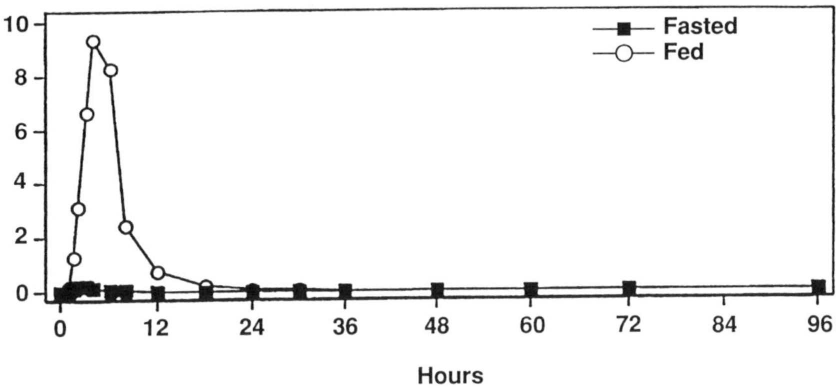

Figure 1. The influence of food con the concentration time profile for a drug currently entering phase II

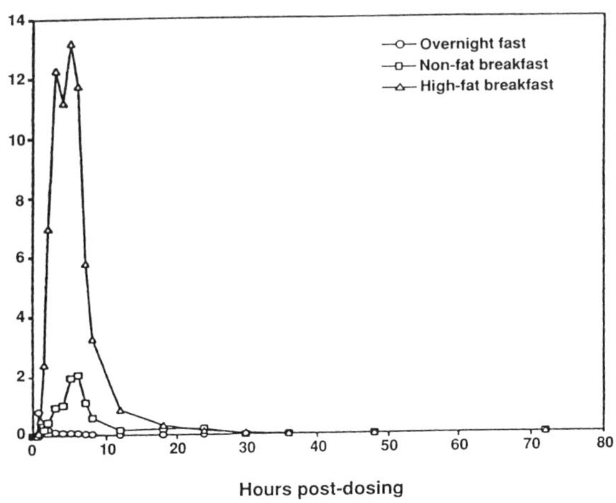

Figure 2. The influence of different types of food on the concentration time profile for a drug currently entering phase II

of 50 and 100 mg were to be compared. For a given dose, the difference in the AUC when taken either with a meal, or in a fasted state, is about 50 fold. Even if the company is correct in that the true difference is less because of the formation of an active metabolite, the probability of finding a difference between the two doses seems small given the influence of food.

Controlling whether the drug should be taken with or without food should minimise inter- and intra-subject variability when a food effect is present. Of clinical interest also is the large difference in effect that different types of meals may have (Figure 2). It seems reasonable to assume that this would result in large intra-individual variability if the drug is recommended to be taken with a meal. Such intra-subject variability could be minimised by giving information as to what types of food should or should not be eaten.

The duration of a food effect has, perhaps, been less acknowledged. The effect of a high fat meal can last for more than four hours. A meal could also influence the absorption of drugs taken during a significant window of time prior to the meal. Hence, depending on the habits of an individual patient it may not be possible to avoid a food effect.

Elimination

Inter-subject variability in drug metabolism is well-known. The fairly continuous variability associated with CYP3A4 activity and the discrete bands of variability in CYP2D6 activity are examples of this. It will be interesting to see how many CYP2D6 substrates will be developed in the future as drug companies try and minimise the inter-subject variability in response to their products. Tolterodine, a recently approved CYP2D6 substrate, is an interesting example because the applicant demonstrated that, due to the formation of an active metabolite, one dose range could be recommended, regardless of metabolic status. Genotypic expression of metabolic status is certainly a determinant of inter-subject variability. The fact that phenotypic expression may vary and thus contribute to intra-subject variability is an area that has not been possible to regulate thus far.

Drug developers should, and in the main, do, determine the major metabolic routes of elimination for a new drug. In this respect *in vitro* data can often be very valuable when deciding which, and then designing, the *in vivo* studies needed prior to registration. Once the metabolic pathways have been identified the sensitivity to inhibition or induction of the pathway can be tested with inhibitors/inducers. In this way, the risk of other drugs influencing the pharmacokinetics of the new drug can be established. Similarly, *in vitro* and *in vivo* data can be used to predict the potential of the new drug to influence the pharmacokinetics of other drugs. For a more extensive discussion of this topic the reader is referred to guidelines on these issues recently released in Europe and the US. It is hoped that these guidelines will help reduce variability in response due to potential drug interactions. It is also hoped that, in the future, more information will be made available to regulatory agencies as to the duration (onset and offset) of drug interaction effects, thus permitting appropriate dosing recommendations to be made and so minimising intra-subject variability.

Studies in patients with decrease organ failure have, for a long time, been a part of a standard drug development program. However, the impression can be gained that these studies are performed only to satisfy regulatory agencies. For example, the value of many studies in patients with decreased liver function could be questioned. It is important that more is learnt about how different enzymes are influenced by different types of liver impairment. The frequently used Child-Pugh scoring system, whilst at least giving some indication as to the degree of impairment, is probably not be the best way to grade the capacity of the different metabolic enzymes and more appropriate methods need to be developed.

The analysis of the results from these studies in organ impairment can also sometimes be questioned. This can be illustrated by that in studies in decreased renal failure, patients are often grouped together in what are fairly arbitrarily chosen ranges. One such example of this is shown in Table 1. When used to stratify patients for dosage recommendations theses ranges are, of course, valuable. However, there is no reason to use such categorisations when analysing the results. Use of the (continuous) individual values for creatinine clearance and the corresponding observed AUC estimates should, in many cases, increase the value of the results.

Table 1.
An example of grouping of patients with impaired organ function into arbitrarily chosen categories.

	Cretatinine Clearance (ml/min)			
Parameter	>90 (n=4)	66-90 (n=4)	41-65 (n=5)	10-40 (n=8)
C_{max}	17±10	24±10	18±12	26±18
AUC_{0-t} (ng.h/ml)	150±57 84-204	148±31 127-193	166±38 108-215	268±152 106-516

The fact of presence or absence of disease in an eliminating organ is a factor determining the magnitude of the inter-subject variability. However, a disease state is a process that may get better, remain the same, or degenerate, all changes which will impact on the intra-subject variability. It is important that the prescriber is given information that will enable doses to be adjusted at appropriate times with respect to degree of impairment.

Patient characteristics

Studies in elderly are often part of a drug development program. Granted the ageing population and their extensive use of drugs, this is not only justifiable but necessary. Given the increase in life expectancy one could sometimes, perhaps, question the value of studies in patients of only 65-75 years of age. Subjects included in these studies are often relatively healthy and probably display only a minor decrease in renal function compared with a younger population. The results obtained will, therefore, underestimate the true impact of age on inter-subject variability.

Potential gender differences should also be studied. Differences are found in the pharmacokinetics between men and women far more often than result in different dosing recommendations. One reason for this could be that the observed difference lacks clinical significance. But how do we know that? Separate dose finding studies are seldom performed and phase III studies are not powered to detect a difference in adverse events or lack of effect between these two groups. Some of the new anti-migraine products are examples of this. The AUC in women is twice that observed in men. This disease is common in women and phase II and III studies often include many women. One can speculate that either the women are given a too high dose or, probably more likely, the men receive too low a dose.

The effect of weight is another often neglected factor. In an recent application for a new AIDS drug it was shown that trough plasma levels above 3.5 M were desirable to maintain the clinical efficacy and to possibly reduce the risk of tolerance development. It is apparent from Table 2 that many patients with an exposure below the desired concentration range were heavier than the groups with higher plasma levels. This was not perceived by the applicant to be of clinical significance. Hence, the company has applied for the same dose for all patients, which is surprising given the seriousness of the indication and the consequences of a sub-optimal treatment.

Table 2.
The relationship between weight and trough plasma concentration for a new AIDS drug.

	Trough concentration windows			
	<3,5 μM	3,5 to 7.0 μM	>7.0 μM	All data
n	32	81	39	152
CL/F (L/h)	16.3±1.6	11.7±1.6	6.8±1.7	11.4±3.6
Weight (kg)	90±17	79±14	75±14	81±16

Age and gender are not usually factors that alter during the course of a single study, and thus contribute more to inter-subject rather than intra-subject variability. This is not the case for weight, where, in serious disease states/processes, it is quite conceivable that a patients' weight may decrease as the condition worsens, or increase as the patient gets better. Should a drugs pharmacokinetics be dependent upon weight, then altering the dose in accordance with weight changes seems a fairly simple way of managing the consequent intra-subject variability.

Social habits

The effect of grapefruit juice on many CYP3A4 substrates has made us aware that dietary habits may influence the response to drug treatment. Smoking is another factor well-known to influence certain drugs. An example of a factor that has been less well studied is pharmacokinetics in vegetarians. All these social factors need not remain constant in a given patient during a course of treatment. An understanding of the impact of these factors is certainly a case where regulators can and do have an impact on minimising intra-subject variability.

APPLICABILITY OF PHASE III DATA

In order to maximise the possibility of achieving conclusive, confirmatory results, phase II and III studies are often designed to minimise the inter-subject variability. One could speculate that the increased number of exclusion criteria observed in clinical trials conducted in Sweden is a result of this (Figure 3). Thus, the studied population is a selection of patients that will not entirely represent the intended target population. Information generated from phase I or pre-clinical studies are later used to generalise the clinical results obtained to the wider group of patients covered by indication applied for.

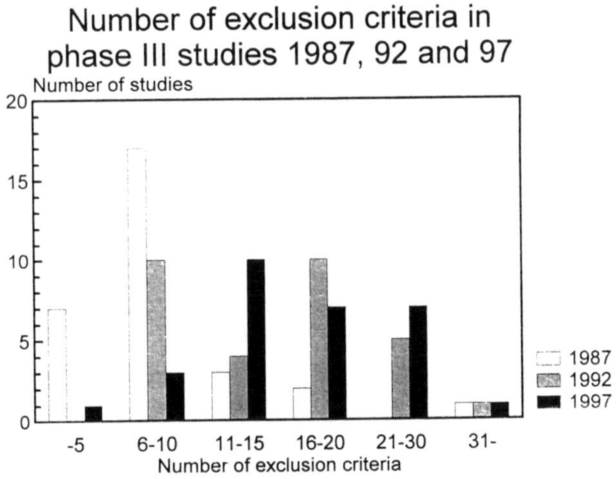

Figure 3. Number of exclusion criteria in protocols for phase III studies 1987, 92 and 97 submitted to the MPA

It appears as if drug developers find it easier to accept corrections for some sources of variability more than others. For example, industry and regulators often accept dose corrections in patients with decreased renal function based on pharmacokinetic data. If it is unknown whether AUC or Cmax (or another composite measure) is best correlated to the dynamic endpoint in question (and one ends up with different dosing recommendations depending on which pharmacokinetic variable chosen), then the risk of sub-therapeutic doses versus the risk of dose-related ADRs has to guide the dose selection.

Despite the arguments presented above, to convince an applicant of the need for a correction for other sources of variability such as gender effects or even food (if such an effect was not considered in the design of the study) is difficult. The applicant often argues that significant results were obtained in the phase III studies without correction for these sources of variability and that there were no differences in adverse events between, for example, men and women. Such an argument does not consider that the study, in this respect, was probably underpowered, and so is unconvincing for the regulatory agencies.

Another consideration seldom (if ever) acknowledged is the possibility of an altered concentration-effect relationship in different patients. The general lack of PK/PD information in the package submitted to the regulatory agencies prevents us from addressing this. In all cases when agencies try and correct for factors that contribute to inter-subject variability, an underlying assumption has to be made that the concentration-effect relationship in the different patient groups is the same. This certainly does not have to be the case. Wade and Sambol (1995) showed that not only do the elderly display increased felodipine plasma levels for a given dose of the drug, but even for the same plasma concentration, a greater response is observed than for a younger patient. Thus providing dosing instructions that correct only for the decrease in clearance observed in the elderly, but do not correct for the attenuated response observed, are clearly not optimal.

DOSE SELECTION

The selection of recommended dose/dose range is often an interesting challenge. The dose proposed by the applicant must be evaluated by the regulatory authority. Some of the new anti-migraine drugs can be used to illustrate this.

For one of the newer "triptans" a five-fold difference was found in the AUC values for a group of healthy volunteers (large inter-subject variability). The estimated (assuming dose-linearity) intra-individual variability was much less. Dose-response studies showed that a doubling of the dose within the suggested dose range increased the number of patients free from pain after 2 hours by only a few percent. The available concentration-effect data indicated that the variability in this relationship was relatively small. Based on these data some argued that the lower dose should be recommended (or even half of it), and possibly, for patients not responding during the first attack, a higher dose could be taken in subsequent attacks. Others believed that the dose related ADRs for the highest dose were acceptable and concluded with the argument that there was an intra-individual variability in the severity of the attacks (and thereby variability in the need of pain-relief), and so the highest dose should be given to all patients.

Regardless of which view one subscribes to, the above discussion illustrates many of the factors that need to considered when deciding upon dosing recommendations.

LABELLING

The documented characteristics of a drug should be described in the SPC. It is important that drug labelling rewards the applicants who <u>have</u> investigated sources of variability and not the opposite. The newly adopted European paediatric guideline allows the inclusion of pharmacokinetic information for children in the SPC, even if there are no, or insufficient, clinical data to include this age group in the indication/posology. It is hoped that this guideline will encourage applicants to perform pharmacokinetic studies in children so that the drug can ultimately be prescribed for this patient group at an earlier point in time than is currently the case. Having said that, contra-indicating patient groups which have not been studied but for whom there is no reason to suspect that they have different pharmacokinetics seems questionable. Such a course of action could put a prescriber with no other treatment options in a difficult position.

On the other hand, there is sometimes a tendency by regulators to pretend that we know more than we do. The often general dosing recommendations for patients with decreased liver function are an example of this It would seem better to avoid general terms such as "moderately impaired liver function" and, instead, describe the actual patients studied in more detail. Similar arguments can be made within the area of drug interactions where it is sometimes difficult to extrapolate to doses other than those studied. Such a course of action could be viewed as the regulatory agencies avoiding their responsibilities, but surely it is preferable that the prescriber, with their more intimate knowledge of the individual patient, makes the best informed decision possible, rather than relying on educated guess work from the regulatory agencies.

CONCLUSION

The aim of this article has been to give a very subjective, but regulatory perspective, on the issue of managing inter- and intra-subject variability. It is recognised that the current health care environment favours a "one dose fits all" situation. However, everybody realises that the response in an individual patient to a given dose depends upon a unique combination of factors that can influence both the pharmacokinetics and pharmacodynamics of the drug. It should be task of all regulatory agencies to encourage the drug developers to identify the factors that are of clinical relevance and so minimise their impact on inter- and intra-subject variability. Furthermore, the information obtained should be described in the SPC and so permit the prescriber to treat each individual patient in the best clinical and, perhaps also, cost-effective manner.

REFERENCES

1. Wade, JR, & Sambol, NC. Felodipine population dose-response and concentration - response in patients with essential hypertension. Clin Pharmacol Ther 1995;57:569-581.

<u>Discussion</u>: Management of variability - Regulatory aspects

A. Breckenridge:

I wonder if you share that, in drug regulation, we tend to concentrate up on factors relating to inter-individual variability and efficacy. Perhaps at the expense of issues concerning safety. This may well be because safety is considered a post-licensing problem, but it does seem that the emphasis is perhaps slightly in the wrong direction.

T. Salmonson:

There are many reasons for that. For example, the assessors are often experts at their own area. They focus on efficacy, because that is what they are interested in. I think one could speculate that one reason why Posicor was so happily accepted in the US and in the rest of Europe was because they already assumed that some of the ongoing trials were coming up favourably. We are focusing a lot on efficacy and not on safety, which is very ridiculous. I believe that we sometimes could leave the efficacy-establishing issue to the clinicians. But to judge for safety, in overall relation you need a larger group of patients and you need a type of qualification and knowledge, which perhaps the prescribing physician does not have.

C. Martínez:

I have a question concerning the study population and target population. And I fully understand that by the selection criteria that we have, the study population would go more away from being representative of the target population, which would probably increase the power of the study because of lower variability. If we go back to the animal studies, what we have are inbred strains of rats, from those we achieve specific conclusions. Do you think we should go back and have a random sample of the rats?

T. Salmonson:

No, I guess not. When in rats you are trying to establish and look at only one thing, it creates no problem. But if you want to look for something that you do not know, like safety for instance, it becomes very difficult to generalise. You can use the same argument when we perform population studies in a group of people, which is not really representative. There are a lot of problems, like the cost-related ones due to the enormous requirements in the development of the new drugs. So it is understandable why they are trying to limit these studies.

H.K. Kroemer:

I am interested in getting a statement on how in the long-term you handle the food issue, because it is turning out to be an important point. I recall a publication from Canada about single-dose administration of propafenone, in which they could show that food made an interaction only in extensive metabolisers, as a result of a CYP2D6 inhibition. When you asked them to do the same in a steady state, they tell you that they did not see any effect, although they never published that. In general, you can have very nice and dramatic effects for single administration, but you may not be able to solve or clarify with other studies. Finally, in real life you never will be able to adjust drug-doses for food intake in all the people. Therefore, I would like to know how you plan in the long term to deal with this issue.

T. Salmonson:

I think you are absolutely right. The food interaction most often decreases when you analyse it under steady state conditions. That is why many companies do it as planned, and if there is still an effect they investigate the effect under steady state conditions. Often there is no way you can practically avoid a food effect, because a food effect is there for a very long time. As we saw in the AIDS example, I would rather say take it with food and have that little restriction.

H.K. Kroemer:

But how do you deal with it in a practical way? People are likely to say to you, like the previous example, that there is an extreme difference, whether you take it with food or not. Is there a point where you would reject a drug, based on data like that?

T. Salmonson:

Yes, there is such a point. We have a recent example where a drug may be rejected because there is a dramatic, clinically relevant food effect. It is a three times daily drug. Some people argue that you cannot launch a drug with that type of characteristics. The extreme example I showed you was a clinical trial, where we just put a question-mark regarding the doubling of the dose and in real life it may be impossible to avoid it regardless how you write the labelling compared to the huge variability that one would expect, given the magnitude of the food effect and the effect of different types of food.

D.A. Smith:

That was the reason why it was something to be dealt with in the design stage, because it is almost impossible once you have put it into development to do anything about it. It is something which is actually doable at that stage, to actually incorporate it in your drug discovery programme. I would just like to throw in the thought that most drugs are not taken individually, but they are normally taken in combination. The biggest disadvantage is when you have to take one drug with food and the other after the food, or three hours after. This is a situation almost impossible to comply, which is the case with AIDS therapy, where you are taking multiple tablets throughout the day.

T. Salmonson:

You are absolutely right. You can have a food effect for four hours after the meal. So, it is impossible to avoid a food effect for a drug that you take three times a day.

Index of authors

Keyword index